Sample Sizes for Clinical, Laboratory and Epidemiology Studies

Sample Sizes for Clinical, Laboratory and Epidemiology Studies

Fourth Edition

David Machin
Leicester Cancer Research Centre
University of Leicester, Leicester, UK
Medical Statistics Group, School of Health and Related Research,
University of Sheffield, Sheffield, UK

Michael J. Campbell
Medical Statistics Group, School of Health and Related Research,
University of Sheffield, Sheffield, UK

Say Beng Tan
SingHealth Duke-NUS Academic Medical Centre, Singapore

Sze Huey Tan
Division of Clinical Trials and Epidemiological Sciences
National Cancer Centre, Singapore

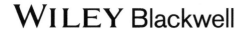

Library of Congress Cataloging-in-Publication Data

Names: Machin, David, 1939– author. | Campbell, Michael J., 1950– author. | Tan, Say Beng, author. | Tan, Sze Huey, author.
Title: Sample Sizes for Clinical, Laboratory and Epidemiology Studies / David Machin, Michael J. Campbell, Say Beng Tan, Sze Huey Tan.
Description: Fourth edition. | Hoboken, NJ : Wiley, [2018]. | Preceded by Sample size tables for clinical studies / David Machin ... [et al.]. 3rd ed. 2009. | Includes bibliographical references and index. |
Identifiers: LCCN 2018001008 (print) | LCCN 2018002299 (ebook) | ISBN 9781118874929 (pdf) | ISBN 9781118874936 (epub) | ISBN 9781118874943 (hardback)
Subjects: | MESH: Research Design | Clinical Studies as Topic | Statistics as Topic | Sample Size | Tables
Classification: LCC R853.C55 (ebook) | LCC R853.C55 (print) | NLM W 20.55.C5 | DDC 615.5072/4–dc23
LC record available at https://lccn.loc.gov/2018001008

Cover design: Wiley
Cover images: © Ralf Hiemisch / Getty Images (Background Abstract Image) © SergeyIT / Getty Images (Crowd Image on Top), © SUWIT NGAOKAEW / Shutterstock (Scientist Image on bottom)

Set in 10/12pt Warnock by SPi Global, Pondicherry, India

10 9 8 7 6 5 4 3 2 1

Contents

Preface

It has been more than thirty years since the original edition of 'Statistical Tables for the Design of Clinical trials' was published. During this time, there have been considerable advances in the field of medical research, including the completion of the Human Genome Project, the growth of personalised (or precision) medicine using targeted therapies, and increasingly complex clinical trial designs.

However, the principles of good research planning and practice remain as relevant today as they did thirty years ago. Indeed, all these advances in research would not have been possible without investigators holding firm to these principles, including the need for a rigorous study design and the appropriate choice of sample size for the study.

This fourth edition of the book features a third change in title. The original title had suggested (although not intentionally) a focus on 'clinical trials', the second saw an extension to 'clinical studies' and now 'clinical, laboratory and epidemiology studies'. Currently, sample size considerations are deeply imbedded in planning clinical trials and epidemiological studies but less so in other aspects of medical research. The change to the title is intended to draw more attention to areas where sample size issues are often overlooked.

This text cannot claim to be totally comprehensive and so choices had to be made as to what to include. In general terms, there has been a major reorganisation and extension of many of the chapters of the third edition, as well as new chapters, and many illustrative examples refreshed and others added. In particular, basic design considerations have been extended to two chapters; repeated measures, more than two groups and cluster designs each have their own chapter with the latter extended to include stepped wedge designs. Also there is a chapter concerning genomic targets and one concerned with pilot and feasibility studies.

In parallel to the increase in the extent of medical research, there has also been a rapid and extensive improvement in capability and access to information technology. Thus while the first edition of this book simply provided extensive tabulations on paper, the second edition provided some basic software on a floppy disc to allow readers to extend the applicability to situations outside the scope of the printed tables. This ability was further enhanced in the third edition with more user-friendly and powerful software on a CD-ROM provided with the book. The book is supported by user-friendly software through the associated Wiley website. In addition, R statistical software code is provided.

Despite these improved software developments, we have still included some printed tables within the text itself as we wish to emphasise that determining the appropriate sample size for a study is not simply a task of plugging some numerical values into a formula with the parameters concerned, but an extensive investigation of what is suitable for the study intended. This would include face-to-face discussions between the investigators and statistical team members, for which having printed tables available can be helpful. The tabulations give a very quick 'feel' as to how sensitive sample sizes can often be to even small perturbations in the assumed planning values of some of the parameters concerned. This brings an immediate sense of realism to the processes involved.

For the general reader Chapters 1 and 2 give an overview of design considerations appropriate to sample size calculations. Thereafter the subsequent chapters are designed to be as self-contained as possible. However, some later chapters, such as those describing cluster and stepped wedge designs, will require sample size formulae from the earlier chapters to complete the sample size calculations.

We continue to be grateful to many colleagues and collaborators who have contributed directly or indirectly to this book over the years. We specifically thank Tai Bee Choo for help with the section on competing risks, Gao Fei on cluster trials and Karla Hemming and Gianluca Baio on aspects of stepped wedge designs.

David Machin, Michael J. Campbell, Say Beng Tan and Sze Huey Tan
July 2017

Dedication

The authors would like to dedicate this book to Oliver, Joshua, Sophie and Caitlin; Matthew, Annabel, Robyn, Flora and Chloe; Lisa, Sophie, Samantha and Emma; Kim San, Geok Yan and Janet.

1

Basic Design Considerations

SUMMARY

This chapter reviews the reasons why sample size considerations are important when planning a clinical study of any type. The basic elements underlying this process include the null and alternative study hypotheses, effect size, statistical significance level and power, each of which are described. We introduce the notation to distinguish the population parameters we are trying to estimate with the study, from their anticipated value at the planning stages and also from their estimated value once the study has been completed. We emphasise for comparative studies that, whenever feasible, it is important to randomise the allocation of subjects to respective groups.

The basic properties of the standardised Normal distribution are described. Also discussed is how, once the effect size, statistical significance level and power for a comparative study using a continuous outcome are specified, the Fundamental Equation (which essentially plays a role in most sample size calculations for comparative studies) is derived.

The Student's *t*-distribution and the Non-central *t*-distribution are also described. In addition the Binomial, Poisson, Negative-Binomial, Beta and Exponential statistical distributions are defined. In particular, the circumstances (essentially large study sizes) in which the Binomial and Poisson distributions have an approximately Normal shape are described. Methods for calculating confidence intervals for a population mean are indicated together with (suitably modified) how they can be used for a proportion or a rate in larger studies. For the Binomial situation, formulae are also provided where the sample size is not large. Finally, a note concerning numerical accuracy of the calculations in the illustrative examples of later chapters is included.

1.1   Why Sample Size Calculations?

To motivate the statistical issues relevant to sample size calculations, we will assume that we are planning a two-group clinical trial in which subjects are allocated at random to one of two alternative treatments for a particular medical condition and that a single endpoint measure has been specified in advance. However, it should be emphasised that the basic principles described, the formulae, sample size tables and associated software included in this book are equally relevant to a wide range of design types covering all areas of medical research ranging from the epidemiological to clinical and laboratory-based studies.

Whatever the field of inquiry the investigators associated with a well-designed study will have considered the research questions posed carefully, formally estimated the required sample size (the particular focus for us in this book), and recorded the supporting reasons for their choice. Awareness of the importance of these has led to the major medical and related journals demanding that a detailed justification of the study size be included in any submitted article as it is a key component for peer

Sample Sizes for Clinical, Laboratory and Epidemiology Studies, Fourth Edition. David Machin, Michael J. Campbell,
Say Beng Tan and Sze Huey Tan.
© 2018 John Wiley & Sons Ltd. Published 2018 by John Wiley & Sons Ltd.

reviewers to consider when assessing the scientific credibility of the work undertaken. For example, the *General Statistical Checklist* of the *British Medical Journal* asks statistical reviewers of their submitted papers 'Was a pre-study calculation of study size reported?' Similarly, many research grant funding agencies such as the Singapore National Medical Research Council now also have such requirements in place.

In any event, at a more mundane level, investigators, grant-awarding bodies and medical product development companies will all wish to know how much a study is likely to 'cost' both in terms of time and resources consumed as well as monetary terms. The projected study size will be a key component in this 'cost'. They would also like to be reassured that the allocated resource will be well spent by assessing the likelihood that the study will give unequivocal results. In particular for clinical trials, the regulatory authorities, including the Committee for Proprietary Medicinal Products (CPMP, 1995) in the European Union and the Food and Drug Administration (FDA, 1988 and 1996) in the USA, require information on planned study size. These are encapsulated in the guidelines of the International Conference on Harmonisation of Technical Requirements for Registration of Pharmaceuticals for Human Use (1998) ICH Topic E9.

If too few subjects are involved, the study is potentially a misuse of time because realistic differences of scientific or clinical importance are unlikely to be distinguished from chance variation. Too large a study can be a waste of important resources. Further, it may be argued that ethical considerations also enter into sample size calculations. Thus a small clinical trial with no chance of detecting a clinically useful difference between treatments is unfair to all the patients put to the (possible) risk and discomfort of the trial processes. A trial that is too large may be unfair if one treatment could have been 'proven' to be more effective with fewer patients as a larger than necessary number of them has received the (now known) inferior treatment.

Providing a sample size for a study is not simply a matter of providing a single number from a set of statistical tables. It is, and should be, a several-stage process. At the preliminary stages, what is required are 'ball-park' figures that enable the investigators to judge whether or not to start the detailed planning of the study. If a decision is made to proceed, then the later stages are used to refine the supporting evidence for the preliminary calculations until they make a persuasive case for the final patient numbers chosen. Once decided this is then included (and justified) in the final study protocol.

After the final sample size is determined and the protocol is prepared and approved by the relevant bodies, it is incumbent on the research team to expedite the recruitment processes as much as possible, ensure the study is conducted to the highest of standards possible, and ensure that it is eventually reported comprehensively.

1.2   Statistical Significance

Notation

In very brief terms the (statistical) objective of any study is to estimate from a sample the value of a population parameter. For example, if we were interested in the mean birth weight of babies born in a certain locality, then we may record the weight of a selected sample of N babies and their mean weight $\bar{w}$ is taken as our estimate of the population mean birth weight denoted ω_{Pop}. The Greek ω distinguishes the population value from its estimate, the Roman $\bar{w}$. When planning a study, we are clearly ignorant of ω_{Pop} and neither do we have the data to calculate $\bar{w}$. As we shall see later, when planning a study the investigators will usually need to provide some value for what ω_{Pop} may turn out to be. This anticipated value is denoted ω_{Plan}. This value then forms (part of) the basis for subsequent sample size calculations.

Outcomes

In any study, it is necessary to define an outcome (endpoint) which may be, for example, the birth weight of the babies concerned, as determined by the objectives of the investigation. In other situations this outcome may be a measure of blood pressure, wound healing time, degree of palliation, a patient reported outcome (PRO) that indicates the level of some aspect of their Quality of Life (QoL) or any other relevant and measureable outcome of interest.

The Effect Size

Consider, as an example, a proposed randomised trial of a placebo (control, C) against acupuncture (A) for the relief of pain in patients with a particular diagnosis. The patients are randomised to receive either A or C (how placebo acupuncture can be administered is clearly an important consideration). In addition, we assume that pain relief is assessed at a fixed time after randomisation and is defined in such a way as to be unambiguously evaluable for each patient as either 'success' or 'failure'. We assume the aim of the trial is to estimate the true difference δ_{Pop} between the true success rate π_{PopA} of A and the true success rate π_{PopC} of C. Thus the key (population) parameter of interest is δ_{Pop} which is a composite of the two (population) parameters π_{PopA} and π_{PopC}.

At the completion of the trial the A patients yield a treatment success rate p_A which is an estimate of π_{PopA} and for C the corresponding items are p_C and π_{PopC}. Thus, the observed difference, $d = p_A - p_C$, provides an estimate of the true difference (the effect size) $\delta_{Pop} = \pi_{PopA} - \pi_{PopC}$.

Significance Tests

In a clinical trial, two or more forms of therapy or intervention may be compared. However, patients themselves vary both in their baseline characteristics at diagnosis and in their response to subsequent therapy. Hence in a clinical trial, an apparent difference in treatments may be observed due to chance alone, that is, we may observe a difference but it may be explained by the intrinsic characteristics of the patients themselves rather than 'caused' by the different treatments given. As a consequence, it is customary to use a 'significance test' to assess the weight of evidence and to estimate the probability that the observed data could in fact have arisen purely by chance.

The Null Hypothesis and Test Size

In our example, the null hypothesis, termed H_{Null}, implies that A and C are equally effective or that $\delta_{Pop} = \pi_{PopA} - \pi_{PopC} = 0$. Even when that null hypothesis is true, at the end of the study an observed difference, $d = p_A - p_C$ other than zero, may occur. The probability of obtaining the observed difference d or a more extreme one, on the *assumption* that $\delta_{Pop} = 0$, can be calculated using a statistical test. If, under this null hypothesis, the resulting probability or p-value is very small, then we reject this null hypothesis of no difference and conclude that the two treatments do indeed differ in efficacy.

The critical value taken for the p-value is arbitrary and is denoted by α. If, once calculated following the statistical test, the p-value $\leq \alpha$ then the null hypothesis is rejected. Conversely, if the p-value $> \alpha$, one does not reject the null hypothesis. Even when the null hypothesis is in fact true there is a risk of rejecting it. To reject the null hypothesis when it is true is to make a Type I error and the associated probability of this is α. The quantity α can be referred to either as the test size, significance level, probability of a Type I error or, sometimes, the false-positive error.

The Alternative Hypothesis and Power

Usually in statistical significance testing, by rejecting the null hypothesis, we do not specifically accept any alternative hypothesis, and it is usual to report the range of plausible population values with a confidence interval (*CI*) as we describe in **Section 1.6**. However, sample size calculations are usually posed in a hypothesis test framework, and this requires us to specify an alternative hypothesis, termed H_{Alt}, that the *true* effect size is $\delta_{Pop} = \pi_{PopA} - \pi_{PopC} \neq 0$.

The clinical trial could yield an observed difference d that would lead to a p-value $> \alpha$ even though the null hypothesis is really *not* true, that is, π_{PopA} truly differs from π_{PopC} and so $\delta_{Pop} \neq 0$. In such a situation, we then *fail* to reject the null hypothesis although it is indeed false. This is called a Type II or false-negative error and the probability of this is denoted by β.

As the probability of a Type II error is based on the assumption that the null hypothesis is *not* true, that is, $\delta_{Pop} \neq 0$, then there are many possible values for δ_{Pop} in this instance. Since there are countless potential values then each would give a different value for β.

The *power* is defined as one minus the probability of a Type II error, $1 - \beta$. Thus 'power' is the probability of what 'you want', which is obtaining a 'significant' p-value when the null hypothesis is *truly* false and so a difference between two interventions may be claimed.

1.3   Planning Issues

The Effect Size

Of the parameters that have to be pre-specified before the sample size can be determined, the true effect size is the most critical. Thus, in order to estimate sample size, one must first identify the magnitude of the difference between the interventions A and C that one wishes to detect (strictly the minimum size of scientific or clinical interest) and quantify this as the (anticipated) effect size denoted δ_{Plan}. Although what follows is couched in terms of planning a randomised control trial, analogous considerations apply to all comparative study types.

Sometimes there is prior knowledge that enables an investigator to anticipate what size of benefit the test intervention is likely to bring, and the role of the trial is to confirm that expectation. In other circumstances, it may be possible to say that, for example, only the prospect of doubling of their median survival would be worthwhile for patients with a fatal disease who are rapidly deteriorating. This is because the test treatment is known to be toxic and likely to be a severe burden for the patient as compared to the standard approach.

One additional problem is that investigators are often optimistic about the effect of test interventions; it can take considerable effort to initiate a trial and so, in many cases, the trial would only be launched if the investigating team is enthusiastic about the new treatment A and is sufficiently convinced about its potential efficacy over *C*. Experience suggests that as trials progress there is often a growing realism that, even at best, the initial expectations were optimistic. There is also ample historical evidence to suggest that trials which set out to detect large effects nearly always result in 'no significant difference was detected'. In such cases there may have been a true and clinically worthwhile, but smaller, benefit that has been missed, since the level of detectable difference set by the design was unrealistically high and hence the sample size too small to detect this important difference.

It is usual for most clinical trials that there is considerable uncertainty about the relative merits of the alternative interventions so that even when the new treatment or intervention under test is thought for scientific reasons to be an improvement over the current standard, the possibility that this is not the case is allowed for. For example, in the clinical trial conducted by Chow, Tai, Tan, *et al* (2002) it was thought, at the planning stage, that high dose tamoxifen would not compromise survival in patients with inoperable hepatocellular carcinoma. This turned out not to be the case and, if anything, tamoxifen was detrimental to their ultimate survival time. This is not an isolated example.

In practice, when determining an appropriate effect size, a form of iteration is often used. The clinical team might offer a variety of opinions as to what clinically useful difference will transpire — ranging perhaps from an unduly pessimistic small effect to the optimistic (and unlikely in many situations) large effect. Sample sizes may then be calculated under this range of scenarios with corresponding patient numbers ranging perhaps from extremely large to relatively small. The importance of the clinical question and/or the impossibility of recruiting large patient numbers may rule out a very large trial but conducting a small trial may leave important clinical effects not firmly established. As a consequence, the team may next define a revised aim maybe using a summary derived from their individual opinions, and the calculations are repeated. Perhaps the sample size now becomes attainable and forms the basis for the definitive protocol.

There are a number of ways of eliciting useful effect sizes using clinical opinion: a Bayesian perspective has been advocated by Spiegelhalter, Freedman and Parmar (1994), an economic approach by Drummond and O'Brien (1993) and one based on patients' perceptions rather than clinicians' perceptions of benefit by Naylor and Llewellyn-Thomas (1994). Gandhi, Tan, Chung and Machin (2015) give a specific case study describing the synthesis of prior clinical beliefs, with information from non-randomised and randomised trials concerning the treatment of patients following curative resection for hepatocellular carcinoma. Cook, Hislop, Altman et al (2015) also give useful guidelines for selection of an appropriate effect size.

One- or Two-Sided Significance Tests

It is plausible to assume in the acupuncture trial referred to earlier that the placebo is in some sense 'inactive' and that any 'active' treatment will have to perform better than the 'inactive' treatment if it is to be adopted into clinical practice. Thus rather than set the alternative hypothesis as H_{Alt}: $\pi_{PopA} \neq \pi_{PopC}$, it may be replaced by H_{Alt}: $\pi_{PopA} > \pi_{PopC}$. This formulation leads to a 1-sided statistical significance test.

On the other hand, if we cannot make this type of assumption about the new treatment at the design stage, then the alternative hypothesis is H_{Alt}: $\pi_{PopA} \neq \pi_{PopC}$. This leads to a 2-sided statistical significance test.

For a given sample size, a 1-sided test is more powerful than the corresponding 2-sided test. However, a decision to use a 1-sided test should never be made after looking at the data and observing the direction of the departure. Such decisions should be made at the design stage, and a 1-sided test should *only* be used if it is *certain* that departures in the particular direction *not anticipated* will always be ascribed to chance and therefore regarded as non-significant, however large they turn out to be.

It is more usual to carry out 2-sided tests of significance *but*, if a 1-sided test is to be used, this should be indicated and justified clearly for the problem in hand. **Chapter 6**, which refers to post-marketing studies, and **Chapter 11**, which discusses non-inferiority trials, give some examples of studies where the use of a 1-sided test size can be clearly justified.

Choosing α and β

It is customary to start by specifying the effect size required to be detected and then to estimate the number of patients necessary to enable the trial to detect this difference if it truly exists. Thus, for example, it might be anticipated that acupuncture could improve the response rate from 20% with *C* to 30% with *A* and, since this is deemed a plausible and medically important improvement, it is desired to be reasonably certain of detecting such a difference if it really exists. 'Detecting a difference' is usually taken to mean 'obtaining a statistically significant difference with the *p*-value < 0.05'; and similarly the phrase 'to be reasonably certain' is usually interpreted to mean something like 'to have a chance of at least 90% of obtaining such a *p*-value' if there really is an improvement from 20 to 30%. This latter statement corresponds, in statistical terms, to saying that the power of the trial should be 0.9 or 90%.

The choice for α is essentially an arbitrary one, the choice being made by the study investigating team. However, practice, accumulated over a long period of time, has established $\alpha = 0.05$ as something of a convention. Thus in the majority of cases, investigators, editors of journals and their readers have become accustomed to anticipate this value. If a different value is chosen then investigators would be advised to explain why.

Convention is not so well established with respect to the size of β, although in the context of a randomised control trial, to set $\beta > 0.2$, implying a power of less than 80%, would be regarded with some scepticism. Indeed, the use of 90% has become more of the norm (however, see **Chapter 16**, concerned with feasibility studies where the same considerations will not apply). In some circumstances, it may be the type of study to be conducted that determines this choice. Nevertheless, it is the investigating team which has to consider the possibilities and make the final choice.

Sample Size and Interpretation of Significance

The results of the significance test, calculated on the assumption that the null hypothesis is true, will be expressed as a '*p*-value'. For example, at the end of the trial if the difference between treatments is tested, then a *p*-value < 0.05 would indicate that so extreme or greater an observed difference could be expected to have arisen by chance alone less than 5% of the time, and so it is quite likely that a treatment difference really is present.

However, if only a few patients were entered into the trial then, even if there really was a true treatment difference, the results are likely to be less convincing than if a much larger number of patients had been assessed. Thus, the weight of evidence in favour of concluding that there is a treatment effect will be much less in a small trial than in a large one. In statistical terms, we would say that the 'sample size' is too small and that the 'power of the test' is very low.

Suppose the results of an *observed* treatment difference in a clinical trial are declared 'not statistically significant'. Such a statement only indicates that there was insufficient weight of evidence to be able to declare that 'the observed difference is *unlikely* to have arisen by chance'. It does *not* imply that there is 'no clinically important difference between the treatments' as, for example, if the sample size was too small the trial might be very unlikely to obtain a significant *p*-value even when a clinically relevant difference is truly present. Hence, it is of crucial importance to consider sample size and power when interpreting statements about 'non-significant' results. In particular, if the power of the statistical test was very low, all one can conclude from a non-significant result is that the question of treatment differences remains unresolved.

1.4   The Normal Distribution

The Normal distribution plays a central role in statistical theory and frequency distributions resembling the Normal distribution form are often observed in practice. Of particular importance is the standardised Normal distribution, which is the Normal distribution that has a mean equal to 0 and a standard deviation (*SD*) equal to 1. The probability density function of such a Normally distributed random variable z is given by

$$\phi(z) = \frac{1}{\sqrt{2\pi}} exp\left(-\frac{1}{2}z^2\right), \qquad (1.1)$$

where π represents the irrational number 3.14159.... The curve described by equation (1.1) is shown in **Figure 1.1**

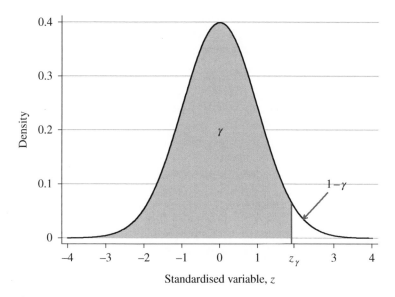

Figure 1.1 The probability density function of a standardised Normal distribution. (*See insert for color representation of the figure.*)

For sample size purposes, we shall need to calculate the area under some part of this Normal curve. To do this, use is made of the symmetrical nature of the distribution about the mean of 0 and the fact that the total area under a probability density function is unity.

Any shaded area similar to that in **Figure 1.1** which has area γ (here $\gamma \geq 0.5$) has a corresponding value of z_γ along the horizontal axis that can be calculated. This may be described in mathematical terms by the following integral:

$$\gamma = \int_{-\infty}^{z_\gamma} \phi(z)dz = \Phi(z_\gamma). \tag{1.2}$$

For areas with $\gamma < 0.5$ we can use the symmetry of the distribution to calculate, in this case, the values for the unshaded area. For example if $\gamma = 0.5$, then one can see from **Figure 1.1** that $z_\gamma = z_{0.5} = 0$. It is also useful to be able to find the value of γ for a given value of z_γ and this is tabulated in **Table 1.1**. For example if $z_\gamma = 1.96$ then **Table 1.1** gives $\gamma = 0.97500$. In this case, the shaded area of **Figure 1.1** is then 0.975 and the unshaded area is $1 - 0.975 = 0.025$.

For purposes of sample size estimation, it is the area in the tail, $1 - \gamma$, that is often needed and so we most often need the value of z for a specified area. In relation to test size, we denote the area by α and **Table 1.2** gives the value of z for differing values of α. Thus for *1-sided* $\alpha = 0.025$ we have $z = 1.9600$. As a consequence of the symmetry of **Figure 1.1**, if $z = -1.9600$ then $\alpha = 0.025$ is also in the lower tail of the distribution. Hence, the tabular value of $z = 1.9600$ also corresponds to *2-sided* $\alpha = 0.05$. Similarly, **Table 1.2** gives the value of z corresponding to the appropriate area under the curve for one- and two-tailed values of $1 - \beta$.

The 'Fundamental Equation'

When the outcome variable of a study is continuous and Normally distributed, the mean, $\bar{x}$, and standard deviation, s, calculated from the data obtained on n subjects provide estimates of the population mean μ_{Pop} and standard deviation σ_{Pop} respectively. The corresponding standard error of the mean is then estimated by $SE(\bar{x}) = \dfrac{s}{\sqrt{n}}$.

In a parallel group trial to compare two treatments, with n patients in each group, the true relative efficacy of the two treatments is $\delta_{Pop} = \mu_{Pop1} - \mu_{Pop2}$, and this is estimated by $d = \bar{x}_1 - \bar{x}_2$, with standard error $SE(d) = \sqrt{\dfrac{s_1^2}{n} + \dfrac{s_2^2}{n}}$. It is usual to assume that the standard deviations are the same in both groups, so $\sigma_{Pop1} = \sigma_{Pop2} = \sigma_{Pop}$ (say). In which case a pooled estimate obtained from the data of both groups is $s = \sqrt{\dfrac{s_1^2 + s_2^2}{2}}$, so that $SE(d) = \sqrt{\dfrac{s^2}{n} + \dfrac{s^2}{n}} = s\sqrt{\dfrac{2}{n}}$.

The null hypothesis of no difference between groups is expressed as H_0: $\delta = \mu_{Pop1} - \mu_{Pop2} = 0$. This corresponds to the left hand Normal distribution of **Figure 1.2** centred on 0. Provided the groups are sufficiently large, then a test of the null hypothesis, H_0: $\delta = 0$, of equal means calculates

$$z = \frac{d - 0}{SE(d)} = \frac{d}{s\sqrt{\dfrac{2}{n}}} \tag{1.3}$$

and, for example, if this is sufficiently large, it indicates evidence against the null hypothesis.

Now if this significance test, utilising the data we have collected, is to be *just* significant at some level α, then the corresponding value of z is $z_{1-\alpha}$ and that of d is denoted d_α. That is, if the observed value d equals or exceeds the critical value d_α, then the result is declared statistically significant at significance level α.

At the planning stage of the study, when we have no data, we would express the conceptual result of equation (1.3) by

$$z_{1-\alpha} = \frac{d_\alpha}{\sigma\sqrt{\frac{2}{n}}} \quad \text{or} \quad d_\alpha = z_{1-\alpha}\sigma\sqrt{\frac{2}{n}}. \tag{1.4}$$

The alternative hypothesis, H_{Alt}: $\delta \neq 0$, where we assume $\delta > 0$ for convenience, corresponds to the right hand Normal distribution of **Figure 1.2** centred on δ. If this were the case then we would expect d to be close to δ, so that $d - \delta$ will be close to zero. To just *reject* the hypothesis that $\delta = \mu_1 - \mu_2 \neq 0$, we require our observed data to provide

$$z = \frac{d - \delta}{SE(d)} = \frac{d - \delta}{s\sqrt{\frac{2}{n}}} = -z_{1-\beta}. \tag{1.5}$$

At the planning stage of the study, when we have no data, we would express this conceptual result by

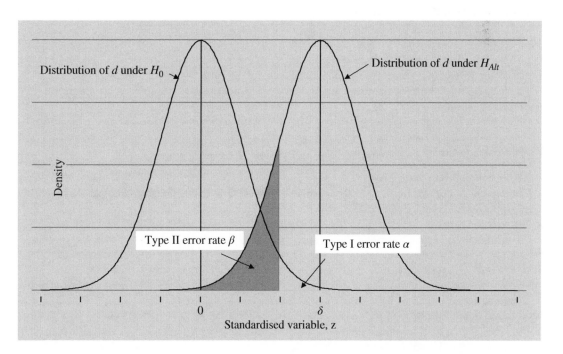

Figure 1.2 Distribution of d under the null ($\delta = 0$) and alternative hypotheses ($\delta > 0$).

$$d_\alpha = \delta - z_{1-\beta}\sigma\sqrt{\frac{2}{n}}. \tag{1.6}$$

Equating (1.4) and (1.6) for d_α, and rearranging, we obtain the total sample size for the trial as

$$N = 2n = \frac{4\left(z_{1-\alpha} + z_{1-\beta}\right)^2}{\left(\delta/\sigma\right)^2} = \frac{4\left(z_{1-\alpha} + z_{1-\beta}\right)^2}{\Delta^2}. \tag{1.7}$$

Here $\Delta = \delta/\sigma$ is termed the standardised effect size. The essential structure of equation (1.7) occurs in many calculations of sample sizes and this is why it is termed the 'Fundamental Equation'.

The use of (1.7) for the case of a *two-tailed* test, rather than the *one-tailed* test discussed previously, involves a slight approximation since d is also statistically significant if it is less than $-d_\alpha$. However, with d positive the associated probability is negligible. Thus, for the more usual situation of a 2-sided test, we simply replace $z_{1-\alpha}$ in (1.7) by $z_{1-\alpha/2}$.

In applications discussed in this book, 2-*sided* α and 1-*sided* β correspond to the most frequent application. A 1-sided α and/or 2-sided β are used less often (see **Chapter 11** concerned with non-inferiority designs, however).

Choice of Allocation Ratio

Even though the Fundamental Equation (1.7) has been derived for comparing two groups of equal size, it will be adapted in subsequent chapters to allow for unequal subject numbers in the comparator groups. Thus, for example, although the majority of clinical trials allocate subjects to the two competing interventions on a 1:1 basis, in many other situations there may be different numbers available for each group so that allocation is planned in the ratio 1: φ with $\varphi \neq 1$.

If equal allocation is used, then $\varphi = 1$, and so equation (1.7) yields N_{Equal} and hence $n_{Equal} = N_{Equal}/2$ per group. However if $\varphi \neq 1$, then '$2n$' is replaced by '$n + \varphi n$' and the '4' by '$(1+\varphi)^2/\varphi$'. This in turn implies $N_{Unequal} = n_{Equal}(1+\varphi)^2/2\varphi$. The minimum value of the ratio $(1+\varphi)^2/2\varphi$ is 2 when $\varphi = 1$. Hence, $N_{Unequal} > N_{Equal}$ and therefore a study using unequal allocation will require a larger number of subjects to be studied.

In order to design a study comparing two groups the design team supplies

- The allocation ratio, φ
- The *anticipated standardised effect size*, Δ, which is the size of the anticipated difference between the two groups expressed in relation to the *SD*.
- The probability of a Type I error, α, of the statistical test to be used in the analysis.
- The probability of a Type II error, β, equivalently expressed as the power $1 - \beta$.

Notation

Throughout this book, we denote a 2-*sided* (or two-tailed) value for z corresponding to a 2-sided significance level, α, by $z_{1-\alpha/2}$ and for a 1-*sided* significance level by $z_{1-\alpha}$. The same notation is used in respect to the Type II error β.

Use of Tables 1.1 and 1.2

Table 1.1
Example 1.1   In retrospectively calculating the power of the test from a completed trial comparing two treatments, an investigator has obtained $z_{1-\beta} = 1.05$ and would like to know the corresponding power, $1 - \beta$.

In the terminology of **Table 1.1**, the investigator needs to find γ for $z_\gamma = 1.05$. Direct entry into the table with $z_\gamma = 1.05$ gives the corresponding $\gamma = 0.85314$. Thus, the power of the test would be approximately $1 - \beta = 0.85$ or 85%.

Table 1.2
Example 1.2   At the planning stage of a randomised trial, an investigator is considering using a one-sided or one-tailed test size α of 0.05 and a power of 0.8. What are the values of $z_{1-\alpha}$ and $z_{1-\beta}$ that are needed for the calculations?

For a one-tailed test one requires a probability of α in one tail of the corresponding standardized Normal distribution. The investigator thus needs to find $z_\gamma = z_{1-\alpha}$ or $z_{0.95}$. A value of $\gamma = 0.95$ could be found by searching in the body of **Table 1.1**. Such a search gives z as being between 1.64 and 1.65. However, direct entry into the second column of **Table 1.2** with $\alpha = 0.05$ gives the corresponding $z = 1.6449$. To find $z_{1-\beta}$ for $1 - \beta = 0.80$, enter the second column to obtain $z_{0.80} = 0.8416$.

At a later stage in the planning, the investigator is led to believe that a 2-sided test would be more appropriate; how does this affect the calculations?

For a two-tailed test with $\alpha = 0.05$, direct entry into the second column of **Table 1.2** gives the corresponding $z_{0.975} = 1.9600$.

1.5   Distributions

Central and Non-Central *T*-Distributions

Suppose we had n Normally distributed observations with mean $\bar{x}$ and SD s. Then, under the null hypothesis, H_0, that the true mean value $\mu = 0$, the function

$$t = \frac{\bar{x} - 0}{s/\sqrt{n}} \tag{1.8}$$

has a Student's t-distribution with degrees of freedom (df) equal to $n - 1$.

Figure 1.3 shows how the central t-distribution is less peaked, with fatter tails, than the corresponding Normal distribution. However, once the df attains 30, it becomes virtually identical to the Normal distribution in shape.

Values of $t_{df,1-\alpha/2}$ are given in **Table 1.3**. For example if $df = 9$ and 2-sided $\alpha = 0.05$ then $t_{9,0.975} = 2.2622$. As the df increase, the corresponding tabular values decrease until, when $df = \infty$, $t_{9,0.975} = 1.9600$. This is now the same as $z_{0.975} = 1.9600$ found in **Tables 1.1** and **1.2** for the Normal distribution.

Under the alternative hypothesis, H_{Alt}, that $\mu \neq 0$, the function

$$t_{Non-Central} = \frac{\bar{x} - \mu}{s/\sqrt{n}} \tag{1.9}$$

has a Non-Central-t (NCT) distribution, with $df = n - 1$ and non-centrality parameter $\psi = \dfrac{\mu\sqrt{n}}{\sigma}$. Thus if μ and σ are fixed, the ψ depends only on the square root of the sample size, n.

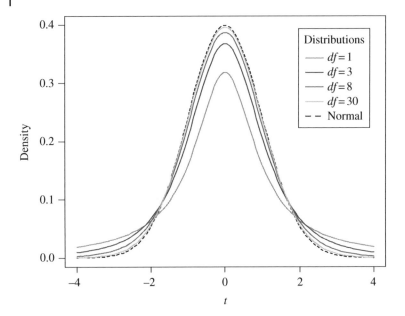

Figure 1.3 Central *t*-distributions with different degrees of freedom (*df*) and the corresponding Normal distribution. (*See insert for color representation of the figure.*)

Figure 1.4 shows the distribution of various NCT distributions with $\mu = \sigma = 1$; $df = 1$, 3, 8 and 30, and hence non-centrality parameter $\psi = \sqrt{2}$, $\sqrt{4}$, $\sqrt{9}$ and $\sqrt{31}$ respectively. In general as ψ increases, the mean of the NCT distribution moves away from zero, the SD decreases and so the distribution becomes less skewed. However, as shown in **Figure 1.4**, even with $n = 31$, the NCT distribution is slightly positively skewed relative to the Normal distribution with the same mean and SD.

The cumulative NCT distribution represents the area under the corresponding distribution to the left of the ordinate x and is denoted by $T_{df}(t|\psi)$. However, in contrast to the value of $z_{1-\alpha/2}$ in **Table 1.1**, which depends only on α, and $t_{df,1-\alpha/2}$ of **Table 1.3**, which depends on α and df, the corresponding $NCT_{1-\alpha/2, df, \psi}$ varies according to the three components α, df and ψ and so the associated tables of values would need to be very extensive. As a consequence, specific computer-based algorithms, rather than tabulations, are used to provide the specific ordinates needed.

Binomial

In many studies the outcome is a response and the results are expressed as the proportion of subjects who achieve this response. As a consequence, the Binomial distribution plays an important role in the design and analysis of the corresponding trials.

For a specified probability of response π, the Binomial distribution is the probability of observing exactly r (ranging from 0 to n) responses in n patients or

$$b\left(r; \pi, n\right) = \frac{n!}{r!(n-r)!}\pi^r \left(1-\pi\right)^{n-r}. \tag{1.10}$$

Here, for example, $n! = n \times (n-1) \times (n-2) \times \ldots \times 2 \times 1$ and $0! = 1$.

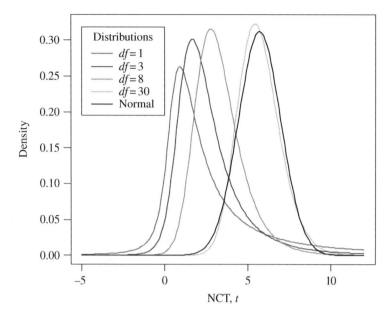

Figure 1.4 Non-central *t*-distributions with $\mu = \sigma = 1$, hence non-centrality parameters $\psi = \sqrt{n}$, with increasing $df = n - 1$ with *n* equal to 2, 4, 9 and 31. For $n = 31$ the corresponding Normal distribution with mean $\sqrt{31} = 5.57$ is added. (*See insert for color representation of the figure.*)

For a fixed sample size *n*, the shape of the Binomial distribution depends only on π. Suppose $n = 5$ patients are to be treated, and it is known that on average 0.25 will respond to this particular treatment. The number of responses actually observed can only take integer values between 0 (no responses) and 5 (all respond). The Binomial distribution for this case is illustrated in **Figure 1.5**. The distribution is not symmetric, it has a maximum at one response, and the height of the blocks corresponds to the probability of obtaining the particular number of responses from the five patients yet to be treated. It should be noted that the mean or expected value for *r*, the number of successes yet to be observed if we treated *n* patients, is $n\pi$. The potential variation of this expectation is expressed by the corresponding $SD(r) = \sqrt{n\pi(1-\pi)}$.

Figure 1.5 illustrates the shape of the Binomial distribution for $\pi = 0.25$ and various *n* values. When *n* is small (here 5 and 10), the distribution is 'skewed to the right' as the longer tail is on the right side of the peak value. The distribution becomes more symmetrical as the sample size increases (here 20 and 50). We also note that the width of the bars decreases as *n* increases since the total probability of unity is divided amongst more and more possibilities.

If π were set equal to 0.5, then all the distributions corresponding to those of **Figure 1.5** would be symmetrical whatever the size of *n*. On the other hand if $\pi = 0.75$, then all the distributions would be skewed to the left.

The cumulative Binomial distribution is the sum of the probabilities of equation (1.10) from $r = 0$ to a specific value of $r = R$, that is

$$B(R; \pi, n) = \sum_{r=0}^{r=R} \frac{n!}{r!(n-r)!} \pi^r (1-\pi)^{n-r}. \tag{1.11}$$

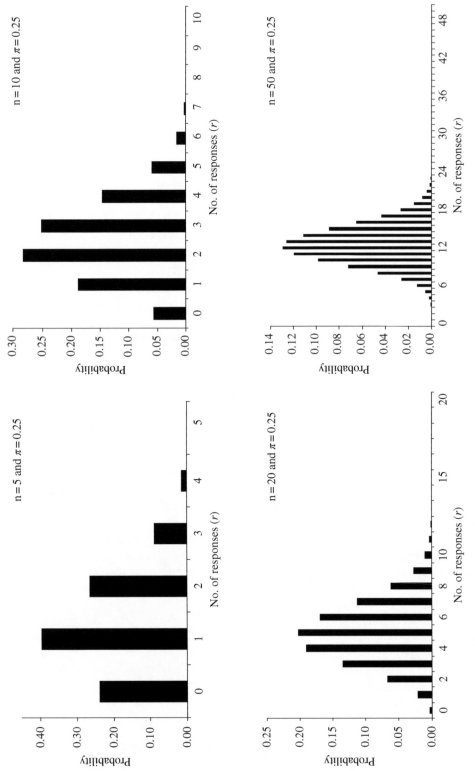

Figure 1.5 Binomial distribution for $\pi = 0.25$ and various values of n (adapted from Campbell, Machin and Walters, 2007).

The values given to r, R, π and n in expressions (1.10) and (1.11) will depend on the context. This expression corresponds to equation (1.2), and the unshaded area in **Figure 1.1**, of the standardised Normal distribution.

Poisson

The Poisson distribution is used to describe discrete quantitative data such as counts that occur independently and randomly in time at some average rate. For example, the number of deaths in a town from a particular disease per day and the number of admissions to a particular hospital casualty department typically follow a Poisson distribution.

Suppose events happen randomly and independently in time at a constant rate. If the events happen with a rate of λ events per unit time, the probability of r events happening in unit time is

$$Poisson(r) = \frac{exp(-\lambda)\lambda^r}{r!}, \tag{1.12}$$

where $exp(-\lambda)$ is a convenient way of writing the exponential constant e raised to the power $-\lambda$. The constant e is the base of natural logarithms which is 2.718281 ....

The mean of the Poisson distribution for the number of events per unit time is simply the rate, λ. The variance of the Poisson distribution is also equal to λ, and so the $SD = \sqrt{\lambda}$.

Figure 1.6 shows the Poisson distribution for four different means $\lambda = 1$, 4, 10 and 15. For $\lambda = 1$ the distribution is very right skewed, for $\lambda = 4$ the skewness is much less, and as the mean increases to $\lambda = 10$ or 15, the distribution is more symmetrical. These look more like the Binomial distribution of **Figure 1.5** and ultimately the Normal distribution shape of **Figure 1.1**.

Negative-Binomial

A key property of the Poisson distribution is that the mean and the variance are both equal to λ. However, there are situations where the mean and variance may be expected to differ. In which case, the Negative-Binomial (NB) distribution which we consider when comparing rates in **Chapter 6** may provide an appropriate description for the resulting data. The distribution is defined by

$$NB(r) = \frac{\Gamma(r+1/\kappa)}{\Gamma(r+1)\Gamma(1/\kappa)} \frac{(\kappa\lambda)^r}{(1+\kappa\lambda)^{r+1/\kappa}}. \tag{1.13}$$

Here the underlying mean rate is λ and the over-dispersion (a variance greater than λ) is accounted for by the parameter κ and implies a variance of $\lambda(1 + \kappa\lambda)$. In equation (1.13) the quantity $\Gamma(r+1)$ represents the gamma function which, when r is a non-negative integer, equals $r!$. Thus if $r = 3$, $\Gamma(4) = 3 \times 2 \times 1 = 6$ while if $r = 4$, $\Gamma(5) = 4 \times 3 \times 2 \times 1 = 24$. However if, for example, $\kappa = 2$ then $\Gamma(r + \frac{1}{2})$ cannot be expressed as a simple product of successive non-negative integers. In fact if $r = 4$, then $\Gamma(4.5) = \int_0^\infty e^{-u}u^{3.5}du \approx 11.63$. As might be expected, this is somewhere between $3! = 6$ and $4! = 24$.

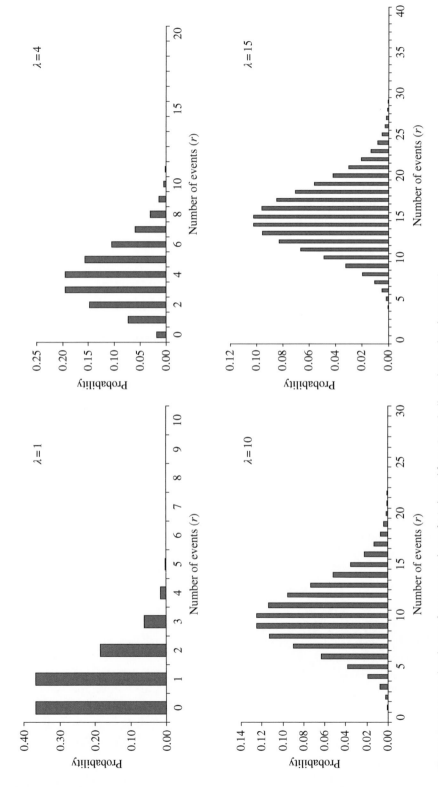

Figure 1.6 Poisson distribution for various values of λ (adapted from Campbell, Machin and Walters, 2007).

Beta

Another distribution that we will utilise when discussing therapeutic exploratory studies including dose-finding studies and phase II trials in **Chapters 17 and 18** is the Beta distribution. This distribution is similar to the Binomial distribution of equation (1.10) but allows non-integer powers of the terms π and $(1 - \pi)$. It takes the form

$$beta(\pi, v, w) = \frac{\pi^{v-1}(1-\pi)^{w-1}}{Beta(v, w)},\tag{1.14}$$

where v and w are usually > 1 for our purpose and $Beta(v, w) = \int_0^1 u^{v-1}(1-u)^{w-1}\,du$. This integral can be solved numerically for a given v and w and its value ensures that the sum (strictly the integral) of all the terms of (1.14) is unity. In contrast to (1.10) the Beta distribution is that of the continuous variable π rather than of the integer r of the Binomial distribution.

In general when planning a study where the outcome of interest is measured as a proportion, the Beta distribution may be used to encapsulate, given our *prior* knowledge about π, the parameter we are trying to estimate with the trial. This prior knowledge may include relevant information from other sources such as the scientific literature or merely reflect the investigator's belief in the ultimate activity of the therapy under test.

Once trial recruitment is complete and r responses from the n subjects concerned are observed, the prior knowledge is then combined with the study data to obtain a *posterior* distribution for π. This is formed from the product of parts of equations (1.14) and (1.10), that is, $\pi^{v-1}(1 - \pi)^{1-w} \times \pi^r(1 - \pi)^{n-r} = \pi^{r+v-1}(1 - \pi)^{n-r+1-w}$. The Beta distribution is chosen as it combines easily with the Binomial distribution in this way. The posterior distribution forms the basis of Bayesian methods and represents our overall belief at the close of the trial about the distribution of the population parameter, π.

Once we have obtained the posterior distribution, we can compute the probability that π falls within any pre-specified region of interest. For example, the investigator might wish to know the probability that the true response proportion exceeds a pre-specified target value. This contrasts with the confidence interval approach of **Section** 1.6, which does not answer this question but provides an estimate of the true response proportion, along with the associated 95% confidence interval (termed Frequentist as opposed to Bayesian). Arguably, in the context of early stage trials discussed in **Chapter 17**, since their main goal is not to obtain a precise estimate of the response rate of the new drug but rather to accept or reject the drug for further testing in a randomised controlled trial, a Bayesian approach seems best. However, the majority of studies are not designed using a Bayesian framework.

Exponential

In survival time studies, such as those describing the subsequent survival experience of a group of patients diagnosed with cancer, if the death rate is constant then the pattern of their deaths follows an Exponential distribution.

If the death rate is θ per unit time, then the proportion of subjects alive at time t is

$$S(t) = e^{-\theta t}.\tag{1.15}$$

This is often written $S(t) = exp(-\theta t)$ and is termed the survival function of the Exponential distribution. More generally the death rate is replaced by the hazard rate as the event of concern may not be

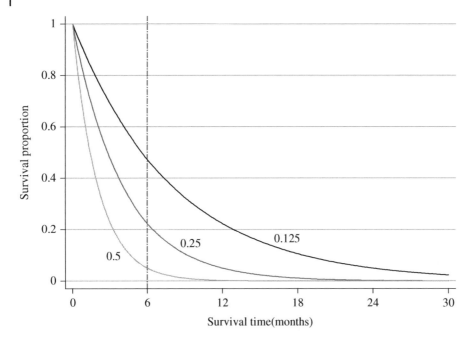

Figure 1.7 The Exponential survival function with constant hazards of $\theta = 0.125$, 0.25 and 0.5. (*See insert for color representation of the figure.*)

death but (say) time to relapse of a disease or the healing time of an ulcer. The constant hazard rate is a unique property of the Exponential distribution. Sample sizes for survival time studies are discussed in **Chapter 7**.

The shape of the Exponential survival distribution of equation (1.15) is shown in **Figure 1.7** for a hazard rate $\theta = 0.25$ per month. It is clear from this graph that only about 0.2 (20%) of the population remains alive at 6 months, less than 10% at 12 months, and very few survivors beyond 18 months. This is not very surprising since the hazard rate tells us that one-quarter of those alive at a given time will die in the following month.

As **Figure 1.7** also shows, with a hazard rate $\theta = 0.125$ the Exponential survival function will lie above that of $\theta = 0.25$ since the death rate is lower, while for $\theta = 0.5$ it falls below since, in this case, the death rate is higher.

A constant value of the hazard rate implies that the probability of death remains constant as successive days go by. This idea extends to saying that the probability of death in any time interval depends only on the width of the interval. Thus the wider the time interval, the greater the probability of death in that interval, but where the interval begins (and ends) has no influence on the death rate.

1.6   Confidence Intervals

When describing the Fundamental Equation (1.7), we have presumed that the study involves two treatment groups and that, once the data are all collated, a statistical significance test of the null hypothesis will be conducted from which a *p*-value will be determined. Whether this is statistically significant or not, a *p*-value alone gives the reader, who wishes to make use of the published results of a particular study, little practical information. As a consequence, it is therefore incumbent on the investigating team to quote the estimated effect (the observed difference between the treatments) together with an indication of the uncertainty attached to this value by the corresponding (usually 95%) confidence interval (*CI*). Together these enable an interested reader of the final report of the study to better judge the relative impact of the alternative interventions.

Even in situations when no comparison is to be made, for example in estimating the prevalence of a particular disease, it remains important to provide the relevant confidence interval.

In general, for the purposes of this book and at the planning stage of a study, discussion is easier in terms of statistical significance but nevertheless we emphasise that key *CIs* should always be quoted in the final report of any study of whatever design.

In the following sections, we give the expressions for standard errors (*SEs*) and *CIs* for some key summary statistics including the mean, proportion, rate and hazard rate corresponding to data obtained from the Normal, Binomial, Poisson and Exponential distributions. Although not detailed here, there are corresponding *CIs* for the appropriate measures of the difference between groups. *CIs* for some of these latter situations are included in **Chapter 9**.

Normal

Confidence interval for a mean
Large samples
The sample mean, proportion or rate is the best estimate we have of the true population mean, proportion or rate. We know that the distribution of these parameter estimates from many samples of the same size will be more or less Normal. As a consequence, we can construct a *CI*—a range of values in which we are confident the true population value of the parameter is likely to lie. Such an interval for the population mean μ_{Pop} is defined by

$$\bar{x} - \left[z_{1-\alpha/2} \times SE(\bar{x})\right] \text{ to } \bar{x} + \left[z_{1-\alpha/2} \times SE(\bar{x})\right], \tag{1.16}$$

where $\bar{x}$ is the mean from a sample of n subjects and $SE(\bar{x}) = \dfrac{\sigma_{Pop}}{\sqrt{n}}$. To calculate the *CI* an estimate, s, of the true *SD* σ_{Pop} has to be obtained from the data. Values of $z_{1-\alpha/2}$ are found from **Table 1.2**, so that for a 95% *CI*, $\alpha = 0.05$ and we have $z_{0.975} = 1.9600$.

Example 1.3 Regional brain volumes in extremely preterm infants
Parikh, Kennedy, Lasky, *et al* (2013) report the mean regional brain volume in 21 high-risk ventilator-dependent infants randomised to receive placebo (*P*) as $\bar{x} = 277.8\,\text{cm}^3$ with *SD* = 59.1. Thus $SE(\bar{x}) = 59.1/\sqrt{21} = 12.90\,\text{cm}^3$. From these the 95% *CI* for the population mean is $277.8 - (1.96 \times 12.90)$ to $277.8 + (1.96 \times 12.90)$ or 252.5 to 303.1 cm^3.

Hence, loosely speaking, we are 95% confident that the true population mean regional brain volume for such preterm infants lies between 253 and 303 cm^3. Our best estimate is provided by the sample mean of 278 cm^3.

Strictly speaking, it is incorrect to say that there is a probability of 0.95 that the population mean birth weight lies between 253 and 303 cm^3 as the population mean is a fixed number and not a random variable and therefore has no probability attached to it. Nevertheless, many statisticians often describe *CI*s in that way. The value of 0.95 is really the probability that the *CI* calculated from a random sample will include the population value. Thus for 95% of the *CI*s it will be true to say that the population mean, μ_{Pop}, lies within this interval. However we only ever have one CI and we cannot know for certain whether it includes the population value or not.

Small samples
Equation (1.16) for the $100(1 - \alpha)\%$ *CI* for a mean strictly only applies when the sample size is relatively large—a guide is if *n*, the number of subjects contributing to the mean, exceeds 25. When sample sizes are smaller, the following expression should be used instead

$$\bar{x} - \left[t_{df,1-\alpha/2} \times SE(\bar{x})\right] \text{ to } \bar{x} + \left[t_{df,1-\alpha/2} \times SE(\bar{x})\right]. \tag{1.17}$$

Here $t_{df,1-\alpha/2}$ replaces $z_{1-\alpha/2}$ of equation (1.16).

Degrees of Freedom (df) Besides depending on α, $t_{df,1-\alpha}$ of equation (1.17) also depends on the degrees of freedom, *df*, utilised to estimate the true standard deviation, σ, in the final analysis of the study. For a single mean, the $df = n - 1$. Values of $t_{df,1-\alpha/2}$ are found from **Table 1.3**. For example, for a sample mean based on $n = 10$ observations, $df = 10 - 1 = 9$. The corresponding 95% *CI* has $\alpha = 0.05$ and so $t_{df,1-\alpha/2} = t_{9,0.975} = 2.2622$, whereas the corresponding $z_{0.975}$ (see the last row of **Table 1.3**) is 1.9600. Thus the small sample leads, for a given α, to a wider *CI*.

Use of Table 1.3

Example 1.4 Regional brain volumes in extremely preterm infants
In the randomised trial of Parikh, Kennedy, Lasky, *et al* (2013) of *Example 1.3*, the reported mean regional brain volume in those receiving *P* was based on $n = 21$ infants, which is not a very large sample size. Thus it is more appropriate to estimate the *CI* of the mean using the *t*-distribution with $df = 21 - 1 = 20$. For a 95% *CI*, **Table 1.3** gives $t_{df,1-\alpha/2} = t_{20,0.975} = 2.0860$ so that equation (1.17) leads to $277.8 - (2.0860 \times 12.90)$ to $277.8 + (2.0860 \times 12.90)$ or 250.9 to $304.7 \, \text{cm}^3$. This *CI* is a little wider than that calculated using the Normal distribution of **Table 1.1**.

Binomial

Confidence interval for a proportion
If *r* is the number of patients who respond out of *n* recruited for a trial, then the response proportion $p = r/n$ is the estimate of the true response rate π_{Pop}. The *SE* of *p* is $SE(p) = \sqrt{\dfrac{p(1-p)}{n}}$ and the corresponding approximate $100(1 - \alpha)\%$ *CI* for π_{Pop} is calculated using the '*traditional*' method by analogy with equation (1.16) as

$$p - \left[z_{1-\alpha/2} \times SE(p)\right] \text{ to } p + \left[z_{1-\alpha/2} \times SE(p)\right]. \tag{1.18}$$

The reason we can do this is provided by the distributions shown in **Figure 1.5** where, as *n* gets larger, the shape of the Binomial distribution comes closer and closer to that of the Normal distribution until they are almost indistinguishable. However, this '*traditional*' approximation of equation

(1.16) should not be used if the proportion responding is either very low or very high or if the numbers of patients involved is small. In these cases we advocate the use of the *'recommended'* method described by Newcombe and Altman (2000), see also Julious (2005), and which is computed as follows.

Calculate $p=\dfrac{r}{n}$, $A=2r+z_{1-\alpha/2}^2$, $B=z_{1-\alpha/2}\sqrt{z_{1-\alpha/2}^2+4r(1-p)}$ and $C=2\left(n+z_{1-\alpha/2}^2\right)$.

The corresponding 2-sided $(1-\alpha)\%$ *CI* is then given by

$$\frac{(A-B)}{C} \quad \text{to} \quad \frac{(A+B)}{C}. \tag{1.19}$$

This method can be used even when no responses occur, that is when $r=0$, and hence $p=0$. In which case the *CI* is

$$0 \quad \text{to} \quad \frac{z_{1-\alpha/2}^2}{\left(n+z_{1-\alpha/2}^2\right)}. \tag{1.20}$$

Furthermore, if all patients respond, $r=n$ so that $p=1$, and the *CI* then becomes

$$\frac{n}{\left(n+z_{1-\alpha/2}^2\right)} \quad \text{to} \quad 1. \tag{1.21}$$

Example 1.5   Carboplatin for metastatic rhabdomyosarcoma

Chisholm, Machin, McDowell, *et al* (2007, Table 2) reported 1 complete and 4 partial responses among 17 children or adolescents with newly diagnosed metastatic rhabdomyosarcoma who had received carboplatin. The corresponding overall response rate was $p=5/17=0.2941$ with

$$SE(p)=\sqrt{\frac{0.2941(1-0.2941)}{17}}=0.1105.$$

Using the *'traditional'* method of equation (1.16) gives a 95% *CI* for π_{Pop} of 0.0775 to 0.5107, whereas using the *'recommended'* method of equation (1.19) results in 0.1328 to 0.5313. These are quite different but only the latter is correct and should be quoted.

As it is usual to quote response rates in percentages, the corresponding trial report would quote for these data: '... the response rate observed was 29% (95% *CI* 13 to 53%).'

Poisson

Confidence interval for a rate

If r events are observed in a very large number of n subjects, then the rate is $R=r/n$ as with the Binomial proportion. However, for the Poisson distribution r is small relative to n, so the standard error of R, is

$$SE(R)=\sqrt{\frac{R(1-R)}{n}}\approx\sqrt{\frac{R}{n}}. \tag{1.22}$$

In this case, the approximate $100(1 - \alpha)\%$ *CI* for the population value of λ_{Pop} is calculated using the '*traditional*' method, by

$$R - \left[z_{1-\alpha/2} \times SE(R) \right] \text{ to } R + \left[z_{1-\alpha/2} \times SE(R) \right]. \qquad (1.23)$$

However, although we refer to the number of events as r, we also add that this is the number of events observed in a '*unit of time*' and it is therefore essentially a rate. Thus the estimated rate for λ is often expressed as $R = r/Y$, where Y is the unit of time concerned. Thus, in *Example 1.6* below, we refer to R as the number of organ donations per day, which is 1.82 as calculated from 1,330 donations over a two year (731 day) period. In such a case n, of equation (1.22), is replaced by Y.

The reason we can use equation (1.23) is provided by the distributions shown in **Figure 1.6** where, as λ gets larger, the shape of the Poisson distribution comes closer and closer to that of the Normal distribution until they are almost indistinguishable. However, this '*traditional*' approximation of equation (1.16) should not be used if R (before division by n or Y as appropriate) is very low or if the numbers of subjects involved small.

Example 1.6 Cadaveric heart donors
The study of Wight, Jakubovic, Walters, *et al* (2004) gave the number of organ donations calculated over a two-year period as $R = 1,330/731 = 1.82$ per day. This is a rate with $SE(R) = \sqrt{\dfrac{1.82}{731}} = 0.05$.

Therefore, using equation (1.23) the 95% *CI* for λ_{Pop} is $1.82 - 1.96 \times 0.05$ to $1.82 + 1.96 \times 0.05$ or 1.72 to 1.92 organ donations per day. This *CI* is quite narrow, suggesting that the true value of (more strictly the range for) λ_{Pop} is well established.

Exponential

Confidence interval for a hazard rate
The hazard rate is estimated by $\theta = D/T$ where D is the number of deaths (or events) while T is the total survival experience in (say) years of the n subjects in the study. When D and/or n is large, an approximate 95% *CI* can be obtained from

$$log\ \theta - \left[1.96 \times SE\left(log\ \theta \right) \right] \text{ to } log\ \theta + \left[1.96 \times SE\left(log\ \theta \right) \right], \qquad (1.24)$$

since $log\ \theta$ often follows more closely a Normal distribution than does θ itself. In this case, $SE(log\theta) = \dfrac{1}{\sqrt{D}}.$

Example 1.7 Glioblastoma
Sridhar, Gore, Boiangiu, *et al* (2009) treated 23 patients with non-extensive glioblastoma with concomitant temozolomide and radiation of whom 18 died in a total of 33.32 years of follow-up while 5 patients remain alive and so provided censored observations. The corresponding hazard rate $\theta = 18/33.32 = 0.5402$ per year.

Substituting $\theta = 0.5402$ in equation (1.24) gives $log\ \theta = -0.6158$, $SE(log\theta) = 1/\sqrt{18} = 0.2357$ and the 95% *CI* for $log\ \theta$ as $-0.6158 - (1.96 \times 0.2357)$ to $-0.6158 + (1.96 \times 0.2357)$ or -1.0778 to -0.1538. If we exponentiate (anti-log) both limits of this interval, we obtain $exp(-1.0778) = 0.3403$ to $exp(-0.1538) = 0.8574$ per year or 34 to 84% for the 95% *CI* for θ.

1.7   Use of Sample Size Tables

Number of Subjects

Before conducting a clinical trial to test the value of acupuncture, a researcher believes that the placebo group will yield a response rate of 30%. How many subjects are required to demonstrate an anticipated response rate for acupuncture of 50% at a given significance level and power?

Power of a Study

A common situation is one where the number of patients that can be recruited for a study is governed by forces such as time, money, human resources, disease prevalence or incidence rather than by purely scientific criteria. The researcher may then wish to know 'What is the probability (the power) of detecting the perceived clinically relevant difference in treatment efficacy if a trial of this given size is conducted?'

Size of Effect

A reasonable power, say 80%, may be fixed and the investigators wish to explore with a particular sample size in mind, what size of effect could be established within this constraint.

1.8   Numerical Accuracy

This book contains formulae for sample size determination for many different situations. If these formulae are evaluated with the necessary input values provided, they will give sample sizes to a mathematical accuracy of a single subject. However, the user should be aware that when planning a study of whatever type, the investigators are planning in the presence of considerable uncertainty with respect to the eventual outcome so it is important not to be misled by this apparent precision.

When calculating sample sizes from the formulae given, as well as in the examples and in the statistical software provided, there may be some numerical differences between what is published and what an investigator may obtain in repeating the calculations.

Such divergences may arise in a number of ways. For example, when a particular calculation is performed there is often a choice of the number of significant figures to be used in the calculation process. Although the final sample size, N, must be integer, such a choice will in general provide non-integer values which are then rounded (usually upwards) to the nearest integer value. To give an extreme example, the use of two significant figure accuracy for the individual components within a sample size calculation may result in $N = 123.99$, whereas four figure accuracy may lead to $N = 124.0001$. Rounding upwards then introduces a discrepancy between 124 and 125. Further, if a 1:1 allocation to the two groups to be compared is required, then the former gives $n = 62$ per group but the latter gives $n = 62.5$, which would be rounded to 63 and hence an upward revised $N = 126$. Depending on the numerical values derived, further discrepancies can occur in circumstances if these calculations use, for example, 123.99/2 or 124.0001/2 rather than 124/2 and 125/2.

However, since investigators are usually planning in situations of considerable uncertainty, these differences will usually have little practical consequence. Also in view of this, it would seem in general rather wise to take, for example, a final N of 100 rather than 98, and certainly 1,000 rather than 998. Indeed, although this will require some judgement, perhaps a calculated N of 90 or 950 may become 100 and 1,000 respectively.

This suggests that, in the majority of applications, the number obtained should be rounded upwards to the nearest 5, 10 or more to establish the required sample size. We advise to round upwards as this gives rise to narrower confidence intervals and hence more 'convincing' evidence.

The above comments clearly make sense when the final sample sizes under discussion are relatively large, but more care will be needed in small and particularly very small sized studies. Also, when discussing the cluster designs of **Chapters 12** and **13**, care is needed. In this context, the final sample size is the product of the total number of clusters, K, and the number of subjects within each cluster, m, so that $N = Km$. Suppose the investigator plans for $m = 45$ per cluster, and the sample size calculations lead to $K = 7.99$ or 8.0001 depending on the number of significant figures used. Then rounding to 8 and 9 respectively and requiring a 1:1 allocation of the intervention to clusters gives $K = 8$ or 10. In which case, automatically rounding 8.0001 upwards to 10 results in 2 extra clusters and hence a study requiring a further 90 subjects. Again, some judgement is now necessary by the investigating team to decide the final choice of study size.

In some cases, statistical research may improve the numerical accuracy of some of the sample size formulae reproduced here which depend on algebraic approximations. However, these improvements are likely to have less effect on the subsequent subject numbers obtained than changes in the planning values substituted into the corresponding formulae.

1.9 Software for Sample Size Calculations

Since sample size determination is such a critical part of the design process, we recommend that all calculations are carefully checked before the final decisions are made. This is particularly important for large and/or resource intensive studies. In-house checking by colleagues is important as well.

Sample size calculations for a number of situations are available in various statistical packages such as SAS, SPSS and Stata. They are also available in a number of propriety packages as listed below.

Borenstein M, Rothstein H and Cohen J (2005). *Power & Precision (Power Analysis): Version 4.* Biostat, Englewood, New Jersey, USA.

Lenth RV (2006-9). *Java Applets for Power and Sample Size.* http://www.stat.uiowa.edu/~rlenth/Power.

NCSS, LC (2017). *Pass 15 Power Analysis and Sample Size Software (PASS 15)*: Kaysville, Utah, USA.

SAS Institute (2004). *Getting Started with the SAS Power and Sample Size Application: Version 9.1,* SAS Institute, Cary, North Carolina.

StataCorp (2014). *Stata Statistical Software: Release 14.* College Station, Texas, USA.

Statistical Solutions (2015). *nQuery Adviser + nTerim: Users Guide.* Cork, Ireland.

References

Technical

Campbell MJ, Machin D and Walters SJ (2007). *Medical Statistics: A Textbook for the Health Sciences,* 4th edn. Wiley, Chichester.

Cook JA, Hislop J, Altman DG, Fayers P, Briggs AH, Ramsay CR, Norrie JD, Harvey IM, Buckley B, Fergusson D, Ford I.(2015). Specifying the target difference in the primary outcome for a randomised controlled trial: guidance for researchers. Trials, **16**, 12.

Drummond M and O'Brien B (1993). Clinical importance, statistical significance and the assessment of economic and quality-of-life outcomes. *Health Economics*, **2**, 205–212.

Gandhi M, Tan S-B, Chung AY-F and Machin D (2015). On developing a pragmatic strategy for clinical trials: A case study of hepatocellular carcinoma. *Contemporary Clinical Trials*, **43**, 252–259.

Julious SA (2005). Two-sided confidence intervals for the single proportion: comparison of seven methods. *Statistics in Medicine*, **24**, 3383–3384.

Naylor CD and Llewellyn-Thomas HA (1994). Can there be a more patients-centred approach to determining clinically important effect size for randomized treatments? *Journal of Clinical Epidemiology*, **47**, 787–795.

Newcombe RG and Altman DG (2000). Proportions and their differences. In Altman DG, Machin D, Bryant TN and Gardner MJ (eds). *Statistics with Confidence*. 2nd edn. British Medical Journal Books, London, pp 45–56.

Regulatory

CPMP Working Party on Efficacy of Medicinal Products (1995). Biostatistical methodology in clinical trials in applications for marketing authorizations for medical products. *Statistics in Medicine*, **14**, 1659–1682.

FDA (1988). *Guidelines for the Format and Content of the Clinical and Statistics Section of New Drug Applications*. US Department of Health and Human Services, Public Health Service, Food and Drug Administration.

FDA (1996). *Statistical Guidance for Clinical Trials of Non Diagnostic Medical Devices (Appendix VIII)*. US Department of Health and Human Services, Public Health Service, Food and Drug Administration. (http://www.fda.gov/RegulatoryInformation/Guidances/ucm106757.htm)

International Conference on Harmonisation of Technical Requirements for Registration of Pharmaceuticals for Human Use (1998). *ICH Harmonised Tripartite Guideline—Statistical Principles for Clinical Trials E9*. (http://www.ich.org/products/guidelines/efficacy/efficacy-single/article/statistical-principles-for-clinical-trials.html).

Examples

Chow PK-H, Tai B-C, Tan C-K, Machin D, Johnson PJ, Khin M-W and Soo K-C (2002). No role for high-dose tamoxifen in the treatment of inoperable hepatocellular carcinoma: An Asia-Pacific double-blind randomised controlled trial. *Hepatology*, **36**, 1221–1226.

Chisholm JC, Machin D, McDowell H, McHugh K, Ellershaw C, Jenney M, Foot ABM (2007). Efficacy of carboplatin in a phase II window study to children and adolescents with newly diagnosed metastatic soft tissue sarcoma. *European Journal of Cancer*, **43**, 2537–2544.

Parikh NA, Kennedy KA, Lasky RE, McDavid GE and Tyson JE (2013). Pilot randomized trial of hydrocortisone in ventilator-dependent extremely preterm infants: effects on regional brain volumes. *The Journal of Pediatrics*, **162**, 685–690.

Sridhar T, Gore A, Boiangiu I, Machin D and Symonds RP (2009). Concomitant (without adjuvant) temozolomide and radiation to treat glioblastoma: A retrospective study. *Journal of Oncology*, **21**, 19–22.

Wight J, Jakubovic M, Walters S, Maheswaran R, White P and Lennon V (2004). Variation in cadaveric organ donor rates in the UK. *Nephrology Dialysis Transplantation*, **19**, 963–968.

Table 1.1 The cumulative Normal distribution function, $\Phi(z)$: The probability that a Normally distributed variable is less than z [Equation (1.2)].

z	0.00	0.01	0.02	0.03	0.04	0.05	0.06	0.07	0.08	0.09
0.0	0.50000	0.50399	0.50798	0.51197	0.51595	0.51994	0.52392	0.52790	0.53188	0.53586
0.1	0.53983	0.54380	0.54776	0.55172	0.55567	0.55962	0.56356	0.56749	0.57142	0.57535
0.2	0.57926	0.58317	0.58706	0.59095	0.59483	0.59871	0.60257	0.60642	0.61026	0.61409
0.3	0.61791	0.62172	0.62552	0.62930	0.63307	0.63683	0.64058	0.64431	0.64803	0.65173
0.4	0.65542	0.65910	0.66276	0.66640	0.67003	0.67364	0.67724	0.68082	0.68439	0.68793
0.5	0.69146	0.69497	0.69847	0.70194	0.70540	0.70884	0.71226	0.71566	0.71904	0.72240
0.6	0.72575	0.72907	0.73237	0.73565	0.73891	0.74215	0.74537	0.74857	0.75175	0.75490
0.7	0.75804	0.76115	0.76424	0.76730	0.77035	0.77337	0.77637	0.77935	0.78230	0.78524
0.8	0.78814	0.79103	0.79389	0.79673	0.79955	0.80234	0.80511	0.80785	0.81057	0.81327
0.9	0.81594	0.81859	0.82121	0.82381	0.82639	0.82894	0.83147	0.83398	0.83646	0.83891
1.0	0.84134	0.84375	0.84614	0.84849	0.85083	0.85314	0.85543	0.85769	0.85993	0.86214
1.1	0.86433	0.86650	0.86864	0.87076	0.87286	0.87493	0.87698	0.87900	0.88100	0.88298
1.2	0.88493	0.88686	0.88877	0.89065	0.89251	0.89435	0.89617	0.89796	0.89973	0.90147
1.3	0.90320	0.90490	0.90658	0.90824	0.90988	0.91149	0.91308	0.91466	0.91621	0.91774
1.4	0.91924	0.92073	0.92220	0.92364	0.92507	0.92647	0.92785	0.92922	0.93056	0.93189
1.5	0.93319	0.93448	0.93574	0.93699	0.93822	0.93943	0.94062	0.94179	0.94295	0.94408
1.6	0.94520	0.94630	0.94738	0.94845	0.94950	0.95053	0.95154	0.95254	0.95352	0.95449
1.7	0.95543	0.95637	0.95728	0.95818	0.95907	0.95994	0.96080	0.96164	0.96246	0.96327
1.8	0.96407	0.96485	0.96562	0.96638	0.96712	0.96784	0.96856	0.96926	0.96995	0.97062
1.9	0.97128	0.97193	0.97257	0.97320	0.97381	0.97441	0.97500	0.97558	0.97615	0.97670
2.0	0.97725	0.97778	0.97831	0.97882	0.97932	0.97982	0.98030	0.98077	0.98124	0.98169
2.1	0.98214	0.98257	0.98300	0.98341	0.98382	0.98422	0.98461	0.98500	0.98537	0.98574
2.2	0.98610	0.98645	0.98679	0.98713	0.98745	0.98778	0.98809	0.98840	0.98870	0.98899
2.3	0.98928	0.98956	0.98983	0.99010	0.99036	0.99061	0.99086	0.99111	0.99134	0.99158
2.4	0.99180	0.99202	0.99224	0.99245	0.99266	0.99286	0.99305	0.99324	0.99343	0.99361
2.5	0.99379	0.99396	0.99413	0.99430	0.99446	0.99461	0.99477	0.99492	0.99506	0.99520
2.6	0.99534	0.99547	0.99560	0.99573	0.99585	0.99598	0.99609	0.99621	0.99632	0.99643
2.7	0.99653	0.99664	0.99674	0.99683	0.99693	0.99702	0.99711	0.99720	0.99728	0.99736
2.8	0.99744	0.99752	0.99760	0.99767	0.99774	0.99781	0.99788	0.99795	0.99801	0.99807
2.9	0.99813	0.99819	0.99825	0.99831	0.99836	0.99841	0.99846	0.99851	0.99856	0.99861
3.0	0.99865	0.99869	0.99874	0.99878	0.99882	0.99886	0.99889	0.99893	0.99896	0.99900
3.1	0.99903	0.99906	0.99910	0.99913	0.99916	0.99918	0.99921	0.99924	0.99926	0.99929
3.2	0.99931	0.99934	0.99936	0.99938	0.99940	0.99942	0.99944	0.99946	0.99948	0.99950
3.3	0.99952	0.99953	0.99955	0.99957	0.99958	0.99960	0.99961	0.99962	0.99964	0.99965
3.4	0.99966	0.99968	0.99969	0.99970	0.99971	0.99972	0.99973	0.99974	0.99975	0.99976
3.5	0.99977	0.99978	0.99978	0.99979	0.99980	0.99981	0.99981	0.99982	0.99983	0.99983
3.6	0.99984	0.99985	0.99985	0.99986	0.99986	0.99987	0.99987	0.99988	0.99988	0.99989
3.7	0.99989	0.99990	0.99990	0.99990	0.99991	0.99991	0.99992	0.99992	0.99992	0.99992
3.8	0.99993	0.99993	0.99993	0.99994	0.99994	0.99994	0.99994	0.99995	0.99995	0.99995
3.9	0.99995	0.99995	0.99996	0.99996	0.99996	0.99996	0.99996	0.99996	0.99997	0.99997
z	0.00	0.01	0.02	0.03	0.04	0.05	0.06	0.07	0.08	0.09

Table 1.2 Percentage points of the Normal distribution for differing α and $1-\beta$.

α		$1-\beta$		
1-sided	2-sided	1-sided	2-sided	z
0.0005	0.001	0.9995	0.999	3.2905
0.0025	0.005	0.9975	0.995	2.8070
0.005	0.01	0.995	0.99	2.5758
0.01	0.02	0.99	0.98	2.3263
0.0125	0.025	0.9875	0.975	2.2414
0.025	0.05	0.975	0.95	1.9600
0.05	0.1	0.95	0.9	1.6449
0.1	0.2	0.9	0.8	1.2816
0.15	0.3	0.85	0.7	1.0364
0.2	0.4	0.8	0.6	0.8416
0.25	0.5	0.75	0.5	0.6745
0.3	0.6	0.7	0.4	0.5244
0.35	0.7	0.65	0.3	0.3853
0.4	0.8	0.6	0.2	0.2533
0.45	0.9	0.55	0.1	0.1257

Table 1.3 Student's t-distribution, $t_{df,1-\alpha/2}$.

df	2-sided α			
	0.20	0.10	0.05	0.01
1	3.0777	6.3138	12.7062	63.6567
2	1.8856	2.9200	4.3027	9.9248
3	1.6377	2.3534	3.1824	5.8409
4	1.5332	2.1318	2.7764	4.6041
5	1.4759	2.0150	2.5706	4.0321
6	1.4398	1.9432	2.4469	3.7074
7	1.4149	1.8946	2.3646	3.4995
8	1.3968	1.8595	2.3060	3.3554
9	1.3830	1.8331	2.2622	3.2498
10	1.3722	1.8125	2.2281	3.1693
11	1.3634	1.7959	2.2010	3.1058
12	1.3562	1.7823	2.1788	3.0545
13	1.3502	1.7709	2.1604	3.0123
14	1.3450	1.7613	2.1448	2.9768
15	1.3406	1.7531	2.1314	2.9467
16	1.3368	1.7459	2.1199	2.9208
17	1.3334	1.7396	2.1098	2.8982
18	1.3304	1.7341	2.1009	2.8784
19	1.3277	1.7291	2.0930	2.8609

Table 1.3 (Continued)

df	2-sided α			
	0.20	0.10	0.05	0.01
20	1.3253	1.7247	2.0860	2.8453
21	1.3232	1.7207	2.0796	2.8314
22	1.3212	1.7171	2.0739	2.8188
23	1.3195	1.7139	2.0687	2.8073
24	1.3178	1.7109	2.0639	2.7969
25	1.3163	1.7081	2.0595	2.7874
26	1.3150	1.7056	2.0555	2.7787
27	1.3137	1.7033	2.0518	2.7707
28	1.3125	1.7011	2.0484	2.7633
29	1.3114	1.6991	2.0452	2.7564
30	1.3104	1.6973	2.0423	2.7500
31	1.3095	1.6955	2.0395	2.7440
32	1.3086	1.6939	2.0369	2.7385
33	1.3077	1.6924	2.0345	2.7333
34	1.3070	1.6909	2.0322	2.7284
35	1.3062	1.6896	2.0301	2.7238
36	1.3055	1.6883	2.0281	2.7195
37	1.3049	1.6871	2.0262	2.7154
38	1.3042	1.6860	2.0244	2.7116
39	1.3036	1.6849	2.0227	2.7079
40	1.3031	1.6839	2.0211	2.7045
41	1.3025	1.6829	2.0195	2.7012
42	1.3020	1.6820	2.0181	2.6981
43	1.3016	1.6811	2.0167	2.6951
44	1.3011	1.6802	2.0154	2.6923
45	1.3006	1.6794	2.0141	2.6896
∞	1.2816	1.6449	1.9600	2.5759

2

Further Design Considerations

SUMMARY
Although **Chapter 1** has outlined some key components of relevance to sample size estimation, each study nevertheless has unique features, so the methods we include in the following chapters may need to be adapted accordingly. Here we describe aspects of how the groups to compare are identified, situations where more than two groups are concerned, some of which may involve identifying systematic trends across the groups, and also factorial designs which can simultaneously investigate different questions within one study. Also examined is the role of covariates and the design consequences of studies in which multiple (rather than single) outcomes are recorded and repeated significance tests are conducted. The chapter also gives some examples of how the study size calculations might be justified and presented for both the initiating study protocol and the final publication of the research findings. There is also a section on ethical issues relevant to sample size calculations.

2.1   Group Allocation

As Machin and Campbell (2005) and many others point out, of fundamental importance to the design of any clinical trial (and to all types of other studies when feasible) is the random allocation of subjects to the options under study. Such allocation safeguards against bias in the estimate of the statistic describing the group. Thus it is as important to allocate laboratory animals randomly to the alternatives in an experiment as it is to allocate patients randomly to the respective medical interventions under test. Nevertheless, there are many circumstances where this may not be feasible and a non-randomised study is entirely appropriate. Clearly in many situations no allocation is made by the investigators themselves as the groups they wish to compare are already established. For example, as part of a larger study, Day, Machin, Aung, *et al* (2011) compare from clinic records 138 patients with primary open angle glioma (POAG) and 105 with primary angle closure glioma (PACG) with respect to the central corneal thickness (CCT) μm at presentation.

Sample Sizes for Clinical, Laboratory and Epidemiology Studies, Fourth Edition. David Machin, Michael J. Campbell, Say Beng Tan and Sze Huey Tan.
© 2018 John Wiley & Sons Ltd. Published 2018 by John Wiley & Sons Ltd.

2.2 More than Two Groups

Regression Model

For any study designed, there will be an underlying statistical model. Thus when comparing two groups, *Standard* (*S*) and *Test* (*T*), the model can be summarised in the form

$$y = \beta_0 + \beta_1 x_1. \tag{2.1}$$

Here we assume that the endpoint *y* concerned is a continuous variable and the two groups are defined by $x_1 = 0$ or 1 for *S* and *T* respectively. For *S*, $x_1 = 0$, and equation (2.1) becomes $y = \beta_0$, so β_0 represents the true or population mean μ_S. In a similar way, for *T*, $x_1 = 1$, and equation (2.1) becomes $y = \beta_0 + \beta_1$. Thus $(\beta_0 + \beta_1)$ represents the true or population mean μ_T. From this we obtain $\delta = \mu_T - \mu_S = \beta_1$. Hence β_1 represents the true difference in means between the two groups. Once the data from the study is obtained, the regression model is fitted to the data to obtain b_0 and b_1 as estimates of β_0 and β_1. The main focus is then on b_1, the estimate of the difference in means between the respective groups. In such a situation, the null hypothesis, H_0, can be expressed as $\delta = \mu_T - \mu_S = 0$ or equivalently $\beta_1 = 0$, and the alternative hypothesis is $H_{Alt}: \beta_1 \neq 0$.

In practice, the outcome concerned may be continuous, ordered categorical, binary, rate or a survival time variable depending on the context.

Unstructured Groups

When there are more than two groups to compare, the situation is more complicated as there is no longer one clear alternative hypothesis. For example, if three groups *A*, *B* and *C* are to be compared then equation (2.1) is extended to

$$y = \beta_0 + \beta_1 x_1 + \beta_2 x_2. \tag{2.2}$$

Here, the three groups are defined by the relevant combinations of x_1 and x_2. Thus we denote $x_1 = 1$ for subjects of group *A* and $x_1 = 0$ for those *not* of group *A*, while $x_2 = 1$ for subjects of *B* and $x_2 = 0$ for those *not* of group *B*. Therefore those subjects who belong to *A* are the combination $(x_1 = 1, x_2 = 0)$, those of *B* are $(x_1 = 0, x_2 = 1)$, and those of *C* are $(x_1 = 0, x_2 = 0)$. In terms of the parameters $(\beta_0, \beta_1, \beta_2)$ of (2.2), the three groups are represented by $(\beta_0 + \beta_1)$, $(\beta_0 + \beta_2)$ and (β_0) respectively. The sample size for the study is then required to be sufficient to estimate both β_1 and β_2 reliably.

However, although there is a single null hypothesis that the population means are all equal and that corresponds to $H_0: \beta_1 = \beta_2 = 0$, there are several potential alternative hypotheses. These include one which postulates that the group means of *A* and *B* are equal but differ from *C*. Another may state that *A*, *B* and *C* all differ from each other, which then leads to comparisons of *A* versus *B*, *B* versus *C*, and *C* versus *A*.

Clearly equation (2.2) can be expanded to include more than three unordered groups, but this will bring further complication to the design choices.

Ordered Groups

Studies with *g* (>2) groups may have some structure embedded in their design. For example, the study may wish to compare increasing (possibly including zero) doses of the same drug or include another type of ordered grouping. Thus, although the null hypothesis would still be that all population means are equal, as when there is no structure, the alternative will now be $H_{Ordered}$, which is either $\mu_{Pop1} < \mu_{Pop2} < ... < \mu_{Popg}$ or $\mu_{Pop1} > \mu_{Pop2} > ... > \mu_{Popg}$. In the simplest case, the group options may be ordered on a numerical (possibly logarithmic) scale, and this may allow $H_{Ordered}$ to be expressed in a linear expression of the form

$$\mu_{Pop} = \beta_0 + \beta_1 x_1. \tag{2.3}$$

The corresponding regression model is then similar to equation (2.1), but x_1 is now a numerical (possibly continuous) variable rather than a binary one, and the sample size is calculated on the basis of an anticipated planning value of β_1, denoted β_{Plan}. The corresponding null hypothesis is H_0: $\beta_1 = 0$. Clearly at the close of the study, if the estimate b_1 of β_1 is close to zero and the null hypothesis is not rejected, then this suggests that the value of x_1 has little or no bearing on the value of μ_{Pop}. Conversely, if the null hypothesis is rejected then we conclude that $\beta_1 \neq 0$ and so x_1 does influence the corresponding value of the population mean at each point.

Factorial Designs

A rather different situation arises with factorial designs. If a 2×2 factorial trial is planned to compare two factors, **A** and **B** each of two levels, then there will be four groups to be compared with n subjects per group. Such a design may be particularly useful in circumstances where (say) factor **A** addresses a major therapeutic question, while factor **B** poses a more secondary one. For example, **A** might be the addition of a further drug to an established combination chemotherapy for a cancer while **B** may be the choice of an anti-emetic delivered with the drugs. For efficient use of such a design, the two main effects, that is the different options within **A** and those within **B**, are each compared using two means with $2n$ subjects in each group. However, this assumes an absence of interaction between the factors, which implies that the effect of **A** remains the same irrespective of which of the options within **B** the patient receives and vice-versa. If this is not the case, we might then wish to estimate the size of this interaction effect and so have a sufficiently large sample size for this purpose.

In planning a 2×2 factorial trial, the first step would be to assume no interaction was present and consider the sample size appropriate for factor **A**. The second step would be to consider the sample size for factor **B**, which may concern a different effect size and use a different power from that of the factor **A** comparison. Clearly, if the resulting sample sizes are similar then there is no difficulty in choosing, perhaps, the larger as the required total sample size. If the sample sizes are very disparate then a discussion would ensue to determine the most important comparison and perhaps a reasonable compromise would be reached. This compromise figure could then be used to check what magnitude of interaction (if present) could be detected with such numbers and may have to be increased if there is a strong possibility of an interaction being present.

If no interaction is present, the corresponding model is similar to equation (2.2) and becomes

$$y = \beta_0 + \beta_A x_A + \beta_B x_B. \tag{2.4}$$

Here $x_A = 1$ represents one level of factor **A** and $x_A = 0$ the other, and the quantity to estimate is β_A with corresponding terminology for factor **B**. If an interaction is thought to be present, then the model is extended to include a term involving the product $x_A \times x_B$ and becomes

$$y = \beta_0 + \beta_A x_A + \beta_B x_B + \beta_{AB} x_A x_B. \tag{2.5}$$

In this case the additional parameter β_{AB} has also to be estimated.

As with the situation when there is no structure between the groups, factorial designs imply a minimum of two significance tests at the analysis stage and hence the possibility of distorted *p*-values resulting and false conclusions being drawn.

2.3   The Role of Covariates

Extending the Design Model

As we have indicated in the preceding section, underlying whichever design is chosen for the study in question is a corresponding regression model that encapsulates the specific design characteristics. The objective of the study is then to estimate the associated regression coefficients such as β_A and β_B of equation (2.4).

In the context of a clinical trial, the investigators may focus on the interventions that will define (say) the two groups but in many situations will also be conscious that specific characteristics of the patients entering the trial are known *a priori* to strongly influence the outcome. Such a characteristic (a covariate) may be the clinical stage of a disease that carries a prognosis known to worsen with increasing stages.

As a consequence, although the purpose of the trial is not to quantify the effect of the covariate(s), their influence may need to be accounted for when assessing the interventions concerned. This requires the design model to be extended to include the covariate. Thus when comparing interventions T and S and taking into account a covariate, v_1, which is either binary or a continuous variable, equation (2.1) is extended to become:

$$y = \beta_0 + \beta_1 x_1 + \gamma_1 v_1. \tag{2.6}$$

In general, the number of x and v terms required in the model will depend on the particular study concerned. Essentially by including v_1, which is known to strongly influence y, we are accounting for an anticipated potential variation which (had v_1 not been included) otherwise would have been ascribed to a random variation and hence would lead to an over-estimation of $SE(\beta_1)$ and therefore be a less sensitive test of the null hypothesis $\beta_1 = 0$. We label the regression coefficient of the covariate as γ_1 to distinguish it from the basic design coefficients such as β_1, as we need to be reminded that it is these latter ones that are the main focus of the study. In broad terms, the sample size formulae given in the following chapters of this book focus on estimating terms such as β_1 and ignoring the possible impact of the covariate v_1. Thus the sample sizes derived may in some circumstances be conservative.

2.4   Multiple Endpoints

We have based the discussion in **Chapter 1** on the assumption that there is a single identifiable endpoint or outcome upon which group comparisons are based. However, often there is more than one endpoint of interest within the same study, such as wound healing time, pain levels and MRSA infection rates. If one of these endpoints is regarded as more important than the others, it can be named as the primary endpoint and sample-size estimates can be calculated accordingly. A problem arises when there are several outcome measures that are all regarded as *equally* important. A commonly adopted approach is to repeat the sample-size estimates for each outcome measure in turn and then select the largest number as this sample size is sufficient to answer *all* the questions posed by the study. Nevertheless, we recommend that as far as possible a single most relevant endpoint should be identified and classified as the primary endpoint of concern.

Ranking the Multiple Endpoints

In practice, it is very unlikely that the anticipated effect sizes for the multiple endpoints would be of the same magnitude or even the same direction. Thus, for example, if $k = 4$ endpoints, denoted (in rank order of importance) by $\Omega_{(1)}$, $\Omega_{(2)}$, $\Omega_{(3)}$ and $\Omega_{(4)}$, that are used separately in four sample size calculations, then four different estimates are likely to result. The final study size is then likely to be a compromise between the sizes so obtained. Whatever the final size, it should be large enough to satisfy the requirements for the endpoint corresponding to $\Omega_{(1)}$ as this is the most important endpoint and hence the primary objective of the trial.

Although applicable in many other areas of investigation, Fayers and Machin (2016) highlight that in studies assessing Patient Reported Outcomes (PROs) with respect to aspects of Quality of Life (QoL) there may be numerous endpoints to consider. They emphasise that, if possible, it is very important to identify a single PRO as the primary QoL endpoint. As we have indicated, when there are additional endpoints, it is advisable to rank these in order of importance. Although this may be a very long list in a QoL context, it is best that formal analysis should be confined to at most four or five of these. The remainder should be confined to exploratory hypothesis-generating analyses or descriptive purposes only. However, if formal comparisons concerning the four or five major endpoint variables are to be made once the study is complete, then some recognition of the multiple statistical testing that will occur should be taken into account at the planning stage.

2.5 Repeated Significance Tests

When a study involves multiple comparisons, multiple endpoints, variable selection in a multiple regression analysis, or a combination of these, then repeated statistical significance tests are usually involved at the analysis stage. The use of the total data, or parts of it, from the same individuals in these repeated tests distorts the *p*-values (and the corresponding confidence intervals) obtained and thereby might lead to drawing false conclusions from the study. In particular, one might falsely claim statistical significance for some of the comparisons made. Although there is no general solution for this problem, if multiple significance tests are to be conducted then a cautious approach is to inflate the planned study's sample size to compensate for this. One method for doing so is to consider reducing the conventional Type 1 errors by using the Bonferroni correction.

Bonferroni Correction

One component of the sample size formulae presented in subsequent chapters arises from specifying a level of statistical significance, α, to be used in the subsequent analysis of the study once the data are collated. This aspect influences the eventual sample size obtained through the corresponding value of $z_{1-\alpha/2}$ obtained from a standard Normal distribution as described in **Section 1.4** and tabulated in **Table 1.1**. A common value is $\alpha = 0.05$, in which case $z_{1-\alpha/2} = z_{0.975} = 1.9600$, which is then included in the numerator of the sample size calculation formula typified by the Fundamental Equation (1.7).

To guard against false statistical significance as a consequence of multiple statistical testing of k different aspects of data from a single study, it is a sensible precaution to consider replacing α itself by an adjusted value using the *Bonferroni correction*, which is

$$\alpha_{Bonferroni} = \alpha/k. \tag{2.7}$$

In these circumstances, $\alpha_{Bonferroni}$ is then substituted in place of α in the sample size formulae described in the respective chapters to follow. For example, if $k = 4$ and $\alpha = 0.05$, then $\alpha_{Bonferroni} = 0.05/4 = 0.0125$ and searching for $1 - 0.0125/2 = 0.99375$ in **Table 1.1** implies the corresponding $z_{0.99375} \approx 2.496$. As this is larger than 1.96, this implies the study sample size will need to be increased over that planned for a single endpoint.

Figure 2.1 shows the multiplication factors that are required so as to compensate for multiple comparisons when using the Bonferroni correction for two-sided $\alpha = 0.05$ and powers of 80% or 90%. This shows that if $k = 4$ the overall sample size must be increased by multiplication factors of about 1.42 and 1.36.

However, the use of the Bonferroni correction remains controversial as it assumes that the statistical tests of the multiple comparisons are independent of each other, which they are clearly not as they will all to some extent use information from the same subjects recruited for the single study. Bonferroni makes the unrealistic assumption that the outcomes are uncorrelated and is therefore an over correction of the p-values to an unknown degree.

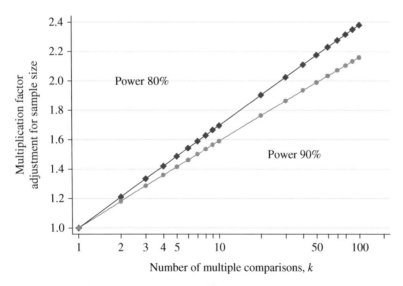

Figure 2.1 Sample size multiplication factors to compensate for k multiple comparisons when applying a Bonferroni correction with two-sided $\alpha = 0.05$ (after Fayers and Machin, 2016, Figure 11.3). (*See insert for color representation of the figure.*)

A compromise approach is, at the analysis stage, to calculate the p-values obtained from the statistical tests of each of the comparisons concerned and then, at the reporting stage, to adopt a cautious approach of only making claims of statistical significance for those with (say) a p-value < 0.01.

2.6 Epidemiological Studies

Although not confined to epidemiological investigations alone, such studies may be prone to issues concerned with repeated significance tests when selecting which of the covariates of possible concern should be included in the final statistical model describing the results of the investigation. For example, in some epidemiological studies to determine (say) potential risk factors for developing a specific disease, there may be no formal design coefficients such as β_1 but only potentially (many) influencing covariates such as v_1. In general, the study design team are interested in the stability of the estimates of the regression coefficients in the ensuing regression model. In such cases, estimating required sample sizes may be quite problematic. One option is for the investigating team to first rank (at least for what are thought likely as major) covariates in terms of their anticipated importance. They then quantify the covariates' impact to obtain corresponding planning values from which sample sizes for each can be determined. On this basis a compromise study size is then agreed upon by the investigating team with a focus on a sample size that will be sufficient to answer the questions relating to the highest ranking covariates.

In our terms, these covariates then define the x's with corresponding β's while the remainder stay as v's with corresponding γ's. The modelling strategy would be to estimate the model containing only the x's and then compare it with models including (some of) the v's.

Approaches to model building using variable selection procedures in such circumstances, all of which involve repeated statistical significance tests, are described by Tai and Machin (2014) who distinguish between design (D), knowingly influential (K), and exploratory or query of uncertain influence (Q) covariates.

In simple terms, if we were estimating a mean then we would consider a sample size of 10 to be rather small for that purpose whereas (and ignoring all else) 25 may be sufficient. If we extend this simplistic view to a regression model containing several x's and/or v's then we might argue that the size of the study should include a minimum of 10 (or maybe 15, or 20, or ...?) subjects for every regression coefficient to be estimated. This is hardly scientific but does suggest a rule-of-thumb against which the planned study size based on other criteria can be compared. Although arbitrary, since there are no effect sizes or power considerations, it can be a useful guide if a preliminary study is planned as a precursor to the main study.

However, this guide is based on the number of subjects recruited and only applies to multiple linear regression in which the endpoint, y, is a continuous (or at least numerical) variable. If the endpoint is binary and (multiple) logistic regression is required for analysis or Cox regression is used for a survival outcome, the rule-of-thumb becomes to plan to observe at least $10r$ events where r is the number of regression parameters to be estimated (including β_0) in the regression model. If 'non-events' are less common than 'events' then 'non-events' replace 'events' here. In general, this will require the number of subjects to be greater than the total number of 'events' or 'non-events' anticipated.

Thus if one had to estimate 6 parameters including the constant term, then one would need at least 60 events to be observed. If one assumed that the event rate was about 50% then this would translate into about 60/0.5 = 120 subjects. However, if the event rate is 90% (rather than 50%), then the corresponding non-event rate is 10%. The study should then aim to observe 60 non-events. This would require approximately 60/0.1 = 600 subjects for the necessary number of 'non-events' to be observed.

This arbitrary rule is based on the number of parameters in the model, not the number of variables. For example, if only a single categorical variable with g categories was fitted, then such a variable adds $g - 1$ parameters to the model.

Whatever the outcome of the planning sample size calculations, these should be cross-checked against the above suggestions.

2.7 The Protocol and Publication

As we have indicated, the justification of sample size in any study is important. This not only gives an indication of the resources required but also forces the research team to think about issues of design carefully. Following are examples of how some resulting sample size calculations were justified.

Example 2.1   Chronic Myelogenous Leukemia
Figure 2.2 gives an early example of the justification for trial size reproduced from that included in the trial protocol of Haanen, Hellriegel and Machin (1979). In retrospect, and taking account of accumulated experience over the years, this summary can be criticised in a number of ways. The first, and most important, is the assumption that in such an aggressive disease a 50% increase in the median disease-free survival time could be anticipated. Had such an advantage been achieved then levamisole would be a wonder drug. The second is that in the years following this publication there was growing realism that many useful therapies were being overlooked since the earlier trials were underpowered and so failed to detect (smaller but important) clinically meaningful differences. Thus, trials with power of 90% have become more the norm.

Further, the calculations assume a one-sided test will be conducted. Also, the rather precise sample size of 76 per treatment group overlooks the uncertainties associated in any sample size calculations. Finally, a source reference for the specific sample size formula used would have been

---

The primary objective of this study is to compare the duration of the disease stage following remission induced by busulfan until onset of metamorphosis. In a pairwise comparison of patients treated with busulfan only after remission and patients treated with busulfan and levamisole, a total of 76 patients followed until relapse is required on each treatment group in order to detect a ratio of 1.5:1 in the median (or mean) remission duration (assumed to follow an exponential distribution) of the two treatment groups (error probabilities $\alpha = 0.05$, $\beta = 0.20$). Thus a total of 152 good-risk patients are to be followed until the onset of the metamorphosis.

Figure 2.2 Sample size for a randomised trial assessing the benefit of adjuvant levamisole added to busulphan for good-risk patients with chronic myelogenous leukaemia (after Haanen, Hellriegel and Machin, 1979).

a useful addition as would the anticipated disease-free survival of those in the control group (busulphan alone).

Example 2.2   Surgical Resection for Patients with Gastric Cancer
Cuschieri, Weeden, Fielding, *et al* (1999) compared two forms of surgical resection for patients with gastric cancer. The primary outcome (event of interest) was time to death. The authors state:
   'Sample size calculations were based on a pre-study survey of 26 gastric surgeons, which indicated that the baseline 5-year survival rate of D_1 surgery was expected to be 20%, and an improvement in survival to 34% (14% change) with D_2 resection would be a realistic expectation. Thus 400 patients (200 in each arm) were to be randomised, providing 90% power to detect such a difference with p-value < 0.05.'

Example 2.3   Steroid or Cyclosporine for Oral Lichen Planus
The protocol of March 1998 of the subsequently published trial conducted by Poon, Tin, Kim, *et al* (2006) to compare steroid with cyclosporine for the topical treatment of oral lichen planus stated:
   'It is anticipated that in patients taking topical *Steroid*, the response rate at 1 month will be approximately 60%. It is anticipated that this may be raised to as much as 80% in those receiving *Cyclosporine*. With two-sided test size 5%, power 80%, then the corresponding number of patients required is approximately 200 (Machin, Campbell, Fayers and Pinol, 1997, Table 3.1).'
   However, despite international collaboration, the trial subsequently recruited only 139 patients and demonstrated little difference at 1 month with a 52% response rate with *Steroid* and 48% with *Cyclosporine*.

Example 2.4   Cardiovascular Guidelines
Figure 2.3 illustrates the very detailed sample size justification for the proposed CLUES study given by Etxeberria, Pérez, Alcorta, *et al* (2013). Their sample size calculations set $\alpha = 0.05$ (with a two-sided test implied) and $1 - \beta = 0.8$ and the recruitment is set to involve 40 primary care units (PCU) each of which will concern patients from 10 clinicians. The design is a cluster randomised clinical trial (see **Chapter 12**) with half the clusters assigned to the *Intervention* and half to *Control*. The aim is to improve the proportion of patients with either diabetes or hypertension who have an appropriate number of annual HbA1c analyses.

Example 2.5   Sequential Hormonal Therapy in Advanced and Metastatic Breast Cancer
Iaffaioli, Formato, Tortoriello, *et al* (2005) conducted two Phase II trials of sequential hormonal therapy with first-line Anastrozole and second-line Exemestane in advanced and metastatic breast cancer. The authors provide their justification for sample size as follows:
   'The sample size calculation for both single-stage studies was performed as proposed by A'Hern (2001), this method being an exact version of the algorithm first presented by Fleming (1982). The Anastrizole evaluation required 93 subjects to decide whether the proportion of patients (P) with a clinical benefit was $\leq 50\%$ or $\geq 65\%$. If the number of patients with clinical benefit was ≥ 55, the hypothesis that $P \leq 50\%$ was rejected with a target error rate of 0.050 and an actual error rate of 0.048. If the number of patients with clinical benefit was ≤ 54, the hypothesis that $P \geq 65\%$ was rejected with a target error rate of 0.100 and an actual error rate of 0.099.'
   A similar justification was provided for the Exemestane component of this study.

Sample size

The following aspects were taken into account when calculating the sample size:

- On average, 45–50% of diabetic patients assigned to a healthcare professional undergo at least two annual HbA1c analyses (standard deviation 15–20%). An annual analysis is requested in around 35% of hypertensive patients. (Data taken from the Provider Agreement, 2007).

- From a clinical and operational viewpoint, an intervention strategy would be worthwhile if these averages could be increased to 55–60% for diabetes and 43% for hypertension.

- The size of the PCUs is similar, with around 10 physicians per PCU, and the number of patients assigned to each clinician is also similar.

- The intracluster correlation coefficient (ICC) is 0.10 [29–31].

In light of these considerations, approximately 100 physicians per group (10 PCUs in each group) would be needed for an α of 0.05 and a β of 0.20. Applying the cluster-related design effect gives a final number of 20 PCUs per group (intervention and control).

Figure 2.3 Sample size for a cluster randomised trial to evaluate cardiovascular guideline implementation in primary care (after Etxeberria, Pérez, Alcorta, *et al*, 2013).

2.8 Ethical Issues and Sample Size

Given the uncertainties that surround the values of the parameters required to make sensible 'guesses' about the size of a projected study, many authors including Campbell (2013) have warned about the dangers of making sample size calculations into a ritual to be observed at the expense of good science. This is particularly true of clinical trials, where treatments can cause death or serious injury to a patient. Here, an underpowered trial is possibly unethical, because it is unable to answer the question posed. Similarly, a trial which is overpowered may be unethical because the answer could have been obtained with fewer patients. In which case, some patients will have been randomised to a treatment known to be inferior.

There are arguments for and against doing trials that are unlikely to achieve high statistical power. In principle, the choice between continuing to use inadequately evaluated treatments haphazardly outside the context of controlled trials or offering them within controlled trials should be easy; one will learn nothing from the former and something from the latter. As Schulz and Grimes (2005) point out, it is almost always unrealistic to expect a single study to answer an important question, while the results of relatively small trials can contribute to meta-analyses from which reliable conclusions may be drawn.

The argument against statistically 'underpowered' trials is that difficulties may arise following 'equivocal' results. There is often an opportune time for a clinical trial to be conducted, when investigators are willing to accept a 'balance of probabilities' in favour of alternative treatments. Imprecise estimates of treatment effects from an underpowered trial may change this balance of probabilities and yet still leave considerable doubt as to the relative efficacy of the treatments compared. This may make it difficult to obtain ethics approval and patient consent for a confirmatory trial addressing the same question. In addition, Campbell (2013) notes that equivocal trials are probably less likely to be submitted and accepted for publication, and so will be less readily available for inclusion in meta-analyses.

Bacchetti, McCulloch and Segal (2005, 2008) have argued that at the planning stage, the projected value of a study (as measured by the size of the effect) decreases as the sample size increases. The projected total burden on participants, however, is proportional to sample size, implying that the ratio of study value to participant burden can only worsen as sample size increases. The diminishing marginal returns imply that ignoring costs when planning sample size, as is routine with conventional power calculations, can lead to very poor cost efficiency, and supposedly underpowered studies can be much more cost efficient.

An additional objection is that the key concept of 'underpowered' is ill defined. For example, Halpern, Karlawish and Berlin (2002) have endorsed the 80% power requirement but cited only 'tradition' as supporting it. Additional ambiguity arises from the fact that, for any sample size, one can always find design assumptions that produce 80% power. Iteratively adjusting assumptions such as the effect size until a desired sample size appears 'adequate' will appear to meet the supposed standard, but it actually does nothing to make the study itself any more ethical.

A strong justification for sample size calculations has been put by Williamson, Hutton, Bliss, *et al* (2000) who pointed out that prior power calculation can be beneficial as it forces investigators, *before the study commences*, to identify the main outcome variable. This can then be verified at the analysis stage in order to protect against data dredging. The authors also noted that it makes clear, *before the results are known*, what the authors considered to be a meaningful effect size so claims for superiority or non-inferiority can be verified. For example, a confidence interval that includes the null hypothesis value of zero as well as an estimated clinically meaningful effect the study remains inconclusive, whereas if it includes zero but excludes a meaningful effect we have grounds for saying that the test treatment is no better, or no worse, than the standard.

An ethical study will have a sample size calculation, although should resources be limited so that it would be impossible to achieve a high power, the investigating team should report the practical constraints, provide the power the study can achieve under these restrictions, and describe these in the associated protocol and the subsequent final report.

References

Technical
A'Hern RP (2001). Sample size tables for exact single stage phase II designs. *Statistics in Medicine*, **20**, 859–866.
Bacchetti P, Wolf LE, Segal MR and McCulloch CE (2005). Ethics and sample size. *American Journal of Epidemiology*, **161**, 105–110.

Bacchetti P, McCulloch CE and Segal MR (2008). Simple, defensible sample sizes based on cost efficiency. *Biometrics*, **64**, 577–585.

Campbell MJ (2013). Doing clinical trials large enough to achieve adequate reductions in uncertainties about treatment effects. *Journal of the Royal Society of Medicine*, **106**, 68–71.

Fayers PM and Machin D (2016). *Quality of Life: The Assessment, Analysis and Reporting of Patient-reported Outcomes*. (3nd edn) Wiley-Blackwell, Chichester.

Fleming TR (1982). One-sample multiple testing procedure for Phase II clinical trial. *Biometrics*, **38**, 143–151.

Halpern SD, Karlawish JHT and Berlin JA (2002). The continuing unethical conduct of underpowered clinical trials. *Journal of the American Medical Association*, **288**, 358–362.

Machin D and Campbell MJ (2005). *Design of Studies for Medical Research*, Wiley, Chichester.

Machin D, Campbell MJ, Fayers PM and Pinol A (1997). *Statistical Tables for the Design of Clinical Studies* (2nd edn). Blackwell Scientific Publications, Oxford.

Schulz KF and Grimes DA (2005). Sample size calculations in randomised trials: mandatory and mystical. *Lancet*, **365**, 1348–1353.

Tai B-C and Machin D (2014). *Regression Methods for Medical Research*. Wiley-Blackwell, Chichester.

Williamson P, Hutton JL, Bliss J, Blunt J, Campbell MJ and Nicholson R (2000). Statistical review by research ethics committees. *Journal of the Royal Statistical Society A*, **163**, 5–13.

Examples

Cuschieri A, Weeden S, Fielding J, Bancewicz J, Craven J, Joypaul V, Sydes M and Fayers P (1999). Patient survival after D1 and D2 resections for gastric cancer: long-term results of the MRC randomized surgical trial. *British Journal of Cancer*, **79**, 1522–1530.

Day AC, Machin D, Aung T, Gazzard G, Husain R, Chew PTK, Khaw PT, Seah SKL and Foster PJ (2011). Central corneal thickness and glaucoma in East Asian people. *Investigative Ophthalmology & Visual Science*, **52**, 8407–8412.

Etxeberria A, Pérez I, Alcorta I, Emparanza JI, Ruiz de Velasco E, Iglesias MT, Orozco-Beltrán D and Rotaeche R (2013). The CLUES study: a cluster randomized clinical trial for the evaluation of cardiovascular guideline implementation in primary care. *BMC Health Services Research*, **13**, 438.

Haanen H, Hellriegel K and Machin D (1979). EORTC protocol for the treatment of good-risk patients with chronic myelogenous leukaemia. *A randomized trial. European Journal of Cancer*, **15**, 803–809.

Iaffaioli RV, Formato R, Tortoriello A, Del Prete S, Caraglia M, Pappagallo G, Pisano A, Fanelli F, Ianniello G, Cigolari S, Pizza C, Marano O, Pezzella G, Pedicini T, Febbraro A, Incoronato P, Manzione L, Ferrari E, Marzano N, Quattrin S, Pisconti S, Nasti G, Giotta G, Colucci G and other Goim authors (2005). Phase II study of sequential hormonal therapy with anastrozole/exemestane in advanced and metastatic breast cancer. *British Journal of Cancer*, **92**, 1621–1625.

Poon CY, Goh BT, Kim M-J, Rajaseharan A, Ahmed S, Thongsprasom K, Chaimusik M, Suresh S, Machin D, Wong H-B and Seldrup J (2006). A randomised controlled trial to compare steroid with cyclosporine for the topical treatment of oral lichen planus. *Oral Surg Oral Med Oral Path Oral Radiol Endod*, **102**, 47–55.

3

Binary Outcomes

SUMMARY
This chapter considers sample-size calculations for comparisons between two groups where the outcome of concern is binary. The anticipated effect size between groups is expressed either as a difference between two proportions or by the odds ratio. The situation in which one of the proportions can be assumed known is described. Attention is drawn to difficulties that may arise if one of the proportions is anticipated to be close to zero or unity.

3.1   Introduction

A binary variable is one that only takes one of two values. For example, the outcome for patients receiving a treatment in a clinical trial may be regarded as a 'success' or 'failure'. Typical examples are cured/ not cured or alive/dead.

Sometimes ordered categorical or continuous data may be dichotomised into binary form for ease of analysis. For example in a trial of diets in obese people, the outcome may be the Body Mass Index (BMI) measured in kg/m^2. Nevertheless, the design, and hence analysis, may be more concerned with the proportion of people no longer obese, where 'obesity' is defined as (say) a BMI greater than $30 kg/m^2$ and which is thought relevant to the study population of concern. However dichotomising in this way is not usually a good idea since information is lost in this process and consequently a larger study may be required to answer the key question (see **Chapters 4 and 5** for categorical and continuous endpoints).

3.2   Comparing Proportions

The data necessary to estimate a proportion are often coded as 0 and 1 and so are essentially binary in form. If two groups are to be compared then the results can be summarised in a 2×2 table as shown in **Figure 3.1** in which $N = n_S + n_T$ patients who are assigned at random to one of the treatments, n_S to *Standard* (S) and n_T to *Test* (T). At the design stage, we may have the option to randomise to the two alternative treatments either equally, 1:1, or with an unequal allocation, 1: φ. In either case, $n_T = \varphi n_S$ as in **Figure 3.1**. The same format also applies to studies other than clinical trials that are designed to compare two groups with respect to a binary outcome.

Sample Sizes for Clinical, Laboratory and Epidemiology Studies, Fourth Edition. David Machin, Michael J. Campbell, Say Beng Tan and Sze Huey Tan.
© 2018 John Wiley & Sons Ltd. Published 2018 by John Wiley & Sons Ltd.

Treatment Group	'Success' Code = 1	'Failure' Code = 0	Total	Observed proportion of successes	Anticipated proportion of successes
Standard (S)	a	c	n_S	a/n_S	π_S
Test (T)	b	d	$n_T = \varphi\, n_S$	b/n_T	π_T
Total	r	s	N		

Figure 3.1 Notation for a clinical study comparing the proportion of successes in two (independent) groups.

The corresponding analysis of the subsequent data from a study compares the observed proportion of successes from the two groups of concern.

Effect Size

At the planning stage of a study, we have to specify the anticipated effect size or anticipated difference in proportions: $\delta_{Plan} = \pi_{PlanT} - \pi_{PlanS}$. Here π_{PlanS} and π_{PlanT} are the anticipated proportion of successes under S and T respectively of **Figure 3.1**.

In some situations it may be difficult to propose a value for the effect size, δ_{Plan}, for which a trial is to be designed to detect. However, since the possibility of success under S is π_S, the odds associated with it are $\pi_S/(1 - \pi_S)$. Similarly, the odds associated with success under T are $\pi_T/(1 - \pi_T)$. From these, the ratio of these odds, termed the odds ratio, is $OR = \dfrac{\pi_T/(1-\pi_T)}{\pi_S/(1-\pi_S)} = \dfrac{\pi_T(1-\pi_S)}{\pi_S(1-\pi_T)}$. The OR can take any positive value and the corresponding value for the null hypothesis H_0: $\pi_T - \pi_S = 0$ is $OR_{Null} = 1$. In this situation, if π_S and OR are stipulated then the planning value π_T is obtained from

$$\pi_T = \frac{OR\pi_S}{\left(1 - \pi_S + OR\pi_S\right)}. \tag{3.1}$$

Thus, rather than pre-specifying both π_{PlanS} and π_{PlanT}, an investigator may pre-specify OR_{Plan} and (say) π_{PlanS} and then use equation (3.1) to obtain the anticipated π_{PlanT}, from which the anticipated value for δ_{Plan} can be obtained.

Analysis

The standard tests for comparing two proportions are either the χ^2 test or the Fisher's Exact test. The latter is well approximated by the χ^2 test with Yates's continuity correction included, which is termed χ_C^2. The choice of the appropriate test influences the sample size required to detect a difference in proportions. Clearly one should use the same test for the planning as for the analysis. At the analysis stage, χ_C^2 is seldom used now as with modern statistical packages the Fisher's Exact test can be readily computed. However, its close approximation to Fisher's test is useful for deriving sample sizes.

χ^2 Test

Sample size

To aid clarity in the following formulae, we use π_S and π_T to represent π_{PlanS} and π_{PlanT}.

The required total sample size, for specified π_S, π_T, with an allocation ratio to the two groups of 1: φ, 2-sided test size α, power $1 - \beta$ and analysis using the χ^2 test, is

$$N = \left(\frac{1+\varphi}{\varphi}\right)\frac{\left\{z_{1-\alpha/2}\sqrt{\left[(1+\varphi)\bar{\pi}(1-\bar{\pi})\right]} + z_{1-\beta}\sqrt{\left[\varphi\pi_S(1-\pi_S) + \pi_T(1-\pi_T)\right]}\right\}^2}{\delta_{Plan}^2}, \tag{3.2}$$

where

$$\bar{\pi} = (\pi_S + \varphi\pi_T)/(1+\varphi). \tag{3.3}$$

Hence the numbers required in each group are $n_S = N/(1+\varphi)$ and $n_T = \varphi N/(1+\varphi)$. Values for $z_{1-\alpha/2}$ and $z_{1-\beta}$ can be obtained from **Table 1.2**. Sample sizes calculated from equation (3.2) for the situation $\varphi = 1$ are given in **Table 3.1**.

If the effect size is expressed as an odds ratio, OR_{Plan}, then not only does π_S have to be specified but π_T needs to be obtained from equation (3.1) and hence $\bar{\pi}$ from equation (3.3). The sample size is determined from

$$N_{OR} = \frac{(1+\varphi)^2}{\varphi}\frac{\left(z_{1-\alpha/2} + z_{1-\beta}\right)^2}{\left(logOR_{Plan}\right)^2 \bar{\pi}(1-\bar{\pi})}, \tag{3.4}$$

and $n_S = N_{OR}/(1+\varphi)$ and $n_T = \varphi N_{OR}/(1+\varphi)$. Sample sizes calculated from equation (3.4) for the situation $\varphi = 1$ are given in **Table 3.2**.

Equation (3.4) is quite different in form to equation (3.2). However, for all practical purposes, it gives very similar sample sizes, with divergent results only occurring for relatively large differences of OR_{Plan} from unity. Nevertheless, we would recommend the routine use of equation (3.2).

Fisher's Exact Test

Sample size

When using the Exact-test for analysis, after first determining N (then n_S) with one of equations (3.2) or (3.4), the required sample size is obtained using

$$n_S^{Exact} = \frac{n_S}{4}\left[1 + \sqrt{1 + \frac{2(1+\varphi)}{\varphi n_S \times \text{abs}(\delta_{Plan})}}\right]^2 \text{ and } n_T^{Exact} = \varphi n_S^{Exact}. \tag{3.5}$$

Since the term within the square root in (3.5) is always >1, $N_{Exact} = n_S^{Exact} + n_T^{Exact} > N$ so that a larger number of subjects is then required. Essentially this acts as a small sample adjustment to the earlier sample size calculation.

Practical note

It is important to note that when either or both of the anticipated proportions are close to 0 or 1 then the design should anticipate that the Fisher's Exact test will be used to compare the two groups. A rule-of-thumb is to be cautious and use equation (3.5) if either one of the planning proportions results in the product $\pi(1 - \pi) < 0.15$.

3.3 One Proportion Known

In some situations one may know, with a fair degree of certainty, the proportion of successes in one of the groups. For example, a large number of very similar clinical trials may have been conducted with a particular drug, showing that the success rate is about 20%. Thus, in a clinical trial to test a new product under identical conditions, it may not seem necessary to treat any patients with the standard drug. In which case, the investigators may only be concerned to know if the response rate on the T is greater than the S.

χ^2 Test

Sample size

In this situation, we assume the success rate π_S ($= \pi_{Known}$) is known. The object of the study is to estimate π_T, which is then compared with π_{Known}. The required number of subjects in the single group, for significance level α and power $1 - \beta$ for comparing the anticipated π_T with the established success rate π_{Known}, is

$$N = \frac{\left\{z_{1-\alpha/2}\sqrt{\left[\pi_{Known}\left(1-\pi_{Known}\right)\right]} + z_{1-\beta}\sqrt{\left[\pi_T\left(1-\pi_T\right)\right]}\right\}^2}{\delta^2}, \tag{3.6}$$

where values for $z_{1-\alpha/2}$ and $z_{1-\beta}$ can be obtained from **Table 1.2**.

In this situation, that is, with one of the proportions assumed known, it may be more appropriate to use a 1-sided test. In such cases, $z_{1-\alpha/2}$ in equation (3.6) is replaced by $z_{1-\alpha}$.

3.4 Bibliography

The Fisher's Exact test and the χ^2-test for a 2 × 2 contingency table are described in many texts including Campbell, Machin and Walters (2007). Equation (3.2) appears in Fleiss, Levi and Paik (2003) while Demidenko (2007, equation 14) gives an alternative expression which gives similar sample sizes. Julious and Campbell (1996) discuss the approximation of equation (3.4). Fleiss, Tytun and Ury (1980) extended the expression given by Casagrande, Pike and Smith (1978) to equation (3.5) which allows for unequal subject numbers in the two groups. Julious and Campbell (2012) provide a comprehensive review of alternative sample-size formulae for testing differences in proportions. Hosmer and Lemeshow (2000) and Novikov, Fund and Freedman (2010) describe an approach to sample size estimates when logistic regression is to be used to take account of a continuous covariate.

Nwaru and Sheikh (2015) provide an example of a survey concerned with hormonal contraceptive use in women and its potential association with physician-diagnosed asthma, in which the ratio of subjects between the participating groups is chosen as 1: 3/7 or 1: 0.4286.

3.5   Examples and Use of the Tables

Table 1.2
For two-sided test size, $\alpha = 0.05$, $z_{0.975} = 1.96$. For one-sided test size, $\alpha = 0.05$, $z_{0.95} = 1.6449$. For one-sided $1 - \beta = 0.80$ and 0.90, $z_{0.8} = 0.8416$ and $z_{0.9} = 1.2816$.

Table 3.1 and Equations 3.2 and 3.3

Example 3.1   Difference in proportions - Lingual retainers for ortodontic retension
Pandis (2012) uses the information from a retrospective study of Lie, Ozcan, Verkerke, *et al* (2008) to illustrate sample size calculations when comparing proportions. The study found that lingual retainers with conventional acid (*Acid*) etching had a failure rate by 2 years of 38% whereas those with self-etching (*Self*) primers had a rate of 23%. If a confirmatory 1: 1 randomised trial is planned, how many patients would be required?

With planning values set at $\pi_{Acid} = 0.38$, $\pi_{Self} = 0.23$ and $\varphi = 1$, equation (3.3) gives $\bar{\pi} = (0.38 + (1 \times 0.23)/(1 + 1) = 0.305$. Then with $\delta_{Plan} = \pi_{Acid} - \pi_{Self} = -0.15$, a 2-sided test size of 5% and power 90%, equation (3.2) gives

$$N = \frac{(1+1)^2}{1} \frac{\left\{ 1.96\sqrt{\left[(1+1) \times 0.305 \times (1-0.305)\right]} + 1.2816\sqrt{\left[1 \times 0.38 \times (1-0.38) + 0.23 \times (1-0.23)\right]} \right\}^2}{-0.15^2}$$

$= 391.82$ or 392 patients are required with 196 per group. Use of $^S\!S_S$ gives $N = 392$.

Pandis (2012) uses an algebraic simplification of equation (3.2) and obtains a very similar value for $N = 386$. The closest entries in **Table 3.1** are $\pi_1 = 0.4$, $\pi_2 = 0.25$ which give, for power 90%, $N = 406$.

Table 3.1 and Equations 3.2, 3.3, 3.4 and 3.5

Example 3.2   Difference in proportions - MRSA infection in patients with severe burns
In a randomised trial by Ang, Lee, Gan, *et al* (2001), the standard wound covering treatment (*S*) was compared with Moist Exposed Burns Ointment (*M*) in patients with severe burns. One objective of the trial was to reduce the methicillin-resistant *staphylococcus aureus* (MRSA) infection rate at 2 weeks post-admission in such patients from 25% to 5%.

With planning values set at $\pi_S = 0.25$, $\pi_M = 0.05$, $\delta_{Plan} = \pi_M - \pi_S = -0.20$ and for a 2-sided test size of 5% and power 80%, equation (3.3) with $\varphi = 1$, gives $\bar{\pi} = [0.25 + (1 \times 0.05)]/(1+1) = 0.015$. With these values equation (3.2) gives

$$N = \left(\frac{1+1}{1}\right) \frac{\left\{ 1.96\sqrt{\left[(1+1) \times 0.15 \times (1-0.15)\right]} + 0.8416\sqrt{\left[1 \times 0.25 \times (1-0.25) + 0.05 \times (1-0.05)\right]} \right\}^2}{-0.2^2}$$

$= 97.68$ or 98 patients implying $n_S = n_M = 49$ per treatment group. Since $\delta_{Plan} < 0$, to use **Table 3.1** the labels for π_2 and π_1 are interchanged which then gives $N = 98$ as does $^S\!S_S$.

Had it been anticipated that the results of the trial planned would be analysed using the Fisher's Exact test, what influence does this have on the number of patients to be recruited?

As previously with $\pi_M = 0.05$, $\pi_S = 0.25$, $\delta_{Plan} = -0.20$ and $\varphi = 1$, for a 2-sided $\alpha = 0.05$, $1 - \beta = 0.8$, the sample size is $N = 98$. Now using equation (3.6) with $abs(\delta_{Plan}) = 0.20$ gives

$$n_S^{Exact} = 49 \times \frac{1}{4}\left[1 + \sqrt{1 + \frac{2 \times (1+1)}{1 \times 49 \times 0.2}}\right]^2 = 49 \times 1.1954 = 58.57 \quad \text{or} \quad 59 \text{ per group. As a consequence}$$

$N_{Exact} = 118$ and which is also given by direct use of $^S\boxed{S_S}$.

As we have noted earlier, if either of the anticipated proportions are close to 0 or 1 then the design should anticipate that the Fisher's Exact test will be used to compare the two groups. In this example, $\pi_T = 0.05$ is close to 0, the rule-of-thumb gives $\pi_T(1 - \pi_T) = 0.0475 < 0.15$, and so a more appropriate trial size is $N_{Exact} \approx 120$ rather than the 98 suggested previously.

Equations 3.2 and 3.5

Example 3.3 Fisher's Exact test - Difference in proportions - Capnographic monitoring during propofol sedation for colonoscopy

Beitz, Riphaus, Meining, *et al* (2012) conducted a randomised trial to investigate the value of capnographic monitoring during propofol sedation for colonoscopy. In their design they anticipated a reduction in the incidence of oxygen desaturation from $\pi_S = 0.12$ (12%) with standard monitoring (S) to $\pi_C = 0.06$ (6%) with additional capnography (C). They further specified a 0.05 2-sided significance level, a power of 80%, equal allocation to each intervention and that a Fisher's Exact test would be used for the analysis. Use of either equations (3.2) and (3.5) or $^S\boxed{S_S}$ gives $n_S = n_C = 389$. In the event, the trial recruited $n_C = 374$ and $n_S = 383$ and surprisingly reported $p_S = 0.532$ and $p_C = 0.389$. Had these values been used for planning purposes, $^S\boxed{S_S}$ gives $n_S = n_C = 204$. In which case a much smaller trial of about half the size actually conducted would have been anticipated.

Table 3.2 and Equations 3.1, 3.2, 3.3 and 3.4

Example 3.4 Change in odds ratio - MRSA infection in severe burns

Suppose in the randomised trial by Ang, Lee, Gan *et al* (2001), the design team had phrased their objectives as reducing the odds of MRSA by use of Moist Exposed Burns Ointment (M) as compared to standard wound covering treatment. In this case with the same MRSA infection rate at 2-weeks post-admission of 25% (odds 25% to 75% or 1:3), we assume that the investigators anticipated this would be reduced to as little as 1:5 by the use of M.

Here the planning $OR_{Plan} = (1/5)/(1/3) = 0.6$, then with $\pi_S = 0.25$ equation (3.1) gives

$$\pi_M = \frac{0.6 \times 0.25}{[1 - 0.25 + (0.6 \times 0.25)]} = 0.1667. \text{ Direct use of equation (3.2) with these values in } ^S\boxed{S_S} \text{ with a}$$

2-sided test size of 5%, power 80% and $\varphi = 1$ gives $N = 744$.

Alternatively from equation (3.3), $\bar{\pi} = (0.25 + 0.1667)/2 = 0.2084$, and with $OR_{Plan} = 0.6$, equation (3.4)

gives $N_{OR} = \dfrac{(1+1)^2}{1} \dfrac{(1.96 + 0.8416)^2}{(log0.6)^2 \times 0.2084 \times (1 - 0.2084)} = 729.40$ or 730.

This is 14 fewer patients than the 744 derived from equation (3.2) and indicates that (3.4) underestimates slightly when the effect size is distant from $OR_{Null} = 1$.

To make use of **Table 3.2**, the inverse of the odds ratio needs to be used and in this case $1/0.6 = 1.67$. The nearest tabular entries, with a test size of 5% and power 80%, for $1 - \pi_S = 0.75$ are $OR = 1.6$ and 1.7 giving $N = 854$ and 680 respectively, suggesting a final sample size of 760 approximately mid-way between these entries.

Equations 3.1, 3.3 and 3.4

Example 3.5   Change in odds ratio – Pre-specified allocation ratio - Physician-diagnosed asthma
Nwaru and Sheikh (2015) reported a survey concerned with hormonal contraceptive use in women and its potential association with physician-diagnosed asthma. They estimated that amongst women between 16-49 years the prevalence of contraceptive use would be 30%. Thus, the ratio anticipated of non-users to users in their design was set at 7:3 or 1: $\varphi = 3/7 = 0.4286$. They also identified the background prevalence of ever having physician-diagnosed asthma to be 20% and the study was designed to detect an OR of 1.4 with 90% power. Thus with $\pi_{\text{User}} = 0.2$ and $OR_{Plan} = 1.4$,

equation (3.1) gives $\pi_{\text{Non-User}} = \dfrac{1.4 \times 0.2}{\left[1 - 0.2 + (1.4 \times 0.2)\right]} = 0.2593$. Hence with $\varphi = 0.4286$, equation (3.3)

gives $\bar{\pi} = [0.2 + (0.4286 \times 0.2593)]/(1 + 0.4286) = 0.2178$. Setting 2-sided $\alpha = 0.05$, $\beta = 0.1$ in equa-

tion (3.4) then gives $N_{OR} = \dfrac{(1 + 0.4286)^2}{0.4286} \dfrac{(1.96 + 1.2816)^2}{(log 1.4)^2 \times 0.2178 \times (1 - 0.2178)} = 2{,}594.3$. Thus, the number

of non-user women to be recruited was $n_{\text{Non-User}} = \dfrac{2594.3}{1 + 0.4286} = 1{,}815.97$ or 1,816 and

$n_{\text{User}} = \dfrac{0.4286 \times 2594.3}{1 + 0.4286} = 778.32$ or 779.

Nwaru and Sheikh (2015) calculated $N_{OR} = 2{,}494$ non-pregnant women who had completed a questionnaire on asthma and respiratory symptoms were required. The associated surveys conducted to identify such women eventually obtained information from 3,257 of whom $n_{\text{Non-User}} = 2{,}252$ and $n_{\text{User}} = 1{,}005$.

Equations 3.2, 3.3 and 3.4

Example 3.6   Case-Control - Change in odds ratio - Single nucleotide polymorphisms and myocardial infarction
In their Introduction, Cheng, Cho, Cen, *et al* (2015) noted that 'Many single nucleotide polymorphisms (SNPs) show correlated genotypes, …, suggesting that only a subset of SNPs (known as … tagSNPs) need to be genotyped for disease association studies.' From Table 2 of their own study, they concluded that the G allele frequency of rs7069102 of 18.3% in the 287 myocardial infarction (*MI*) patients was significantly higher than the 13.8% from the 654 in the hospital controls group (*HC*).

Suppose a group of investigators wish to conduct a similar study in a different region in China. What would be a reasonable sample size for such a confirmatory study?

When expressed as a difference between proportions, $d = 0.183 - 0.138 = 0.045$ with a corresponding

$OR = \dfrac{0.183/(1 - 0.183)}{0.138/(1 - 0.138)} = 1.3991$. Either d or OR might then be used as potential planning values. The

earlier study had a ratio of *HC* to *MI* of 654:287 or 1: 0.44 and therefore the new investigators assume a similar ratio of 2: 1. Thus with $\pi_{HC} = 0.138$, $\pi_{MI} = 0.183$ and $\varphi = 0.5$, equation (3.3) gives $\bar{\pi} = [0.138 + (0.5 \times 0.183)] / (1 + 0.5) = 0.153$. Further setting 2-sided $\alpha = 0.05$ and $\beta = 0.1$, equation (3.2) gives

$$N = \left(\frac{1+0.5}{0.5}\right) \frac{\left\{1.96\sqrt{[(1+0.5) \times 0.153 \times 0.847]} + 1.2816\sqrt{[0.5 \times 0.138 \times 0.862 + 0.183 \times 0.817]}\right\}^2}{0.045^2}$$

$= 3,114.97$ or $3,115$. Thus $n_{HC} = \dfrac{3114.97}{1+0.5} = 2,077$ and $n_{MI} = \dfrac{0.5 \times 3114.97}{1+0.5} = 1,039$.

Alternatively with $OR_{Plan} = 1.3991$, equation (3.4) gives $N_{OR} = \dfrac{(1+0.5)^2}{0.5} \dfrac{(1.96 + 1.2816)^2}{(log 1.3991)^2 \times 0.153 \times 0.847}$

$= 3,235.19$ or $3,236$, implying $n_{HC} = 2,157$ and $n_{MI} = 1,079$.

With the same planning values used, $\boxed{^SS_S}$ also gives $N = 3,116$, and $N_{OR} = 3,236$. The two methods differ because of approximations made in the derivation of equation (3.4).

As covariates are often present, logistic regression analysis is likely to be used, resulting in adjusted estimates for the OR, so that the larger sample size might be chosen. In fact, Cheng, Cho, Cen, *et al* (2014, Table 2) quoted an $OR = 1.57$ after adjusting for eight (an unusually large number) covariates using logistic regression.

Equation 3.6

Example 3.7 Comparison with historical control - Wound infection
The rate of wound infection over 1 year in an operating theatre was 10%. This figure has been confirmed from several other operating theatres with the same scrub-up preparation. If an investigator wishes to test the efficacy of a new scrub-up preparation, how many operations does he need to examine in order to be 90% confident that the new procedure only produces a 5% infection rate?

Here $\pi_{Test} = 0.05$, $\pi_{Known} = 0.10$, power $1 - \beta = 0.90$ and, if we set *1-sided* $\alpha = 0.05$, equation (3.6) yields

$$N = \frac{\left\{1.6449\sqrt{0.1 \times 0.9} + 1.2816\sqrt{0.05 \times 0.95}\right\}^2}{(0.1 - 0.05)^2} = 238.84 \text{ or } 240 \text{ operations.}$$

However, if this is compared with the more usual situation when both proportions are to be estimated, then a 2-sided test would be required. Entry into **Table 3.1** for $1 - \beta = 0.9$ with $\pi_1 = 0.05$ and $\pi_2 = 0.10$ gives $N = 1,164$ operations, which is almost five times that of the 1-sided situation.

Example 3.8 Comparison with a standard - Spinal anaethesia for caesarean section
Sng, Wang, Assam and Sia (2015) assess the incidence of hypotension, defined as systolic pressure < 80% baseline, in women undergoing spinal anaethesia for caesarean section. The authors justified their study size as follows: 'To evaluate a 20% reduction in the incidence of hypotension from a baseline of 60% with 80% power and a type-1 error rate of 5%. 48 women were required. We aimed for 60 women to allow for a 20% drop-out rate.'

Here $\pi_{Test} = 0.4$, $\pi_{Known} = 0.6$, power $1 - \beta = 0.8$ and, if we set *1-sided* $\alpha = 0.05$, equation (3.7) yields

$$N = \frac{\left\{1.6449\sqrt{0.6 \times 0.4} + 0.8416\sqrt{0.4 \times 0.6}\right\}^2}{(0.6 - 0.4)^2} = 37.10 \text{ or } 38 \text{ women.}$$ Allowing a 20% drop-out rate,

increase this to 46 women. It appears therefore that Sng, Wang, Assam and Sia (2015) assumed a 2-sided hypothesis whereas a 1-sided alternative seems more appropriate.

References

Technical

Campbell MJ, Machin D and Walters SJ (2007). *Medical Statistics: A Textbook for the Health Sciences*, (4th edn.) Wiley, Chichester.

Casagrande JT, Pike MC and Smith PG (1978). An improved approximate formula for comparing two binomial distributions. *Biometrics*, **34**, 483–486.

Demidenko E (2007). Sample size determination for logistic regression revisited. *Statistics in Medicine*, **26**, 3385–3397.

Fleiss JL, Levin B and Paik MC (2003). *Statistical Methods for Rates and Proportions*. Wiley, Chichester.

Fleis JL, Tytun A and Ury HK (1980). A simple approximation for calculating sample sizes for comparing independent proportions. *Biometrics*, **36**, 343–346.

Hosmer DW and Lemeshow S (2000). *Applied Logistic Regression*. (2nd edn.) Wiley, Chichester.

Julious SA and Campbell MJ (1996). Sample size calculations for ordered categorical data (letter). *Statistics in Medicine*, **15**, 1065–1066.

Julious SA and Campbell MJ (2012). Tutorial in biostatistics: sample sizes for parallel group clinical trials with binary data. *Statistics in Medicine*, **31**, 2904–2936.

Novikov I, Fund N and Freedman LS (2010). A modified approach to estimating sample size for simple logistic regression with one continuous covariate. *Statistics in Medicine*, **29**, 97–107.

Examples

Ang ES-W, Lee S-T, Gan CS-G, See PG-J, Chan Y-H, Ng L-H and Machin D (2001). Evaluating the role of alternative therapy in burn wound management: randomized trial comparing Moist Exposed Burn Ointment with conventional methods in the management of patients with second-degree burns. *Medscape General Medicine, **3**, 3.

Beitz A, Riphaus A, Meining A, Kronshage T, Geist C, Wagenpfeil S, Weber A, Jung A, Bajbouj M, Pox C, Schneider G, Schmid RM, Wehrmann T and von Delius S (2012). Capnographic monitoring reduces the incidence of arterial oxygen desaturation and hypoxemia during propofol sedation for colonoscopy: A randomized, controlled study (ColoCap Study). *The American Journal of Gastroenterology*, **107**, 1205–1220.

Cheng J, Cho M, Cen J-M, Cai M-Y, Xu S, Ma Z-W, Liu X, Yang X-L, Chen C, Suh Y and Xiong X-D (2015). A tagSNP in *SIRT1* gene confers susceptibility to myocardial infarction in a Chinese Han population. PLoS ONE, **10**,e.

Lie S-FDJ, Ozcan M, Verkerke GJ, Sandham A and Dijkstra PU (2008). Survival of flexible, braided, bonded stainless steel lingual retainers: a historic cohort study. *European Journal of Orthodontics*, **30**, 199–204.

Nwaru BI and Sheikh A (2015). Hormonal contraceptives and asthma in women of reproductive age: analysis of data from serial national Scottish Health Surveys. *Journal of the Royal Society of Medicine*, **108**, 358–371.

Pandis N (2012). Sample calculations for comparing proportions. *American Journal of Orthodontics and Dentofacial Orthopedics*, **141**, 666–667.

Sng BL, Wang H, Assam PN and Sia AT (2015). Assessment of an updated double-vasopressor automated system using Nexfin™ for the maintenance of haemodynamic stability to improve peri-operative outcome during spinal anaesthesia for caesarean section. *Anaesthesia*, **70**, 691–698.

Table 3.1 Sample size for the comparison of two proportions – two sided $\alpha = 0.05$ and power, $1 - \beta = 0.8$ [Equation (3.2) with $\varphi = 1$].
Each cell gives the total sample size, *N*, for a study assuming equal numbers, *N/2*, are included in each group.

	2-sided $\alpha = 0.05$; Power $1 - \beta = 0.8$									
	First Proportion, π_1									
π_2	0.05	0.1	0.15	0.2	0.25	0.3	0.35	0.4	0.45	0.5
0.1	870	–	–	–	–	–	–	–	–	–
0.15	282	1372	–	–	–	–	–	–	–	–
0.2	152	398	1812	–	–	–	–	–	–	–
0.25	98	200	500	2188	–	–	–	–	–	–
0.3	72	124	242	588	2502	–	–	–	–	–
0.35	54	86	146	276	658	2754	–	–	–	–
0.4	44	64	98	164	304	712	2942	–	–	–
0.45	36	50	72	108	178	326	712	3068	–	–
0.5	30	40	54	78	116	186	340	776	3130	–
0.55	24	32	44	58	82	122	192	346	784	3130
0.6	22	28	34	46	62	84	124	194	346	776
0.65	18	22	28	36	48	62	86	124	192	340
0.7	16	20	24	30	38	48	62	84	122	186
0.75	14	16	20	24	30	38	48	62	82	116
0.8	12	14	16	20	24	30	36	46	58	78
0.85	10	12	14	16	20	24	28	34	44	54
0.9	8	10	12	14	16	20	22	28	32	40
0.95	8	8	10	12	14	16	18	22	24	30

	2-sided $\alpha = 0.05$; Power $1 - \beta = 0.8$								
	First Proportion, π_1								
π_2	0.5	0.55	0.6	0.65	0.7	0.75	0.8	0.85	0.9
0.55	3130	–	–	–	–	–	–	–	–
0.6	776	3068	–	–	–	–	–	–	–
0.65	340	752	2942	–	–	–	–	–	–
0.7	186	326	712	2754	–	–	–	–	–
0.75	116	178	304	658	2502	–	–	–	–
0.8	78	108	164	276	588	2188	–	–	–
0.85	54	72	98	146	242	500	1812	–	–
0.9	40	50	64	86	124	200	398	1372	–
0.95	30	36	44	54	72	98	152	282	870

Table 3.1 (Continued)

π_2	0.05	0.1	0.15	0.2	0.25	0.3	0.35	0.4	0.45	0.5
	2-sided $\alpha=0.05$; Power $1-\beta=0.9$									
	First Proportion, π_1									
0.1	1164	–	–	–	–	–	–	–	–	–
0.15	376	1836	–	–	–	–	–	–	–	–
0.2	202	532	2424	–	–	–	–	–	–	–
0.25	130	266	670	2928	–	–	–	–	–	–
0.3	94	164	322	784	3348	–	–	–	–	–
0.35	72	114	194	370	880	3684	–	–	–	–
0.4	56	84	130	218	406	954	3938	–	–	–
0.45	46	66	94	144	236	434	1006	4106	–	–
0.5	38	52	72	104	154	248	454	10389	4190	–
0.55	32	42	56	78	108	162	256	462	1048	4190
0.6	28	34	46	60	80	112	164	260	462	1038
0.65	24	30	38	48	62	82	114	164	256	454
0.7	20	24	30	38	48	62	82	112	162	248
0.75	16	20	26	32	38	48	62	80	108	154
0.8	14	18	22	26	32	38	48	60	78	104
0.85	12	14	18	22	26	30	38	46	56	72
0.9	10	12	14	18	20	24	30	34	42	52
0.95	8	10	12	14	16	20	24	28	32	38

π_2	0.5	0.55	0.6	0.65	0.7	0.75	0.8	0.85	0.9
	2-sided $\alpha=0.05$; Power $1-\beta=0.9$								
	First Proportion, π_1								
0.55	4190	–	–	–	–	–	–	–	–
0.6	1038	4106	–	–	–	–	–	–	–
0.65	454	1006	3938	–	–	–	–	–	–
0.7	248	434	954	3684	–	–	–	–	–
0.75	154	236	406	880	3348	–	–	–	–
0.8	104	144	218	370	784	2928	–	–	–
0.85	72	94	130	194	322	670	2424	–	–
0.9	52	66	84	114	164	266	532	1836	–
0.95	38	46	56	72	94	130	202	376	1164

Table 3.2 Sample size for the comparison of two proportions using the odds ratio (*OR*) – two sided $\alpha = 0.05$ and power, $1 - \beta = 0.8$ [Equation (3.4) with $\varphi = 1$].

Each cell gives the total sample size, *N*, for a study assuming equal numbers, *N/2*, are included in each group. The corresponding values for an *OR* < 1 are determined by entering the table with 1/*OR* and $(1 - \pi_1)$ replacing π_1.

Odds Ratio OR	2-sided $\alpha = 0.05$, $1 - \beta = 0.8$ π_1									
	0.05	0.1	0.15	0.2	0.25	0.3	0.35	0.4	0.45	0.5
1.2	18266	9740	6046	5590	4818	4342	4048	3872	3790	3786
1.3	8484	4548	3260	2636	2282	2068	1936	1860	1828	1834
1.4	4972	2680	1930	1568	1364	1242	1166	1126	1110	1118
1.5	3306	1792	1296	1060	926	846	798	772	764	772
1.6	2380	1296	944	774	680	622	590	574	570	578
1.7	1808	990	724	598	526	484	460	450	448	454
1.8	1430	788	578	480	424	392	374	366	366	372
1.9	1164	644	476	396	352	326	312	306	306	314
2	972	540	402	336	298	278	266	262	264	270
3	308	182	140	122	112	108	106	106	108	112
4	166	102	82	72	68	66	66	68	70	72
5	108	70	58	52	50	50	50	50	52	56
10	38	28	26	24	24	24	26	26	28	30

Odds Ratio OR	2-sided $\alpha = 0.05$, $1 - \beta = 0.8$ π_1								
	0.55	0.6	0.65	0.7	0.75	0.8	0.85	0.9	0.95
1.2	3860	4016	4274	4670	5274	6234	7888	11266	21520
1.3	1876	1958	2092	2294	2600	3082	3912	5606	10738
1.4	1148	1202	1288	1418	1610	1916	2438	3500	6722
1.5	796	836	898	990	1130	1346	1716	2470	4752
1.6	596	628	676	748	854	1020	1304	1880	3622
1.7	470	498	536	594	680	814	1042	1504	2904
1.8	386	408	442	490	562	674	864	1248	2414
1.9	326	346	374	416	478	574	736	1066	2060
2	282	298	324	362	414	498	640	928	1796
3	118	128	140	156	182	220	284	412	802
4	78	84	92	104	120	146	190	276	536
5	60	64	70	80	92	112	146	214	414
10	32	34	38	42	50	60	78	114	222

Table 3.2 (Continued)

Odds Ratio OR	2-sided $\alpha=0.05$, $1-\beta=0.9$ π_1									
	0.05	0.1	0.15	0.2	0.25	0.3	0.35	0.4	0.45	0.5
1.2	24452	13038	9298	7482	6448	5814	5418	5184	5074	5070
1.3	11356	6088	4364	3528	3056	2768	2590	2490	2446	2454
1.4	6654	3586	2584	2100	1826	1662	1562	1506	1486	1496
1.5	4424	2398	1736	1418	1238	1132	1068	1034	1024	1034
1.6	3184	1734	1262	1036	908	834	790	768	7621	772
1.7	2420	1326	970	798	704	648	616	600	598	608
1.8	1914	1054	774	642	568	524	500	490	488	4989
1.9	1558	864	638	530	470	436	418	410	410	420
2	1300	724	536	448	400	372	358	352	352	360
3	414	242	188	162	150	142	140	140	144	150
4	220	126	110	98	92	88	88	90	92	98
5	146	94	76	70	66	66	66	68	70	74
10	52	38	34	32	32	34	34	36	36	40

Odds Ratio OR	2-sided $\alpha=0.05$, $1-\beta=0.9$ π_1								
	0.55	0.6	0.65	0.7	0.75	0.8	0.85	0.9	0.95
1.2	5166	5376	5720	6252	7062	8344	10560	15082	28808
1.3	2510	2622	2800	3070	3480	4126	5238	7504	14374
1.4	1536	1610	1724	1898	2156	2564	3262	4686	9000
1.5	1064	1120	1202	1326	1512	1800	2298	3306	6362
1.6	798	840	906	1000	1144	1366	1744	2516	4848
1.7	630	666	718	796	910	1090	1394	2014	3886
1.8	516	546	592	656	752	902	1156	1672	3230
1.9	436	462	502	558	640	768	984	1426	2758
2	376	400	434	484	556	666	858	1242	2404
3	158	170	186	210	242	292	378	552	1072
4	104	112	122	138	160	196	252	368	718
5	78	86	94	106	124	150	196	284	554
10	42	46	50	58	66	80	104	152	296

4

Ordered Categorical Outcomes

SUMMARY
This chapter extends the sample-size calculations for comparisons between groups where the outcome of concern is binary to when the outcome is an ordered categorical variable. The corresponding summary for a single group will be the proportion of subjects falling into each of the categories. When planning a comparative two-group study, the anticipated proportions falling within one group may be postulated and the anticipated effect size between groups is expressed by the odds ratio. Alternatively, anticipated proportions falling within both groups may be postulated.

4.1 Introduction

Some endpoint variables in clinical studies simply assign unordered categories to people, such as whether they are of a particular blood group: O, A or AB. In other circumstances when there are more than two categories of classification, it may be possible to order them in some logical way. For example: After treatment a patient may be either (i) improved, (ii) the same, or (iii) worse; A woman may have either (i) never conceived, (ii) conceived but spontaneously aborted, (iii) conceived but had a late abortion, or (iv) given birth to a live infant; A patient with rheumatoid arthritis may be asked to order or rank his preference between four aids designed to assist with his dressing. In each case, numerical values may be assigned to rank the possible outcomes. Outcomes such as these are known as *ordered categorical* or *ordinal* data. Studies involving quality of life and patient self-reported outcomes often use instruments which contain items that take an ordered categorical form.

4.2 Ordered Categorical Data

Mann-Whitney U-Test

A study may be undertaken where the outcome measure of interest is an ordered scale, such as a measure of opinion, say, which used a Likert scale with the ordered categories: Strongly disagree, Disagree, Agree and Strongly agree. For an ordered variable it makes sense to describe one subject as being in a higher (or lower) category than another. The statistical test used to compare groups in this instance is the Mann-Whitney U-test with allowance for ties as described by, for example, Campbell, Machin and Walters (2007).

Sample Sizes for Clinical, Laboratory and Epidemiology Studies, Fourth Edition. David Machin, Michael J. Campbell, Say Beng Tan and Sze Huey Tan.
© 2018 John Wiley & Sons Ltd. Published 2018 by John Wiley & Sons Ltd.

Playfulness	Category i	Number of children		Proportion of children		Cumulative proportion		
		(C)	(P)	(C) $p_{C,i}$	(P) $p_{P,i}$	(C) $Q_{C,i}$	(P) $Q_{P,i}$	OR
Normal	1	3	6	0.14	0.27	0.14	0.27	2.272
Slightly listless	2	5	9	0.24	0.41	0.38	0.68	3.467
Moderately listless	3	5	5	0.24	0.23	0.62	0.91	6.197
Very listless	4	8	2	0.38	0.09	1.00	1.00	-
	Total	21	22	1.00	1.00		OR_{GM}	3.65

Figure 4.1 Playfulness in feverish children following treatment with paracetamol (*P*) and without (Control, *C*) (data from Kinmonth, Fulton and Campbell, 1992).

With only two categories in the scale, we have the binary situation as described in **Chapter 3**. For study size purposes, we need to specify an anticipated effect size and an odds ratio (*OR*) can be used in this context. The investigator may postulate that on the *Test* (*T*) intervention a patient is, say, twice as likely to have a higher score than on the *Standard* (*S*) and so the anticipated *OR* = 2. Alternatively, an investigator may know the proportions expected for *S* and then propose the corresponding proportions in each category that are likely, or of clinical importance, with *T*.

Illustration

In a randomised controlled trial comparing paracetamol (*P*) with a placebo (*C*) for the treatment of feverish children, Kinmonth, Fulton and Campbell (1992) categorised playfulness on a scale from Normal (1) to Very listless (4). A total of 43 children were recruited and the results, with the proportions falling in each playfulness category together with the corresponding cumulative proportions, are given in **Figure. 4.1**.

In this example, every child is categorised at the end of the trial and the number of children falling into the respective categories in each treatment are noted. The individual category proportions are then calculated by dividing these by the corresponding numbers in each treatment group.

Planning Values

For planning purposes, the first requirement is to specify the proportion of subjects anticipated, in each category of the scale, for one of the groups (say *C*). Suppose we have κ ordered categories, for example in **Figure 4.1** $\kappa = 4$, and the planning proportions in *C* are $\pi_{C1}, \pi_{C2}, \ldots, \pi_{C\kappa}$ respectively with $\pi_{C1} + \pi_{C2} + \ldots + \pi_{C\kappa} = 1$. Further, if $Q_{C1}, Q_{C2}, \ldots, Q_{C\kappa}$ are the corresponding cumulative proportions, so that $Q_{C1} = \pi_{C1}$, $Q_{C2} = \pi_{C1} + \pi_{C2}$, and so on until $Q_{C\kappa} = \pi_{C1} + \pi_{C2} + \ldots + \pi_{C\kappa} = 1$. A similar notation applies for *P*.

The *OR* is the relative odds of a subject being in a given category or higher in one group compared to the same categories in the comparator group. For category i, which takes values from 1 to $\kappa - 1$, it is given by

$$OR_i = \frac{Q_{Pi} / (1 - Q_{Pi})}{Q_{Ci} / (1 - Q_{Ci})} \qquad (4.1)$$

For example if $i = 3$ in **Figure 4.1**, $Q_{C3} = 0.62$, $Q_{P3} = 0.91$ so $OR_3 = \dfrac{0.91 / (1 - 0.91)}{0.62 / (1 - 0.62)} = 6.197$.

Sample Size

Proportional Odds

Given the planning proportions $\pi_{C1}, \pi_{C2}, \ldots, \pi_{C\kappa}$ in each category of C, the assumption of proportional odds specifies that the OR_i (similar to those calculated in **Figure 4.1**) will be the same for all categories, from $i = 1$ to $i = \kappa - 1$, and this is equal to OR_{Plan}. In this case, the anticipated values for P can then be calculated using the expression

$$Q_{Pi} = \frac{Q_{Ci} OR_{Plan}}{(1 - Q_{Ci}) + Q_{Ci} OR_{Plan}}. \qquad (4.2)$$

The process begins with $Q_{C1} = \pi_{C1}$ to obtain $Q_{P1} = \pi_{P1}$. Then $Q_{C2} = \pi_{C1} + \pi_{C2}$ to give Q_{P2}, from which $\pi_{P2} = Q_{P2} - \pi_{P1}$ and so on until the anticipated values in each category of P are obtained.

Alternatively, the proportions in each category of the two groups, C and P, can be specified and from these the OR_i, where $i = 1$ to $\kappa - 1$, can be calculated and the OR_{Plan} taken as (say) the geometric mean (*GM*) of these values. For example, with the data of **Figure 4.1**, $OR_1 = 2.272$, $OR_2 = 3.467$ and $OR_3 = 6.197$ and their geometric mean, $GM = (2.272 \times 3.467 \times 6.197)^{1/3} = 3.65$ gives a value for the corresponding OR_{Plan}.

Following either approach, the average proportion of subjects anticipated in category i, that is, $\bar{\pi}_i = (\pi_{Ci} + \pi_{Pi})/2$, is calculated. Then for a 2-sided test size α, power $1 - \beta$, and the groups allocated in the ratio $1:\varphi$, the required total sample size is

$$N_\kappa = \Gamma \times \frac{(1 + \varphi)^2}{\varphi} \frac{(z_{1-\alpha/2} + z_{1-\beta})^2}{(logOR)^2}, \qquad (4.3)$$

where

$$\Gamma = \frac{3}{1 - \sum_{i=1}^{\kappa} \bar{\pi}_i^3}. \qquad (4.4)$$

The resulting sample sizes in each group are $n_C = N_\kappa/(1 + \varphi)$ and $n_P = \varphi N_\kappa/(1 + \varphi)$ respectively.

In fact, the calculation is quite robust to the specification of the proportions. Thus, rather than use the average of the C and P proportions as just described, one can use the C proportions alone.

The assumption of constant *OR* implies that it is justified to use the Mann-Whitney *U*-test in this situation. It also means that one can use the anticipated *OR* from *any* pair of adjacent (broad) categories for planning purposes. Thus, after examining the range of *OR*s given in **Figure 4.1**, the investigators may consider an *OR* closer to 2.5 for planning purposes rather than assume $OR_{Plan} = 3.65$.

Approximate formulae

If the number of categories is large, it is clearly difficult to postulate the proportion of subjects who would fall into a given category. What is more, the Γ of equation (4.4) is quite complex to evaluate. However, there are a number of ways that it can be simplified:

i) Binary situation, $\kappa = 2$

When $\kappa = 2$, equation (4.4) becomes $\Gamma = \dfrac{1}{\pi(1-\pi)}$. Hence equation (4.3) becomes

$$N_2 = \frac{1}{\pi(1-\pi)} \frac{(1+\varphi)^2}{\varphi} \frac{\left(z_{1-\alpha/2} + z_{1-\beta}\right)^2}{(logOR)^2}, \tag{4.5}$$

which is that given for a binary endpoint of equation (3.4).

In this situation the worst-case scenario, in the sense of the largest resulting study size, is when $\bar{\pi} = 0.5$ as, in which case, $\Gamma = \dfrac{1}{0.5 \times 0.5} = 4$ is the maximum value that Γ can take.

ii) All $\bar{\pi}_i$ approximately equal

In particular, if the mean proportions $\bar{\pi}_i$ in each category are (approximately) equal, $\bar{\pi}_i \approx 1/\kappa$, and

$$\Gamma = \frac{3}{1 - \sum_{i=1}^{\kappa} \pi_i^3} = \frac{3}{1 - 1/\kappa^2}. \tag{4.6}$$

The value of Γ now depends only on the number of categories, κ, concerned. If $\kappa = 3$, and therefore all $\bar{\pi}_i \approx 1/3$, $\Gamma = 3/[1 - (1/3)^2] = 27/8 = 3.375$ while for $\kappa = 4$ and 5, Γ diminishes from $48/15 = 3.2$ to $75/24 = 3.125$ respectively.

iii) $\kappa > 5$

If the number of categories *exceeds* five, then $\Gamma \approx 3$ so that

$$N_\kappa \approx \frac{3(1+\varphi)^2}{\varphi} \frac{\left(z_{1-\alpha/2} + z_{1-\beta}\right)^2}{(logOR)^2}. \tag{4.7}$$

Comment

From a practical perspective, if a simple dichotomy of the anticipated data had first been used to determine an *interim* value for the sample size, N_{Binary}, using equation (4.5) with $\bar{\pi} = 0.5$ then we know by comparison with equation (4.7) that the *eventual* sample size chosen could be reduced by a factor of, at most, 3/4 if more categories are introduced. Such a reduction in sample size may represent a considerable saving of resources.

Non-Proportional Odds (NPO)

If proportional odds cannot be assumed then the sample size necessary, when making comparisons using the Mann-Whitney U-test, is given by

$$N_{NPO} = \frac{(1+\varphi)^2}{12\varphi} \frac{(z_{1-\alpha/2} + z_{1-\beta})^2 \left[1 - \frac{1}{(1+\varphi)^3} \sum_{i=1}^{\kappa} \{\varphi\pi_{Si} + \pi_{Ti}\}^3 \right]}{\left[\sum_{i=2}^{\kappa} \left(\pi_{Si} \sum_{j=1}^{i-1} \pi_{Tj} \right) + 0.5 \left(\sum_{i=1}^{\kappa} \pi_{Si}\pi_{Ti} \right) - 0.5 \right]^2}, \tag{4.8}$$

where π_{Si} are the anticipated proportions within each category of the *Standard* (*S*) group and π_{Ti} are the corresponding values with the *Test* (*T*).

4.3   Bibliography

Whitehead (1993, equation 10) describes sample-size calculations for ordered categorical data assuming proportional odds. This assumes that wherever a binary cut is made of the categories, the *OR* will be of the same magnitude. However, he points out that provided the different *OR*s resulting from different binary cuts are all directionally the same, that is all $OR > 1$ or all $OR < 1$, then equation (4.3) still applies. He also points out that there is little increase in power to be gained by increasing the number of categories beyond five. Equation (4.8) is given by Zhao, Rahardja and Qu (2008, equation 12) and this provides a method of calculating sample sizes for the Mann-Whitney U-test, which allows for tied observations (this essentially concerns categorical data as a special example) and does not assume proportional odds. Fayers and Machin (2016) highlight the importance of sample-size methods for ordinal data when conducting studies of patient-reported outcomes often concerned with aspects of health-related quality of life.

4.4   Examples

Table 1.2
For two-sided test size, $\alpha = 0.05$, $z_{0.975} = 1.96$.   For one-sided $1 - \beta = 0.8$ and 0.9, $z_{0.8} = 0.8416$ and $z_{0.9} = 1.2816$.

Equations 4.2, 4.3 and 4.4

Example 4.1   Varying number of categories - Feverish children

Suppose a confirmatory trial is planned in which we wish to replicate the results of the randomised controlled trial of paracetamol (*P*) for the treatment of feverish children conducted by Kinmonth, Fulton and Campbell (1992) and summarised in **Figure 4.1**. We will assume the distribution of children with (Control) *C* and *P* is anticipated to be about the same as found previously so that an $OR_{Plan} = 3.65$ in favour of P is anticipated. Using the C proportions as in **Figure 4.1**, but now applying $OR_{Plan} = 3.65$ at each dichotomy we can calculate the anticipated cumulative proportions for P using equation (4.2). Thus, the proportion expected in the first category of P is $Q_{P1} = 3.65 \times 0.14 / [1 - 0.14 + (3.65 \times 0.14)] = 0.3727$. The cumulative proportion expected in the second category is $Q_{P2} = 3.65 \times 0.38 / [1 - 0.38 + (3.65 \times 0.38)] = 0.6911$, and similarly $Q_{P3} = 0.8562$ and $Q_{P4} = 1$. The actual proportions anticipated are therefore 0.3727, $(0.6911 - 0.3727) = 0.3184$, $(0.8562 - 0.6911) = 0.1651$ and $(1 - 0.8562) = 0.1438$. The proportions averaged across each C and P category are then $(0.14 + 0.3727)/2 = 0.2564$, $(0.24 + 0.3184)/2 = 0.2792$, 0.2056 and 0.2619 respectively. From these, part of equation (4.4) gives $(1 - \sum \bar{\pi}_i^3) = 1 - 0.0649 = 0.9351$.

For 80% power, 5% significance level and $OR_{Plan} = 3.65$, equation (4.3) gives, for $\kappa = 4$ and $\varphi = 1$,

$$N_4 = \frac{3}{0.9351} \frac{(1+1)^2}{1} \frac{(1.96 + 0.8416)^2}{(\log 3.65)^2} = 60.09.$$ Thus 60 children would be randomised equally to C and P.

As pointed out earlier, it is simpler to use the C proportions alone. In this example therefore, equation (4.4) is used with proportions 0.14, 0.24, 0.24 and 0.38 to give $\Gamma = 0.9147$ and from equation (4.3), $N_4 = 60.91$.

Alternatively, given that the proportions 0.2569, 0.2792, 0.2182 and 0.2463 in each of the $\kappa = 4$ categories are approximately equal at 0.25, we can use equation (4.5) to obtain $\Gamma = 3/[1 - (1/4)^2] = 16/5 = 3.2$. Then using this in equation (4.3), the sample size would be obtained as $N_4 = 59.93$, which would be rounded up to 60 children as above.

Alternatively, if we had pooled subjects in categories 1-2 and those of categories 3-4 of **Figure 4.1**, rather than keeping them distinct, we would be designing a study with $\pi_C = 0.38$ and $OR_{Plan} = 3.65$. Use of **Chapter 3**, equation (3.4), with ${}^SS_S$ would then result in $N_2 = 76$ patients. Thus, use of all four categories, rather than simply pooling into two, yields a reduction in recruitment of $76 - 60 = 16$ children. This might result in a substantial savings in time and resources allocated to the study.

Equations 4.2, 4.3 and 4.4

Example 4.2 Equal allocation - Type 2 diabetes mellitus
Zinman, Harris, Neuman, *et al* (2010) conducted a double-blind randomised trial comparing a combination of rosiglitazone and metformin (RM) with placebo (P) in patients with impaired glucose tolerance with the objective of prevention of subsequent type 2 diabetes mellitus. **Figure 4.2** summarises the weight changes of the participants over the trial period. Although not conducted by the authors, a test of significance using the Mann-Whitney U-test gives a p-value = 0.38 and an analysis using ordered logistic regression estimates the $OR = 1.2517$ with 95% CI 0.49 to 1.31.

A new trial is planned using the same proportions as those observed with P, after noting the geometric mean $OR_{GM} = 1.2537$ (which is remarkably close to the OR estimated by the logistic regression), with $OR_{Plan} = 1.25$. Then with ${}^SS_S$, using equations (4.2), (4.3) and (4.4), with 90% power and 5% 2-sided significance level, gives $N_5 = 2,708$.

Suppose the investigators were considering a new formulation of the RM combination which was thought likely to be more effective and considered a revised $OR_{Plan} = 2$. With the same conditions as were previously used, ${}^SS_S$ now gives $N_5 = 282$.

	Weight change (kg)	Placebo (P)	Rosiglitazone/ Metformin (RM)	Estimated OR at each binary split
		Number of subjects (%)	Number of subjects (%)	
Gain	> 3	22 (21.15)	22 (21.36)	1.0126
	> 2 to 3	11 (10.58)	8 (7.77)	0.8717
No change	2 gain to 2 loss	32 (30.77)	46 (44.66)	1.6883
Loss	> 2 to 3	8 (7.69)	6 (5.83)	1.6582
	> 3	31 (29.81)	21 (20.39)	
	Total	104	103	$OR_{GM} =$
				1.2537

Figure 4.2 Weight change in patients with impaired glucose tolerance following treatment with placebo or combination of rosiglitazone and metformin (data from Zinman, Harris, Neuman, *et al*, 2010, Table 2).

Equations 4.2, 4.3 and 4.4

Example 4.3   Ordinal outcome - Intimate partner violence
Assume that investigators plan a trial with women who have experienced intimate partner violence on the basis of the information of **Figure 4.3** obtained from the S group of the WEAVE trial of Hegarty, O'Doherty, Taft, *et al* (2013). For the new trial they set an anticipated effect size $OR_{Plan} = 1.5$ in favour of a new intervention strategy, T. In which case, $\log OR_{Plan} = 0.4055$ and, following the calculations of **Figure 4.3**, equation (4.4) gives $\Gamma = 3.5129$. Finally, the investigators set $\varphi = 1$, 2-sided $\alpha = 0.05$, $\beta = 0.2$ and obtain from equation (4.3) that $N_4 = 3.5129 \times \left[\dfrac{(1+1)^2}{1} \right] \dfrac{(1.96 + 0.8416)^2}{(0.4055)^2} =$ 670.74 or approximately 680 women.

Equations 4.2, 4.3 and 4.4

Example 4.4   Equal allocation - Stroke
Chen, Young, Gan, *et al* (2013) reported the results of a double-blind, placebo (P) controlled, randomised trial of a Chinese medicine neuroaid (*MLC601*) on stroke recovery in which the modified Rankin scale (mRS) was used to assess the patients at 3 months post-randomisation. Their results are summarised in **Figure 4.4**. Calculating the OR at each binary split commencing with Score 5 versus Scores 0-4 combined, the Scores 4-5 versus Scores 0-3 combined, and so on, gives the corresponding values in the final column of the table. The geometric mean of these 5 quantities suggested an overall $OR = 0.9$.

	As a result of participating in the trial, I see the quality of my life as …				
G	Better 0	Somewhat better 1	About the same as before 2	Somewhat worse 3	
Standard (S) $P_{Sg} = s_g/n_S$ Planning	$s_0 = 15$ $p_{S0} = 0.1579$ $\pi_{S0} = 0.1579$	$s_1 = 27$ $p_{S1} = 0.2842$ $\pi_{S1} = 0.2842$	$s_2 = 50$ $p_{S2} = 0.5263$ $\pi_{S2} = 0.5263$	$s_3 = 3$ $p_{S3} = 0.0316$ $\pi_{S3} = 0.0316$	$n_S = 95$
Q_{Sg}	$Q_{S0} = \pi_{S0}$ $= 0.1579$	$Q_{S1} = \pi_{S0} + \pi_{S1}$ $= 0.4421$	$Q_{S2} = \pi_{S0} + \pi_{S1} + \pi_{S2}$ $= 0.9684$	$Q_{S3} = \pi_{S0} + \pi_{S1} + \pi_{S2} + \pi_{S3}$ $= 1$	
Test (T) Q_{Tg}	Q_{T0} $= 0.2195$	Q_{T1} $= 0.5431$	Q_{T2} $= 0.9787$	Q_{T3} $= 1$	
π_{Tg} $(\pi_{Sg} + \pi_{Tg})^3$	$\pi_{T0} = 0.2195$ $[(0.1579 + 0.2195)/2]^3$ $= 0.0067$	$\pi_{T1} = 0.3236$ $[(0.2842 + 0.3236/2])^3$ $= 0.0281$	$\pi_{T2} = 0.4356$ $[(0.5263 + 0.435/2]^3$ $= 0.1113$	$\pi_{T3} = 0.0213$ $[(0.0316 + 0.0213)/2]^3$ $= 0.0000$	Total 0.1461 $\Gamma = 3/[1 - 0.1461] = 3.5129$

Figure 4.3 Deriving the anticipated proportions within each category for the *Test* intervention calculated from that anticipated for women who have experienced intimate partner violence in the *Standard* group with an assumed planning odds ratio, $OR_{Plan} = 1.5$ (data from Hegarty, O'Doherty, Taft, *et al*, 2013).

Modified Rankin Scale		Placebo	ML601	Estimated OR at each binary split
Score	Disability	Number of subjects (%)	Number of subjects (%)	
0	No symptoms	82 (15.4)	79 (14.9)	1.0426
1	No significant	156 (29.4)	172 (32.5)	0.9029
2	Slight	125 (23.5)	119 (22.5)	0.9344
3	Moderate	95 (17.9)	91 (17.2)	0.9391
4	Moderately severe	50 (9.4)	52 (9.8)	0.7319
5	Severe	23 (4.3)	17 (3.2)	
	Total	531	530	$OR_{GM} = 0.9043$

Figure 4.4 Modified Rankin scale at month 3 following treatment with Placebo or MLC601 (data from Chen, Young, Gan, *et al*, 2013, Figure 2).

On the basis of this information a repeat trial is planned, but with a different formulation of Chinese medicine, with a 1:1 randomisation, 2-sided $\alpha = 0.05$ and $\beta = 0.2$, direct use of $^{SS}_S$ requires stipulating the proportions in each *mRS* score group with P, commencing with that of Score 5, together with the anticipated $OR_{Plan} = 0.9$. This gives the sample size per group as $n_P = n_{MLC601} = 4,466$ or a total of $N = 8,932$ or 9,000 post-stroke patients. Alternatively, the proportions in each *mRS* category for both P and *MLC601* respectively can be stipulated.

The investigators consider this sample size too large and enquire, given the same $\alpha = 0.05$ and $\beta = 0.2$, what size of OR_{Plan} would provide a similar sample size to the $N = 1,060$ in the trial conducted by Chen, Young, Gan, *et al* (2013). By investigating a range of planning options using $^{SS}_S$, it turns out that the rather large effect size (that is distant from the null hypothesis value of unity), $OR_{Plan} = 0.735$, requires $N = 1,050$ patients. Consequently, the investigators have to discuss whether such a value is a feasible possibility with the new formulation that they wish to evaluate.

Equations 4.3, 4.4 and 4.6

Example 4.5 Unequal allocation - Stroke

Broderick, Palesch, Demchuk, *et al* (2013) also used the modified Rankin Score (*mRS*) when comparing patients with stroke randomised in a 1:2 ratio to intravenous t-PA (a tissue plasminogen activator) alone (*IV*) and endovascular therapy after intravenous t-PA (*EndIV*) in patients with moderate-to-severe acute ischaemic stroke. The trial was closed early with 629 patients, of the 900 planned, recruited. Some of their results are summarised in **Figure 4.5**.

If these results were to be used to plan a trial but with an improved endovascular therapy, then using equation (4.4) with $\kappa = 7$ categories gives $\Gamma = 3/[1 - (0.1085^3 + 0.1740^3 + ... + 0.2120^3)] = 3.0815$. This is numerically very close to the value from equation (4.6) which results in $\Gamma = 3/[1 - (1/7)^2] = 3.0625$ and justifies the use of this approximation in the planning process. Further, although the first trial

Modified Rankin Score	IV		EndIV		$\bar{\pi}$	Estimated OR at each binary split
	n	π	n	π		
0	19	0.089	53	0.128	0.1085	1.50
1	39	0.182	69	0.166	0.1740	1.12
2	28	0.131	55	0.133	0.1320	1.19
3	35	0.164	71	0.171	0.1675	1.14
4	30	0.140	64	0.154	0.1470	1.26
5	15	0.070	20	0.048	0.0590	1.15
6	48	0.224	83	0.200	0.2120	-
Total	214	1.000	415	1.000		$OR_{GM} = 1.22$

Figure 4.5 Distribution of modified Rankin scores according to intervention received (adapted from Broderick, Palesch, Demchuk, *et al*, 2013, Figure 1).

suggests an $OR \approx 1.2$ in favour of *EndIV*, it is thought a value of $OR_{Plan} = 1.5$ is appropriate. The investigators also discuss the possibility of retaining the $\varphi = 2$ of the previous trial and retain the 2-sided test size of 5% and power 80%.

Use of equations (4.3) and (4.4) give the number of subjects required as

$$N_7 = 3.0625 \times \frac{(1+2)^2}{2} \frac{(1.96 + 0.8416)^2}{(\log 1.5)^2} = 657.83 \text{ or } 660, \text{ which is divisible by } (1 + \varphi) = 3. \text{ Thus, the}$$

number to be recruited to the two treatments is $n_{IV} = 220$ and $n_{EndIV} = 440$. This compares with a smaller $N_7 = 586$, hence $n_{IV} = n_{EndIV} = 293$, had $\varphi = 1$ been assumed.

In fact for the Broderick, Palesch, Demchuk, *et al* (2013) trial itself, the sample size calculation was based on a difference between two proportions rather than taking account of the anticipated outcomes of the individual categories. This binary approach is likely to overestimate the size of the planned trial. They assumed a good outcome as a modified Rankin score of ≤ 2 and this would be achieved in 40% of patients receiving *IV* with an anticipated improvement to 50% with *EndIV*. Thus with a 2-sided test size of 5% and power 80% and $\varphi = 2$, using the methods of our **Chapter 3** $^{S_{Ss}}$ gives $N = 876$, which to allow for non-compliance was increased to 900. Hence $n_{IV} = 300$ and $n_{EndIV} = 600$.

Equation 4.8

Example 4.6 Non-proportional odds - Retinopathy and smoking
Mühlhauser, Bender, Bott, *et al*, (1996) published a study on the influence of smoking history on development of retinopathy in 613 patients with diabetes mellitus. Their results, given in **Figure 4.6**, indicate similar proportions of smokers in those without and with advanced retinopathy with a larger proportion among the non-proliferative group. This profile suggests that using proportional odds is

Retinopathy Status	Number of Subjects		Proportion of smokers
	Non-Smoker (%)	Smoker (%)	
None	191 (66.32)	197 (60.62)	0.51
Non-proliferative	42 (14.58)	76 (23.38)	0.64
Advanced	55 (19.10)	52 (16.00)	0.49
Total	288	325	0.53

Figure 4.6 Retinopathy status by smoking status in patients with diabetes mellitus (data from Mühlhauser, Bender, Bott, *et al*, 1996).

not tenable in this case. A statistical comparison between these groups using the Mann-Whitney U-test, adjusted for ties, gives $z = -0.89$, p-value $= 0.37$.

As the assumption of proportional odds is not appropriate, equation (4.8) is required to estimate sample size.

If the proportions of patients in the non-smoker and smoker groups of **Figure 4.5** are used as planning values for a future repeat study, then S_S with 2-sided $\alpha = 0.05$ and $1 - \beta = 0.8$ and, assuming $\varphi = 1$, suggests $N_{NPO} = 6,022$ patients with diabetes mellitus would be required. Such a study is unlikely to be viable and so the investigators may have to reconsider whether the chosen dichotomy for smoking status, the retinopathy grading or both need to be revised for their future study.

Also, the calculations appear very sensitive to the proportions in the different categories, so that if the percentages are rounded to two figures, for example 66.32% is considered as 66% and so on, then $N_{NPO} = 8,342$ patients so that the methodology may not be very robust. This clearly needs further investigation.

References

Technical

Campbell MJ, Machin D and Walters SJ (2007). *Medical Statistics: A Textbook for the Health Sciences*. (4th edn) Wiley, Chichester.

Fayers PM and Machin D (2016). *Quality of Life: The assessment, analysis and interpretation of patient-reported outcomes*. (3rd edn) Wiley-Blackwell, Chichester.

Whitehead J (1993). Sample size calculations for ordered categorical data. *Statistics in Medicine*, **12**, 2257–2272.

Zhao YD, Rahardja D and Qu Y (2008). Sample size calculation for the Wilcoxon-Mann-Whitney test adjusting for ties. *Statistics in Medicine*, **27**, 462–468.

Examples

Broderick JP, Palesch YY, Demchuk AM, Yeatts SD, Khatri P, Hill MD, Jauch EC, Jovin TG, Yan B, Silver FL, von Kummer R, Molina CA, Demaerschalk BM, Budzik R, Clark WM, Zaidat OO, Malisch TW, Goyal M, Schonwille WJ, Mazighi M, Engelter ST, Anderson G, Spilker J, Carrozzella J, Ryckborst KJ,

Janis LS, Martin RH, Foster LD and Tomsick TA (2013). Endovascular therapy after intravenous t-PA versus t-PA alone for stroke. *New England Journal of Medicine*, **368**, 893–903.

Chen CLH, Young SHY, Gan HH, Singh R, Lao AY, Baroque AC, Chang HM, Hiyadan JHB, Chua CL, Advincula JM, Muengtaweeppongsa S, Chan BPL, de Silva HA, Towanabut S, Suwawela NC, Poungvarin N, Chankrachang S, Wong L, Eow GB, Navarro JC, Venketasubramanian N, Lee CF, Wong L and Bousser M-G (2013). Chinese medicine neuroaid efficacy on stroke recovery: A double-blind, placebo controlled, randomized study. *Stroke*, **44**, 2093–2100.

Hegarty K, O'Doherty L, Taft A, Chondros P, Brown S, Valpied J, Astbury J, Taket A, Gold L, Feder G and Gunn J (2013). Screening and counselling in the primary care setting for women who have experienced intimate partner violence (WEAVE): a cluster randomised controlled trial. *Lancet*, **382**, 249–258.

Kinmonth A-L, Fulton Y and Campbell MJ (1992). Management of feverish children at home. *British Medical Journal*, **305**, 1134–1136.

Mühlhauser I, Bender R, Bott U, Jörgens V, Grüsser M, Wagener W, Overmann H and Berger M (1996). Cigarette smoking and progression of retinopathy and nephropathy in type 1 diabetes. *Diabetic Medicine*, **13**, 536–543.

Zinman B, Harris SB, Neuman J, Gerstein HC, Retnakaran RR, Raboubd J, Qi Y and Hanley AJG (2010) Low-dose combination therapy with rosiglitazone and metformin to prevent type 2 diabetes mellitus (CANOE trial): a double-blind randomised controlled study. *Lancet*, **376**, 103–111.

5

Continuous Outcomes

SUMMARY
This chapter considers sample-size calculations for comparisons between means of groups where the outcome of concern is continuous. The situations when the data can be assumed to have a Normal distribution form, and when they do not, are described. The problem of comparing an estimated mean from one group with an assumed known mean in the other is described.

5.1 Introduction

A continuous variable is one that, in principle, can take any value within a range of values. For example, in a trial comparing anti-hypertensive drugs, one might record the level of blood pressure once a course of treatment has been completed and use this measure to compare different treatments. Continuous variables may be distributed Normally, meaning they have a characteristic bell-shaped curve which is completely determined by the mean and standard deviation. In such cases, groups are compared using the respective means and the corresponding t-test. In some situations, although the data may not be Normally distributed, they can be rendered Normal by a suitable transformation of the data. For example, this can be done by replacing the variable x by its logarithm, $y = logx$, and regarding y as having a Normal distribution. If this is not possible then comparisons may be made using the Wilcoxon-Mann-Whitney U-test. Alternatively, the data may be grouped into two or more categories and the sample size may be determined by the methods of **Chapters 3** and **4**.

5.2 Comparing Means

If the data collected are from a continuous outcome variable plausibly sampled from a Normal distribution, then the appropriate summary statistic is the mean, and the usual test to compare the (independent) groups is the two-sample t-test which assumes the two groups have the same variance. If the variances differ, then Satterthwaite's modification to the t-test is required. If the observations are not Normally distributed, then a suitable test for a shift of location is the Wilcoxon-Mann-Whitney U-test.

Sample Sizes for Clinical, Laboratory and Epidemiology Studies, Fourth Edition. David Machin, Michael J. Campbell, Say Beng Tan and Sze Huey Tan.
© 2018 John Wiley & Sons Ltd. Published 2018 by John Wiley & Sons Ltd.

Effect Size

If we assume the purpose of the study comparison is to compare a *Standard* (*S*) and *Test* (*T*) group with population means μ_S and μ_T respectively, then the corresponding null hypothesis to be tested is H_0: $\delta = \mu_T - \mu_S = 0$. Here δ is known as the effect size. If we further assume the standard deviation (SD), σ, is the same within each group, then the standardised effect size is

$$\Delta = \frac{\delta}{\sigma}. \tag{5.1}$$

As the purpose of a study will be to estimate δ and σ then, at the design stage, the investigators will need to stipulate the corresponding planning values δ_{Plan} and σ_{Plan}, although only Δ_{Plan} is strictly necessary. Indeed in many practical situations, one is more likely to have a feel for Δ_{Plan} rather than the individual component values. In practical terms, a realistic range of Δ_{Plan} is from 0.1 to 1.0. A 'small' effect, that is a stringent planning criterion, might be $\Delta_{Plan} = 0.2$, a 'moderate' one $\Delta_{Plan} = 0.5$ and a 'large' effect, that is a liberal criterion, $\Delta_{Plan} = 0.8$.

In other situations the investigator may know the likely range of the measurements, even though a planning value for the SD is not immediately available. On the assumption that the data will follow a Normal distribution, one can find a ballpark figure for σ_{Plan} by dividing the likely range, that is, the largest likely observation minus the smallest likely observation, of the data by 4. This is because most (approximately 95%) of a Normal distribution is included within 2SDs below the mean and 2SDs above the mean.

Two-Sample *T*-Test

Sample size – equal variances in each group

Following a study to compare two means, designed on the basis of effect size $\Delta_{Plan} = \delta_{Plan}/\sigma_{Plan}$, it is usual to base the analysis on a Student *t*-test. However, to calculate the total sample size, $N = n_S + n_T$, requires an expression for the power of the test under the alternative hypothesis, H_{Alt}. This involves the *non-central t*-distribution (NCT distribution) of **Figure 1.4** which, as pointed out there, is related to the (central) *t*-distribution, but with an extra non-centrality parameter, ψ. For allocation to groups on a 1: φ basis, $n_S = N/(1 + \varphi)$ and $n_T = \varphi N/(1 + \varphi)$ respectively, and the non-centrality parameter is given by

$$\psi = \frac{\Delta_{Plan}}{\sigma_{Plan}\sqrt{\dfrac{(1+\varphi)^2}{\varphi N}}}. \tag{5.2}$$

The corresponding power for a 2-sided test α is given by

$$1 - \beta = 1 - T_{N-2}\left(t_{1-\alpha/2} \mid \psi\right) + T_{N-2}\left(-t_{1-\alpha/2} \mid \psi\right), \tag{5.3}$$

where $T_{N-2}(x|\psi)$ is the cumulative value of the NCT distribution at ordinate x with $N - 2$ degrees of freedom and non-centrality parameter ψ. Here n, μ and σ components of ψ given in **Chapter 1** are respectively replaced by N, δ_{Plan} and $\sigma_{Plan}\sqrt{\dfrac{(1+\varphi)^2}{\varphi}}$.

For a pre-specified β, an iterative computer program is required to search equation (5.3) for the appropriate sample size N.

However, the non-central t-distribution approaches the Normal distribution quite rapidly as the degrees of freedom increase (see **Figure 1.4**) and a very accurate approximation which does not require iteration is available. Thus, for a 2-sided test size α and power $1 - \beta$, the number of subjects required is

$$N = \left[\frac{(1+\varphi)^2}{\varphi} \right] \left[\frac{(z_{1-\alpha/2} + z_{1-\beta})^2}{(\delta_{Plan}/\sigma_{Plan})^2} \right] + \left[\frac{z_{1-\alpha/2}^2}{2} \right].$$

(5.4)

Values for $z_{1-\alpha/2}$ and $z_{1-\beta}$ can be obtained from Table 1.2

It should be noted that when $\varphi = 1$, equation (5.4) is simply the 'Fundamental Equation' (2.6) with an additional term. This last term compensates for the fact that, in practice, the Student's t-test replaces the z-test, as the variance as well as the means have to be estimated from the data. If 2-sided $\alpha = 0.05$, $z_{0.975} = 1.96$, then the last term of equation (5.4) is $\dfrac{1.96^2}{2} \sim 2$. Hence in this situation the extra term increases the total sample size by 2, which will only be of importance in small studies.

Sample sizes calculated from equation (5.4) for $\varphi = 1$ are given in **Table 5.1**.

Optimal allocation of subjects to interventions

If $\varphi = 1$ then equation (5.4), omitting the additional term, gives the sample size $N_{Equal} = 4 \times \dfrac{(z_{1-\alpha/2} + z_{1-\beta})^2}{(\delta_{Plan}/\sigma_{Plan})^2}$.

Alternatively, if $\varphi \neq 1$ then $N_{Unequal} = \left[\dfrac{(1+\varphi)^2}{\varphi} \right] \dfrac{(z_{1-\alpha/2} + z_{1-\beta})^2}{(\delta_{Plan}/\sigma_{Plan})^2}$. Combining these two expressions we have

$$N_{Unequal} = \frac{(1+\varphi)^2}{4\varphi} N_{Equal}.$$

(5.5)

Since $\varphi > 0$, the minimum value of $\dfrac{(1+\varphi)^2}{4\varphi}$ is 1 and this occurs when $\varphi = 1$. This indicates that the optimal ratio of subjects in the two groups is therefore 1:1 and the minimum sample size is N_{Equal} as we highlighted in **Chapter 1**.

Sample size – unequal variances

If it is postulated that the variance in the S group is $\sigma_S^2 = \sigma_{Plan}^2$ but in group T it differs such that $\sigma_T^2 = \tau \sigma_{Plan}^2$, then Satterthwaite's modification to the t-test is required, and the total sample size required is now

$$N_{Satt} = \left(\frac{1+\varphi}{\varphi} \right) \left\{ \left[\frac{(\tau+\varphi)\sigma_{Plan}^2}{\delta_{Plan}^2} \times (z_{1-\alpha/2} + z_{1-\beta})^2 \right] + \left[\frac{(\tau^2+\varphi^3)z_{1-\alpha/2}^2}{2(\tau+\varphi)^2} \right] \right\}.$$

(5.6)

In this situation, the optimal ratio for the number of subjects in each group will depend on τ. Sample sizes calculated from equation (5.6) when $\varphi = 1$ are given in **Table 5.2**.

Wilcoxon-Mann-Whitney U-Test

Sample size

If the outcome variable is continuous but has a distribution which is not Normal and a suitable transformation cannot be found, a Wilcoxon-Mann-Whitney U-test may be used to compare the two groups. If $F_S(x)$ and $F_T(x)$ are the probabilities of an outcome being less than a particular value (x) under options S and T respectively, then a non-parametric test has, as null hypothesis H_0, $F_S(x) = F_T(x)$. The alternative hypothesis H_{Alt} is $F_S(x) \leq F_T(x)$ with strict inequality for at least one value of x. A simple alternative hypothesis is one which assumes that $F_S(x) = F_T(x - \delta)$ for some $\delta > 0$. Here δ represents a shift in location between the two groups under consideration. An approximate formula for the sample size to give a 2-sided significance level α and power $1 - \beta$ is given by

$$N = f \times \left[\frac{(1+\varphi)^2}{\varphi} \right] \left[\frac{(z_{1-\alpha/2} + z_{1-\beta})^2}{(\delta_{Plan} / \sigma_{Plan})^2} + \frac{z_{1-\alpha/2}^2}{2} \right] \tag{5.7}$$

where f depends on the particular form of the distributions $F_S(x)$ and $F_T(x)$.

To calculate f it is necessary to derive the cumulative distribution of the difference of two independent random variables under the null hypothesis assumption that $F_S(x) = F_T(x)$. The quantity f is the first derivative of the derived distribution evaluated at $x = 0$. If we assume the underlying distributions are Normal then

$$f = \frac{\pi}{3} = 1.0472, \tag{5.8}$$

where the π represents the irrational number 3.14159....Since $f > 1$, this implies that equation (5.7) gives larger sample sizes than equation (5.4) for which Normal distributions are assumed.

If the formula for the distribution of the data cannot be reliably obtained, then an alternative approach is to divide the outcome variable of concern into (a maximum of five) categories and use the methods for ordinal data described in **Chapter 4**.

A further option for the calculation of the total sample size, when no ties are anticipated, is to calculate

$$N = \frac{(1+\varphi)^2 (z_{1-\alpha/2} + z_{1-\beta})^2}{12\varphi(P - 0.5)^2}, \tag{5.9}$$

where P is the probability that a randomly selected observation from a subject receiving intervention T is greater than that of a randomly selected observation from a subject receiving S.

One difficulty is providing a suitable planning value for P. However, for a study involving two Normally distributed variables X and Y with a given standardised effect size, it can be shown that

$$P = \text{Prob}(Y > X) = \Phi(\Delta / \sqrt{2}), \tag{5.10}$$

where $\Phi(.)$ is the cumulative Normal distribution of **Table 1.1**. It may seem odd to invoke the Normal distribution when trying to find values of P (since we are assuming the data do not have Normal distributions) so, if a planning value can be identified from other sources, it should be used. Nevertheless, equation (5.9) may be useful as a starting point for sample size calculations.

Table 5.3 gives values of P for selected values of Δ.

5.3 One Mean Known

One-Sample *T*-Test

Sample size

In this situation, we require the number of subjects, N, necessary to show that a given mean μ_T differs from a target value μ_{Known}. Given a 2-sided significance level α (although 1-sided is often used in this situation) and a power $(1 - \beta)$ against the specified alternative μ_T, then the number of subjects required in the group concerned is

$$N = \frac{\left(z_{1-\alpha/2} + z_{1-\beta}\right)^2}{\Delta^2} + \frac{z_{1-\alpha/2}^2}{2}, \tag{5.11}$$

where $\Delta = (\mu_T - \mu_{Known})/\sigma_{Plan}$. Sample sizes calculated from equation (5.11) are given in **Table 5.4**.

5.4 Bibliography

Schouten (1999) derived equation (5.2), which generalised the result of Guenther (1981) to allow for unequal allocation, and equation (5.6), which considers the situation when the variances in the two groups to be compared are unequal. Chow, Shao and Wang (2002) comment on the use of the non-central *t*-distribution of equation (5.3). Lehman (1975) gives a derivation leading to equations (5.7) and (5.8) for use with the Wilcoxon-Mann-Whitney *U*-test. Equation (5.9) was given, for equal size groups, by Noether (1987) and was shown by Zhao, Rahardja and Qu (2008) to be a simplification of their formula for tied data, which we give as equation (4.8). Guenther (1981) gives equation (5.11). A review of sample size determination for non-parametric tests has been given by Rahardja, Zhao and Qu (2012).

Cohen (1988) suggests that a range of plausible values for the standardised effect size, Δ, is from 0.1 to 1.0.

5.5 Examples

Table 1.2
For one-sided test size, $\alpha = 0.05$, $z_{0.95} = 1.6449$.
For two-sided test size, $\alpha = 0.05$, $z_{0.975} = 1.96$.
For one-sided, $1 - \beta = 0.8$, 0.9 and 0.95, $z_{0.8} = 0.8416$, $z_{0.9} = 1.2816$ and $z_{0.95} = 1.6449$.

Table 5.1 and Equation 5.4

Example 5.1   Equal group sizes and equal standard deviations - Foetal compromise
The GRIT Study Group (2004) conducted a clinical trial in which pregnant women with foetal compromise were randomised to either delivering early (E) or delaying birth for as long as possible (D). In a sub-group of women at 24-30 weeks gestation, it was anticipated that the Griffiths full scale development quotient (DQ) at 2 years would be improved by 10 points. They also anticipated that the DQ scores would have $SD = 10$ units.

If a trial is designed on the basis of these, then $\delta_{Plan} = \mu_D - \mu_E = 10$, $\sigma_{Plan} = 10$ and therefore $\Delta_{Plan} = 10/10 = 1.0$. This may be considered as a 'large' effect size. Further assuming $\varphi = 1$, $\alpha = 0.05$ (2-sided) and $1 - \beta = 0.9$, equation (5.4) gives $N = \left[\frac{(1+1)^2}{1} \right] \left[\frac{(1.96+1.2816)^2}{1.0^2} \right] + \left[\frac{1.96^2}{2} \right] =$ $42.03 + 1.92 = 43.95$ or 44. Thus pregnant women who are eligible for the trial would be randomised as 22 to E and 22 to D. **Table 5.1** also gives $N = 44$ as does $^S S_S$.

If Δ_{Plan} is reduced to 0.75 and 0.5 the total sample sizes increase to 78 and 172 pregnant women respectively. Increasing the power to $1 - \beta = 0.95$ increases these three estimates of sample size to 54, 96 and 210.

Table 5.1 and Equation 5.4

Example 5.2   Equal group sizes and equal standard deviations - cartilage repair
Nejadnik, Hui, Choong, *et al* (2011) compared autologous bone marrow-derived mesenchymal stem cells (BMSC) with autologous chondrocyte implantation (ACI) for knee cartilage repair in a non-randomised cohort study. One of the assessments utilised was the International Knee Documentation Committee (IKDC) score, which at 3 months post operatively indicated an advantage to BMSC of about 5.5 units.

A confirmatory randomised trial is considered with the assumption that a $\delta_{Plan} = 5$ is thought to be the clinically worthwhile minimum difference. The investigators consider a design with $\varphi = 1$, 2-sided $\alpha = 0.05$ but with high power, $1 - \beta = 0.95$. The earlier report suggests that IKDC at 3 months can range over the whole of the 0 to 100 possible scores. As a consequence the design team considers a range of options for σ_{Plan} from 10 to 20 units.

Use of equation (5.4) or **Table 5.1** for values of Δ_{Plan} equal to $5/10 = 0.5$, $5/15 \approx 0.3$ and $5/20 = 0.25$ give successive values of the total number of subjects N as 210, 580 and 834. Realising that trials of this size may not be feasible, the investigators lower their power requirements to $1 - \beta = 0.90$, consider $\sigma_{Plan} = 15$ units, agree a revised $\delta_{Plan} = 7.5$ units, give $\Delta_{Plan} = 0.5$ and hence obtain $N = 172$. After further discussion, the investigators conclude that a trial size of 200 patients, 100 per cartilage repair group, is a feasible proposition.

Equation 5.4

Example 5.3   Choice of outcome measures - recovery post colorectal surgery
Fiore, Faragher, Bialocerkowski, *et al* (2013) estimate the sample sizes required using length of stay (LOS) as compared to time-to-readiness for discharge (TRD) as outcomes for potential randomised trials concerned with evaluating alternative options following colorectal surgery. From what appears to be 70 patients, TRD and LOS were both assessed and the corresponding SDs calculated. **Figure 5.1** presents their results together with potential sample sizes for future randomised comparative trials

Outcome measure	SD	Total sample size, N	
		$\delta_{Plan} = 1$	$\delta_{Plan} = 2$
LOS	3.95	492	126
TRD	3.45	376	96

Figure 5.1 Sample size estimates for randomised controlled trials (RCT) using LOS and TRD as outcome measures of short-term recovery post colorectal surgery (after Fiore, Faragher, Bialocerkowski, *et al*, 2013).

using TRD or LOS endpoints. The scenarios presented relate to anticipated effect sizes of δ_{Plan} of 1 and 2 days between the interventions under investigation on the assumption that 2-sided $\alpha = 0.05$, $\beta = 0.2$ and with equal numbers per intervention.

From this information the authors concluded: 'Because TRD is a more precise measure (that is it has lower standard deviation), RCTs using TRD require approximately 23% fewer participants to become adequately powered regardless of the effect size.'

Equation 5.4

Example 5.4 Complex outcome measure - juvenile idiopathic arthritis
Ilisson, Zagura, Zilmer, *et al* (2015) describe a study comparing carotid artery intima-media thickness and myeloperoxidase levels in 39 newly diagnosed juveniles with idiopathic arthritis with 27 healthy controls. The measure considered for sample size determination was the adjusted augmentation index (AIx) defined as follows:

'The AIx was calculated as the difference between the second and the first systolic peaks, divided by pulse pressure and expressed in percentages [Reference given by authors]. The AIx values were adjusted to a heart rate of 75 beats/min (AIx@75) using a built in algorithm in the Sphygmo-Cor Px system (AtCor Medical).'

This is clearly a very complicated measure indeed. The stability of such a measure will depend in a complex way on the reliability of the estimates of its components. In general, simple endpoint measures are preferable in comparative studies.

The authors then used a planning difference in AIx@75 between groups of $\delta_{Plan} = 4.953U$ (rather too precise for this purpose) with $\sigma_{Plan} = 10U$. Then with power of 80% and 2-sided 0.05 significance level concluded:

'A total of 66 persons were targeted to enter this two group study.'

However, this calculation assumes 33 juveniles are to be recruited in each group, and unfortunately use of equation (5.4) gives $N = 130$ (65 per group) as the total number of children that would be required, that is, the sample size the authors give should have been *per intervention*.

This example highlights, for any design, how important it is to have careful verification of the sample size chosen whenever possible.

Table 5.2 and Equation 5.6

Example 5.5 Equal group sizes but unequal standard deviations - intermolar width
In a study reported by Pandis, Polychronopoulou and Eliades (2007) comparing conventional (*CL*) and self-ligating (*SL*) brackets for the treatment of mandipular crowding, the final mean intermolar width in 27 patients assigned *CL* was 44.6 mm ($\sigma_{CL} = 2.7$) whereas in 27 patients assigned to *SL* this was greater at 46.2 mm ($\sigma_{SL} = 1.7$).

Allocation Ratio	Block Size		Power 1−β					
			0.8			0.9		
		φ	n_{CL}	n_{SL}	N	n_{CL}	n_{SL}	N
1 : 1	2	1	33	33	66	43	43	86
5 : 4	9	0.8	35	28	63	50	40	90
3 : 2	5	0.6667	**39**	**26**	**65**	**51**	**34**	**85**
2 : 1	3	0.5	42	21	63	56	28	84

Figure 5.2 Variation in sample size with changing 1: φ allocation and accounting for block size assuming 2-sided α=0.05.

Suppose a confirmatory trial is planned with the investigators having taken note of the differential in the SDs reported for each group. Taking $\sigma_{Plan}=\sigma_{CL}=2.7$, then with $\delta_{Plan}=46.2-44.6=1.6$ mm, the standardised effect size $\Delta_{Plan}=1.6/2.7=0.5926$. Also $\tau_{Plan}=\dfrac{\sigma_{SL}^2}{\sigma_{CL}^2}=\dfrac{1.7^2}{2.7^2}=0.3964$. Assuming $\varphi=1$,

$\alpha=0.05$ (2-sided), $1-\beta=0.8$, equation (5.6) gives $N=\left(\dfrac{1+1}{1}\right)\left\{\left[\dfrac{(0.3964+1)\times2.7^2}{1.6^2}\times\left(1.96+0.8416\right)^2\right]\right.$

$\left.+\left[\dfrac{\left(0.3964^2+1^3\right)\times1.96^2}{2\left(0.3964+1\right)^2}\right]\right\}=64.70$ or 66 to allow equal subject numbers in each group. If the power

is increased to 90% then $N=86$ are required. $^{S}S_{S}$ also gives these values.

However, if we are to use **Table 5.2** for this example, some reformatting is required. Thus $\tau=1/\tau_{Plan}=1/0.3964=2.52$, $\sigma_{Plan}=\sigma_{SL}=1.7$ so that $\Delta=1/\Delta_{Plan}=1.6/1.7=0.94$. The nearest tabular entries are for $\tau=2.5$ and $\Delta=0.9$, which, for power 80% and 90%, give the total sample sizes required as $N=72$ and 94 respectively.

Although we have used $\varphi=1$ in this example, since the $\sigma_{CL}=2.7$ is larger than $\sigma_{SL}=1.7$, it may be preferable to allocate a greater proportion to CL. However, if this is in the context of clinical trials then the allocation possibilities need to allow for blocks of a convenient size to facilitate the randomisation process. For example, if $\varphi=0.8$ then this implies a 5 : 4 ratio and hence a block size of 9. Thus, the final sample size chosen, N, needs to be divisible by 9. **Figure 5.2** shows the sample sizes for various block sizes and indicates that, for this example, the 3: 2 allocation with $\varphi=2/3$ results in the smallest study size. In this case, when $1-\beta=0.8$, $n_{CL}=39$, $n_{SL}=26$ and $N=65$ while for equal allocation $n_{CL}=n_{SL}=33$ and $N=66$. For $1-\beta=0.9$ the comparable numbers are $n_{CL}=51$, $n_{SL}=34$ and $N=85$ and for equal allocation $n_{CL}=n_{SL}=43$ and $N=86$. It should be noted that the numerical rounding from the (usually non-integer) sample size given by the respective equation is taken to the next integer value divisible by the block size. Note that $^{S}S_{S}$ does not do follow this blocking process, so it is left to the investigator to implement this strategy if appropriate.

Table 5.3 and Equations 5.7, 5.8 and 5.9

Example 5.6 Non-Normal data and unequal group sizes - photo-aged skin
Although no justification of the sample size is provided, Watson, Ogden, Cotterell *et al* (2009) randomised 60 patients with photo-aged skin to receive either an anti-ageing (*A-A*) product or merely the vehicle (*V*) used in the manufacture of the product. The deposition of fibrillin-1 in the

skin was assessed after 6 months of treatment. Their results gave the mean and SD values for V as 1.84 and 1.64 and for A-A 2.57 and 1.04. Such relatively large SDs compared to their corresponding means suggest the data are rather skewed. Suppose a repeat trial is planned, but in view of the apparent skewness of the earlier data, the investigators plan an analysis using the Wilcoxon-Mann-Whitney U-test and they wish to recruit relatively more patients to the A-A group and so choose a 2:3 allocation, thus $\varphi = 3/2 = 1.5$.

From the previous trial the investigators note that $d = \bar{x}_{A-A} - \bar{x}_V = 2.57 - 1.04 = 1.43$. However, for them a smaller difference would be clinically important, and so they choose $\delta_{Plan} = 1.2$. They also note the pooled estimate of the SD as $s_{Pool} = \sqrt{\dfrac{1.64^2 + 1.04^2}{2}} = 1.37$ but are concerned it may be somewhat larger with their patients, so they choose a greater $\sigma_{Plan} = 1.45$.

Finally, assuming a 2-sided $\alpha = 0.05$ and $1 - \beta = 0.90$, equation (5.7) combined with equation (5.8) gives the sample size required as $N = 1.0472 \times \left[\dfrac{(1+1.5)^2}{1.5}\right] \left[\dfrac{(1.96+1.2816)^2}{(1.2/1.45)^2} + \left[\dfrac{1.96^2}{2}\right]\right] = 68.86$. However, to enable a 2:3 randomisation, the final number of patients required should be divisible by the block size 5, hence $N = 70$ with $n_V = 28$ and $n_{A-A} = 42$ allocated to the respective agents.

If we use the approach of equation (5.9), then the standardised effect size required is $\Delta = 1.2/1.45 = 0.828$ and the nearest entry for Δ in **Table 5.3** is 0.85. This leads to $P = 0.726$ and so

$$N = \frac{(1+1.5)^2}{12 \times 1.5} \frac{(1.96+1.2816)^2}{(0.726-0.5)^2} = 71.43 \text{ or, in order to be divisible by 5, set as 75. From which}$$

$n_V = 75/2.5 = 30$ and $n_{A-A} = 75 \times (1.5)/2.5 = 45$.

These subject numbers are somewhat larger than those obtained previously by using the simple adjustment, f, as this latter approach requires fewer assumptions.

Table 5.3 and Equations 5.9 and 5.10

Example 5.7 Non-Normally distributed data - health-related quality of life measures
Walters (2009, p63) shows that the Physical Functioning (PF) dimension of the SF36 score was not Normally distributed. He describes a randomised controlled trial of a daily exercise regime for a year to improve quality of life and suggests that a clinically important effect size for any SF36 dimension is a score difference of 10. He gives the SD as about 30 units. This leads $\Delta = 10/30 = 0.33$ and from **Table 5.3** to a value of $P(X > Y)$ between 0.584 and 0.598, or approximately 0.591. Thus from equation (5.9), assuming a 2-sided $\alpha = 0.05$, $1 - \beta = 0.90$ and $\varphi = 1$, we obtain $N = \dfrac{4(1.96+1.2816)^2}{12(0.593-0.5)^2} = $ 404.98 or approximately 400 patients, implying 200 per intervention would be required.

Table 5.4 and Equation 5.11

Example 5.8 Target mean established - systolic blood pressure in patients with chronic kidney disease
Palacios, Haugen, Thompson, *et al* (2016) conducted a retrospective study of 380 patients > 60 years with stages 1–5 pre-dialysis chronic kidney disease and found a mean systolic blood pressure (SBP) of 130.7 mmHg (SD = 12.4). Further, the 68 (17.9%) patients with SBP < 120 mmHg had a relatively worse outcome in terms of subsequent mortality. Suppose an intervention study is planned with the hope to raise the observed mean to 135 mmHg in a similar group of patients.

This specification implies $\mu_{Known} = 130$ and $\Delta_{Plan} = \delta_{Plan}/\sigma_{Plan} = (135 - 130)/12.4 = 0.40$. How many patients should be recruited?

The test to use is the one-sample t-test. If the clinical team specifies $\alpha = 0.05$ for a 2-sided test and a power $1 - \beta = 0.8$, then, with $\Delta = 0.4$, equation (5.11) gives $N = \dfrac{(1.96 + 0.8416)^2}{0.4^2} + \dfrac{1.96^2}{2} = 50.98$ or 51. Alternatively this value can be found from **Table 5.4** or $\boxed{{}^{S}\!S_{S}}$.

On the other hand, if the concern was solely to demonstrate an increased SBP of 5 mmHg, then a 1-sided test size would be appropriate. In this circumstance, the sample size required is reduced to $N = \dfrac{(1.6449 + 0.8416)^2}{0.4^2} + \dfrac{1.6449^2}{2} = 39.99$ or 40 patients.

If a mean of 135 mmHg could be established then, assuming SBP follows a Normal distribution with mean and SD of 135 and 12.4 respectively, the proportion of patients < 120 mmHg is likely to fall from the observed 17.9% to approximately 11%.

References

Technical

Chow SC, Shao J and Wang H (2002). A note on sample size calculations for mean comparisons based on non central t-statistics. *Journal of Pharmaceutical Statistics*, **12**, 441–456.

Cohen J (1988). *Statistical Power Analysis for the Behavioral Sciences*. (2nd edn) Lawrence Erlbaum, New Jersey.

Guenther WC (1981). Sample size formulas for normal theory *t*-tests. *The American Statistician*, **35**, 243–244.

Lehman EL (1975). *Nonparametric Statistical Methods Based on Ranks*. Holden-Day, San Francisco.

Noether GE (1987). Sample size determination for some common nonparametric tests. *Journal of the American Statistical Association*, **82**, 645–647.

Rahardja D, Zhao YD and Qu Y (2012). Sample size determination for the Wilcoxon-Mann-Whitney test. A comprehensive review. *Statistics in Pharmaceutical Research*, **1**, 317–322.

Schouten HJA (1999). Sample size formula with a continuous outcome for unequal group sizes and unequal variances. *Statistics in Medicine*, **18**, 87–91.

Examples

Fiore JF, Faragher IG, Bialocerkowski A, Browning L and Denehy L (2013). Time to readiness for discharge is a valid and reliable measure of short-term recovery after colorectal surgery. *World Journal of Surgery*, **37**, 2927–2934.

Ilisson J, Zagura M, Zilmer K, Salum E, Heilman K, Piir A, Tillmann V, Kals J, Zilmer M and Pruunsild C (2015). Increased carotid artery intima-media thickness and myeloperoxidase level in children with newly diagnosed juvenile idiopathic arthritis. *Arthritis Research & Therapy*, **17**, 180.

Nejadnik H, Hui JH, Choong EPF, Tai B-C and Lee EH (2011). Autologous bone marrow-derived mesenchymal stem cells versus autologous chondrocyte implantation: An observational cohort study. *The American Journal of Sports Medicine*, **38**, 1110–1116.

Palacios CRF, Haugen EN, Thompson AM, Rasmussen RW, Goracke N and Goyal P (2016). Clinical outcomes with a systolic blood pressure lower than 120 mmHg in older patients with high disease burden. *Renal Failure*, **38**, 1364–1369.

Pandis N, Polychronopoulou A and Eliades T (2007). Self-ligating vs conventional brackets in the treatment of mandibular crowding: a prospective clinical trial of treatment duration and dental effects. *American Journal of Orthodontics and Dentofacial Orthopedics*, **132**, 208–215.

The GRIT Study Group (2004). Infant wellbeing at 2 years of age in the Growth Restriction Intervention Trial (GRIT): multicentred randomised controlled trial. *Lancet*, **364**, 513–520.

Walters SJ (2009). *Quality of Life Outcomes in Clinical Trials and Health Care Evaluation*. Wiley, Chichester.

Watson REB, Ogden S, Cotterell LF, Bowden JJ, Bastrilles JY, Long SP and Griffiths CEM (2009). A cosmetic 'anti-aging' product improves photoaged skin: a double-blind, randomized controlled trial. *British Journal of Dermatology*, **161**, 419–426.

Table 5.1 Sample sizes for the two sample *t*-test with 2-sided $\alpha = 0.05$ [Equation (5.4) with $\varphi = 1$].
Each cell gives the total sample size, *N*, for a study assuming equal numbers, *N/2*, are included in each group.

Standardised effect size	Power		
Δ	0.80	0.90	0.95
0.15	1,398	1,870	2,314
0.20	788	1,054	1,302
0.25	506	676	834
0.30	352	470	580
0.35	260	346	428
0.40	200	266	328
0.45	158	210	260
0.50	128	172	210
0.55	106	142	174
0.60	90	120	148
0.65	78	102	126
0.70	66	88	108
0.75	58	78	96
0.80	52	68	84
0.85	46	62	74
0.90	42	54	68
0.95	38	50	60
1.0	34	44	54
1.1	28	38	46
1.2	24	32	40
1.3	22	28	34
1.4	18	24	30
1.5	16	22	26

Table 5.2 Sample sizes for the two sample *t*-test with unequal variances for 2-sided $\alpha = 0.05$, power $1 - \beta = 0.8$ [Equation (5.6) with $\varphi = 1$].
Each cell gives the total sample size, *N*, for a study assuming equal numbers, *N*/2, are included in each group.

	Variance ratio, τ					
Δ	1.5	2	2.5	3	4	5
0.15	1,748	2,096	2,446	2,794	3,492	4,190
0.20	984	1,180	1,376	1,574	1,966	2,358
0.25	630	756	882	1,008	1,260	1,510
0.30	440	526	614	702	876	1,050
0.35	324	388	452	516	644	772
0.40	248	298	346	396	494	592
0.45	196	236	374	314	392	468
0.50	160	192	224	254	318	380
0.55	132	158	184	210	264	316
0.60	112	134	156	178	222	266
0.65	96	114	134	152	190	226
0.70	48	100	116	132	164	196
0.75	72	86	100	116	144	172
0.80	64	76	90	102	126	150
0.85	58	68	80	90	112	134
0.90	52	62	72	80	100	120
0.95	46	56	64	72	90	108
1.0	42	50	58	66	82	98
1.1	36	42	48	56	68	82
1.2	30	36	42	48	58	70
1.3	26	30	36	40	50	60
1.4	24	28	32	36	44	52
1.5	20	24	28	32	38	46

	Variance ratio, τ					
Δ	1.5	2	2.5	3	4	5
0.15	2,338	2,806	3.272	3,740	4,674	5,608
0.20	1,316	1,580	1,842	2,104	2,630	3,156
0.25	844	1,012	1,180	1,348	1,684	2,022
0.30	586	704	820	938	1,172	1,404
0.35	432	518	604	690	862	1,034
0.40	332	398	462	528	660	792
0.45	262	314	366	418	522	626
0.50	214	256	298	340	424	508
0.55	176	212	246	282	350	420
0.60	148	178	208	236	296	354
0.65	128	152	178	202	252	302
0.70	110	132	154	174	218	262
0.75	96	116	134	152	190	228

(Continued)

Table 5.2 (Continued)

Δ	Variance ratio, τ					
	1.5	2	2.5	3	4	5
0.80	86	102	118	134	168	200
0.85	76	90	106	120	150	178
0.90	68	80	94	108	134	160
0.95	62	72	84	96	120	144
1.0	56	66	76	88	108	130
1.1	46	56	64	72	90	108
1.2	40	46	54	62	76	92
1.3	34	40	46	54	66	78
1.4	30	36	40	46	58	68
1.5	26	32	36	40	50	60

Table 5.3 Prob $(Y > X)$ when X and Y are Normally distributed for standardised difference Δ [Equation (5.10)].

Δ	$P(Y > X)$	Δ	$P(Y > X)$	Δ	$P(Y > X)$
0.05	0.514	0.55	0.651	1.05	0.771
0.10	0.528	0.60	0.664	1.10	0.782
0.15	0.542	0.65	0.677	1.15	0.792
0.20	0.556	0.70	0.690	1.20	0.802
0.25	0.570	0.75	0.702	1.25	0.812
0.30	0.584	0.80	0.714	1.30	0.821
0.35	0.598	0.85	0.726	1.35	0.830
0.40	0.611	0.90	0.738	1.40	0.839
0.45	0.625	0.95	0.749	1.45	0.847
0.50	0.638	1.00	0.760	1.50	0.856

Table 5.4 Sample sizes for the one sample *t*-test with 1- and 2-sided $\alpha = 0.05$ [Equation (5.11)].

Standardised effect size	Power: $1 - \beta$					
	0.80		0.90		0.95	
	Test Size: $\alpha = 0.05$					
Δ	1-sided	2-sided	1-sided	2-sided	1-sided	2-sided
0.05	2,475	3,142	3,427	4,205	4,331	5,200
0.10	620	787	858	1,053	1,084	1,302
0.15	277	351	382	469	483	580
0.20	156	199	216	265	272	327
0.25	101	128	139	171	175	210
0.30	71	90	97	119	122	147
0.35	52	66	72	88	90	108
0.40	40	51	55	68	69	84
0.45	32	41	44	54	55	67
0.50	27	34	36	44	45	54
0.55	22	28	30	37	38	45
0.60	19	24	26	32	32	39
0.65	16	21	22	27	27	33
0.70	14	18	19	24	24	29
0.75	13	16	17	21	21	26
0.80	12	15	15	19	19	23
0.85	10	13	14	17	17	20
0.90	9	12	12	15	15	18
0.95	9	11	11	14	14	17
1.0	8	10	10	13	13	15
1.1	7	9	9	11	11	13
1.2	6	8	8	10	9	11
1.3	6	7	7	9	8	10
1.4	5	6	6	8	7	9
1.5	5	6	6	7	7	8

6

Rate Outcomes

SUMMARY

This chapter considers sample-size calculations for comparisons between two groups where the outcome of concern is a count which is then expressed as a rate per unit of time. The anticipated effect size between groups is expressed either as a difference between the two rates or by the risk ratio. Also included are sample size expressions for some single or two-group designs which are often referred to as post-marketing studies. Thus once a drug or medical device has been approved for use by the regulatory authorities, it will then go into routine clinical use. This will usually cover a wider pool of patient types than those recruited to the clinical trial(s) demonstrating their efficacy, and so there may be real concerns about the immediate and longer term consequences of their wider use.

6.1 Introduction

Chapter 1 describes the Poisson distribution as a limit of the Binomial distribution when the proportion of events, π, is small and when the number of subjects, n, is large. In such situations, the number of events observed, r, in a single group study is often expressed as an incidence rate, $R = r/Y$, where Y represents the exposure, that is, the unit of time over which the possibility of the occurrence of the event is monitored. Thus rather than specifically note the occurrence of an event in n subjects, to estimate a *proportion* by $R = r/n$, a period of time Y may be specified and the *rate* estimated by $R = r/Y$. Another option is to recruit n subjects and follow each for a fixed period y in which case the rate is estimated by $R = r/ny$. Alternatively, each of the n subjects may have individual follow-up times, say, y_i, in which case the incidence rate is $R = r/Y$, where $Y = \sum_i y_i$ is the anticipated total follow-up time recorded in the group. In each situation R is the estimate of the population parameter λ. In practice, the incidence rate may be expressed as per-person, per-100-person or per-1000-person days, years or other time frames depending on the context.

A key property of the Poisson distribution of equation (1.12) is that the mean and the variance, V, are both equal to λ. However, in some situations it turns out V is greater than the rate λ, and 'over-dispersion' is designated. In which case, the Negative-Binomial distribution of equation (1.13) may provide an appropriate description for the resulting data.

Although comparing rates is a common topic in epidemiological studies, it also has an important role in pharmaco-epidemiology studies of post-marketing surveillance. For example, after a drug or medical device has been accepted for general use, it may be prudent to survey the subsequently

Sample Sizes for Clinical, Laboratory and Epidemiology Studies, Fourth Edition. David Machin, Michael J. Campbell, Say Beng Tan and Sze Huey Tan.
© 2018 John Wiley & Sons Ltd. Published 2018 by John Wiley & Sons Ltd.

treated patients to identify the type, and quantify the scale, of any adverse effects. In some circumstances it is possible that only one adverse reaction, such as a drug-related death, would be necessary for the drug to be considered unacceptable and withdrawn from a prescription list. In other situations a single adverse occurrence of a particular event would be put down to chance and several occurrences are required to confirm a suspicion about the drug. In most situations the specific adverse reactions of concern may also occur in patients not receiving the drug in question. For example, in an elderly population, deaths are likely to occur in any event. Also, many common adverse reactions such as nausea, drowsiness and headache are prevalent in the general population, and we may need to know whether the drug has provoked an increase in incidence of such adverse reactions over this background rate. If the background incidence is known, then only those receiving the specific drug or device need to be monitored. If, as is more usual, the incidence is not known, then a control population might also be monitored for comparison purposes.

6.2   Comparing Rates

The data necessary to estimate a rate are the number of events observed, 0, 1, 2, 3, … and the relevant denominator Y. The corresponding analysis of the subsequent data from a study compares the observed rates from the two groups of concern.

Effect Size

At the planning stage of a study, we have to specify the anticipated effect size as the anticipated difference in rates $\delta_{Plan} = \lambda_{PlanT} - \lambda_{PlanS}$, where λ_{PlanS} and λ_{PlanT} (abbreviated to λ_S and λ_T in the following) are the anticipated rates under the *Standard* (*S*) and *Test* (*T*) groups respectively. Alternatively, the effect size may be expressed in terms of the risk ratio or relative risk as $RR_{Plan} = \dfrac{\lambda_T}{\lambda_S}$, which can take any positive value. The corresponding null hypotheses are expressed in terms of the population values of the respective rates by $H_0: \delta = \lambda_T - \lambda_S = 0$ or equivalently $H_0: R = \dfrac{\lambda_T}{\lambda_S} = 1$.

In some situations, rather than setting anticipated values for λ_S and λ_T, an investigator may prespecify RR_{Plan} and (say) λ_S. In this later case λ_T (or λ_S as appropriate) is obtained using the general expression

$$\lambda_T = RR\lambda_S. \tag{6.1}$$

Sample size – Poisson distribution

The required total exposure in per-person units, PU, for a specified λ_S, λ_T, with allocation ratio to the two groups as 1: φ, 2-sided test size α, power $1 - \beta$, is given by

$$PU = \left(\frac{1+\varphi}{\varphi}\right)\left(z_{1-\alpha/2} + z_{1-\beta}\right)^2 \frac{\left(\lambda_T + \varphi\lambda_S\right)}{\left(\lambda_T - \lambda_S\right)^2}. \tag{6.2}$$

If the effect size is expressed by the risk ratio, RR_{Plan}, then either λ_S or λ_T has to be specified and equation (6.2) can then be alternatively expressed as

$$PU = \left(\frac{1+\varphi}{\varphi}\right)\left(z_{1-\alpha/2} + z_{1-\beta}\right)^2 \frac{\left(\varphi + RR_{Plan}\right)}{\lambda_S\left(1 - RR_{Plan}\right)^2}. \tag{6.3}$$

The exposures required in each group are $pu_S = PU/(1 + \varphi)$ and $pu_T = \varphi PU/(1 + \varphi)$. Values for $z_{1-\alpha/2}$ and $z_{1-\beta}$ can be obtained from **Table 1.2**.

Sample Size – Negative-Binomial distribution

If the number of counts per individual over a specific time interval cannot be assumed to follow a Poisson distribution then the Negative-Binomial distribution, as described in **Chapter 1**, may be appropriate. In which case the parameter κ as well as λ has to be pre-specified, and the total number of subjects required is given by

$$N = (1+\varphi)V\frac{\left(z_{1-\alpha/2} + z_{1-\beta}\right)^2}{\left[log\left(\frac{\lambda_T}{\lambda_S}\right)\right]^2}. \tag{6.4}$$

Here

$$V = \frac{1}{\tau}\left(\frac{1}{\lambda_S} + \frac{1}{\varphi\lambda_T}\right) + \frac{\kappa(1+\varphi)}{\varphi}, \tag{6.5}$$

and τ is the assumed mean exposure time of all subjects subsequently recruited.

6.3 Post-Marketing Surveillance

In general, the rates λ in post-marketing surveillance studies are very low so that the sample size formulae of equations (6.2) and (6.3) are no longer reliable. Also, single-group studies and non-randomised comparative studies are often undertaken.

Single Group Studies

No comparison group

Suppose the anticipated rate of adverse reactions is λ, the number of occurrences of a particular adverse reaction is r and the number of patients required to be monitored is N. If the incidence of adverse reactions is reasonably low then one might assume that they follow the Poisson distribution of equation (1.12), with λ replaced by $N\lambda$, thus, $P(r) = exp(-N\lambda)\frac{(N\lambda)^r}{r!}$, where $r = 0, 1, 2, 3, \ldots$ .With this assumption and defining γ as the probability that, for a given λ_{Plan}, we will find *less* than a adverse reactions when conducting a study, then N is the solution of the following

$$exp(-N\lambda_{Plan}) \times \sum_{r=0}^{a-1} \frac{(N\lambda_{Plan})^r}{r!} = \gamma. \tag{6.6}$$

Thus in a study, we want a high probability that we can exclude the possibility of more than a adverse reactions and so set $(1 - \gamma)$ to be relatively large.

For $a = 1$, when the particular adverse reaction needs occur in only one or more patients, equation (6.6) becomes $P(0) = \exp(-N\lambda_{Plan}) \dfrac{(N\lambda)^0}{0!} = \exp(-N\lambda_{Plan}) = \gamma$, from which

$$N = \frac{-\log\gamma}{\lambda_{Plan}}. \tag{6.7}$$

For $a > 1$ there is no simple expression for the solution to equation (6.6), but the equation can be solved using numerical methods and some resulting solutions are given in **Table 6.1**.

Known background incidence

If λ_{Back} is the known background incidence of the adverse reaction and ε_{Plan} is the anticipated additional incidence caused by use of the particular drug under study, then a 1-sided test is appropriate. The sample size for given 1-sided α and power $1 - \beta$ is

$$N = \frac{\left[z_{1-\alpha}\sqrt{\lambda_{Back}} + z_{1-\beta}\sqrt{\lambda_{Back} + \varepsilon_{Plan}} \right]^2}{\varepsilon_{Plan}^2}. \tag{6.8}$$

When both λ_{Back} and ε_{Plan} are very small, this is an equivalent expression to equation (3.6) with $\pi_{Known} = \lambda_{Back}$ and $\pi_T = \lambda_{Back} + \varepsilon_{Plan}$. Values of N are given in **Table 6.2**.

Comparative Studies

If the background incidence is unknown then a *Control* (*C*) group is needed to establish this. In this situation also, a 1-sided test is likely to be the most appropriate as one only becomes concerned if the rate with *T* is *greater* than that with *C*. However, it is important to emphasise that a post-marketing study monitors groups whose therapeutic approaches are not allocated at random.

Also in contrast to randomised clinical trials, it is more usual in post-marketing surveillance when comparing *C* and *T* groups to have an allocation ratio $k: 1$ which favours *C* although $k \geq 1$ need not be an integer. This is because in relative terms the numbers taking the drug of concern are perhaps limited and, in these circumstances, the statistical efficiency of the design can be improved if relatively more subjects are monitored in group *C*.

For planning purposes we need to anticipate the background incidence, λ_{BackC} (denoted λ_C for brevity), and postulate the additional incidence that would be regarded as that needed to be detected, ε_{Plan}. For a 1-sided α and power $1 - \beta$, the total number of subjects receiving *T* to be monitored is

$$n_T = \frac{\left\{ z_{1-\alpha}\sqrt{(k+1)\bar{\lambda}(1-\bar{\lambda})} + z_{1-\beta}\sqrt{\lambda_C(1-\lambda_C) + k(\lambda_C + \varepsilon)(1 - \lambda_C - \varepsilon_{Plan})} \right\}^2}{k\varepsilon^2}, \tag{6.9}$$

where

$$\bar{\lambda} = \frac{\left[k\lambda_C + (\lambda_C + \varepsilon_{Plan}) \right]}{k+1}. \tag{6.10}$$

The corresponding $n_C = kn_T$ and hence the total sample size is $N = (k + 1)n_T$.

As sample sizes in post-marketing surveillance studies are often very large, the numbers necessary for *T*, the smaller group, rather than the total sample size *N*, are given by equation (6.9) and in the associated **Table 6.3**.

Matched Case-Control Studies

An alternative to the use of cohort studies for post-marketing surveillance purposes is first to identify those patients experiencing the adverse event, perhaps over a pre-defined period, obtain matched controls who have not experienced the event and ascertain how many in each group have been exposed to the particular substance (drug) under scrutiny. As each individual case is matched to one or more controls, then the allocation ratio of cases to controls is usually stated as $1 : m$, where m is an integer greater than or equal to 1. Thus, each matched unit comprises $(1 + m)$ individuals. Such a design leads to data for which a matched-pair analysis is appropriate.

For planning purposes we need to anticipate the current background incidence which is essentially that anticipated for the controls, λ_C, and postulate the additional incidence that would be regarded as that needed to be detected, ε_{Plan}. For a 1-sided α and power $1 - \beta$, the total number of units to be monitored is

$$U = \frac{1}{m(\lambda_C - \Omega)^2} \left\{ z_{1-\alpha} \sqrt{(1+m)\Pi(1-\Pi)} + z_{1-\beta} \sqrt{\lambda_C(1-\lambda_C) + m\Omega(1-\Omega)} \right\}^2, \tag{6.11}$$

Where

$$\Pi = \frac{\lambda_C}{1+m}\left(m + \frac{\Omega}{\lambda_C}\right) \quad \text{and} \quad \Omega = \frac{\lambda_C + \varepsilon_{Plan}}{1 + \varepsilon_{Plan}}. \tag{6.12}$$

Thus, the number of cases is $n_{Cases} = U$ while $n_{Controls} = mU$. Values of U are given in **Table 6.4**.

Several Independent Reactions

In practice, several adverse reactions to a particular drug are often monitored simultaneously. For planning purposes these are often assumed all to have approximately the same incidence and to act independently of each other. If s reactions are being monitored simultaneously, then to avoid getting many false positive results, the significance level is changed from α to α/s to implement the Bonferroni correction of equation (2.7). Thus the only change required is to replace $z_{1-\alpha}$ by $z_{1-\alpha/s}$ in these equations.

6.4 Bibliography

Equation (6.2) for calculating sample sizes for studies comparing differences in rates in parallel groups of equal size is given by Smith and Morrow (1996). Zhu and Lakkis (2012) describe equation (6.4) for sample sizes using the Negative-Binomial distribution which extends the earlier work of Keene, Jones and Lane (2007) to include a $1: \varphi$ allocation ratio. The expression for V given in equation (6.5) is one of three possibilities suggested. We have included only this one as it appears to be the most conservative and therefore results in somewhat larger sample sizes. For the situation of $\varphi = 1$, this was first given by Keene, Jones, Lane and Anderson (2007) following earlier work by Brooker, Bethony, Rodrigues, *et al* (2005).

The focus on the design of post-marketing surveillance studies was highlighted by Lewis (1981, 1983) while Tubert-Bitter, Begaud, Moride and Abehaim (1994) describe the situations corresponding to equations (6.6) and (6.8). Sample-size issues concerned with case-control designs are discussed by Edwardes (2001) and by Strom (2013) who gives equation (6.12).

6.5 Examples and Use of the Tables

Table 1.2

For 2-sided test size, $\alpha = 0.05$, $z_{0.975} = 1.96$.

For 1-sided test size, $\alpha = 0.05$, $z_{0.95} = 1.6449$.

For $\alpha = 0.05$ and $s = 2$, $\alpha/s = 0.025$ and for 1-sided test, $z_{0.975} = 1.96$.

For 1-sided $1 - \beta = 0.80$ and 0.90, $z_{0.80} = 0.8416$ and $z_{0.90} = 1.2816$.

Equation 6.2

Example 6.1   Unequal group size - Lingual retainer bond failure in dental care

In a retrospective cohort study, Lie, Ozcam, Verkerke, *et al* (2008) reported a lingual retainer failure rate of 0.23 per-person years in a patient group in which conventional etching (*C-E*) had been used. Pandis and Machin (2012) used this information to illustrate sample size calculations by assuming that a proposed randomised trial using self-etching (*S-E*) would reduce this failure rate by 25%. Thus planned values suggested are $\lambda_{C-E} = 0.23$ and $\lambda_{S-E} = 0.75 \times 0.23 = 0.1725$. Then with $\varphi = 1$, 2-sided $\alpha = 0.05$ and $1 - \beta = 0.90$, equation (6.2) gives $PY = \left(\dfrac{1+1}{1} \right)(1.96 + 1.2816)^2 \times \dfrac{0.1725 + (1 \times 0.23)}{(0.1725 - 0.23)^2} = 2,558.32$.

If patients were followed for $y = 3$ years, then the number of patients required, $N_3 = 2,558.32/3 = 852.77$ or 854, with 427 in each monitoring group. The corresponding calculations using $\boxed{S_{Ss}}$ confirm these sample sizes.

   If a randomised control trial is planned to confirm the Lie, Ozcam, Verkerke, *et al* (2008) findings then, for practical purposes, a 1:1 randomisation would generally be advised. However, as shown in **Figure 6.1**, the *PY* required changes with changing φ. It is a minimum at about $\varphi = 0.875$ with $PY = 2,546$ but that is only marginally smaller than when $\varphi = 1$ and $PY = 2,559$. However, there is now quite a disparity between the two groups with $PY_{C-E} = 1,358$ (453 *Standard*) while $PY_{S-E} = 1,188$ (396 *Test*).

   Although not usually advised for randomised controlled trials, if this comparison was to be made using a non-randomised epidemiological cohort design, it may be practical to find subjects in the ratio 1: 0.875 and thereby achieve the same efficiency as a 1:1 design but with fewer participants in the *S-E* group.

Equation 6.2

Example 6.2   Unequal group sizes - Tardive dyskinesia in patients with schizophrenia

In a study conducted by Chong, Tay, Subramaniam, *et al* (2009) the mortality rates among hospitalised patients with schizophrenia were compared in those who had severe tardive dyskinesia (*Severe*) on examination and those who did not (*Absent*). The total follow-up time in 562 patients was 4,094 years and the death rates were $\lambda_{Absent} = 0.96$ and $\lambda_{Severe} = 2.49$ per 100 years. Were the study to be repeated in another location with the rates observed used as planning values then equation (6.2) with 2-sided $\alpha = 0.05$, $1 - \beta = 0.8$ and $\varphi = 1$, gives $PU = 23.135$. However, the unit of concern is 100 years so this implies that an accumulated total of $Y = 2,314$ years of collective follow-up is required.

   The planning team for the proposed study also noted that the earlier study had recruited *Absent* and *Severe* patients in the ratio 4:3 or 1:0.75. Recalculating therefore with $\varphi = 0.75$ they obtained, from

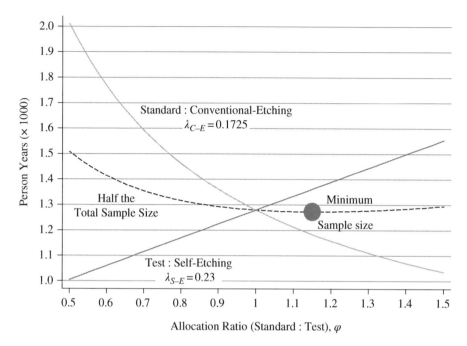

Figure 6.1 Changing number of person-years per group with varying allocation ratio 1: φ for planning values $\lambda_{C-E}=0.23$ and $\lambda_{S-E}=0.1725$, for a 2-sided $\alpha=0.05$ and $1-\beta=0.90$ [Equation 6.2]. (*See insert for color representation of the figure.*)

equation (6.2), $PU=25.113$ and so planned for a somewhat larger study with $Y=2,511$ or approximately 2,500 years of collective follow-up. The corresponding calculations using ^SS_S confirm these sample sizes.

Equations 6.4 and 6.5

Example 6.3   Over-dispersion - Asthma exacerbations

Zhu and Lakkis (2012) describe a suggested trial of 1-year duration in which a new long-acting anticholinergic ($LAMA$) is to be compared with a placebo (P) with the aim of reducing asthma exacerbations in patients taking a combination of long-acting beta-2 agonists and inhaled glucocorticoids for their asthma. Using examples from the clinical literature, they deduce that the Negative-Binomial parameter $\kappa_{Plan}=0.8$, anticipate $\lambda_P=0.66$ will be reduced by 20% to $\lambda_{LAMA}=0.528$ and

assume the mean exposure time will be $\tau_{Plan}=0.9$ years. With equal numbers per intervention, $\varphi=1$,

equation (6.5) gives $V=\dfrac{1}{0.9}\left(\dfrac{1}{0.66}+\dfrac{1}{(1\times0.528)}\right)+\dfrac{0.8\times(1+1)}{1}=5.3879$. Then with 2-sided $\alpha=0.05$

and $1-\beta=0.9$, equation (6.4) becomes $N=(1+1)\times5.3879\times\dfrac{(1.96+1.2816)^2}{\left[log(0.66/0.528)\right]^2}=2,273.92$ or $2,274$

with 1,137 patients per treatment group.

Negative binomial	Mean patient exposure, τ		
parameter, κ	0.8	0.9	1.0
0.7	2,390	2,190	2,030
0.8	2,474	2,274	2,116
0.9	2,560	2,360	2,200

Figure 6.2 Variation in the required total number of patients with asthma required for a comparative trial according to the assumptions for the mean patient exposure, τ, and the Negative-Binomial distribution parameter, κ. [Equations 6.4 and 6.5].

As one would expect, **Figure 6.2** shows that the sample size obtained for the trial varies according to the assumptions made regarding τ and κ. In this example, as τ increases the sample size reduces whereas as κ increases the sample size also increases.

Table 6.1 and Equation 6.6

Example 6.4 Single group - Restricted study size - Cardiac arrhythmia
In a previous survey, a hypertensive drug produced cardiac arrhythmias in about one in 10,000 people. A researcher decides that if a new hypertensive drug produces three such arrhythmias then the drug will have to be withdrawn pending further research. He wishes to detect the possibility of three or more events with a 99% probability of success.

For this problem equation (6.6) has to be solved for N when $\lambda_{Plan} = 1/10,000 = 0.0001$, $a = 3$ and $1 - \gamma = 0.99$. For these values **Table 6.1** gives $N = 84,060$ subjects as does $^{S}S_{S}$. Thus approximately 85,000 subjects are required.

If, on the other hand, the maximum number of subjects was restricted to $N_{Maximum} = 30,000$ then, by scanning **Table 6.1**, the entry with $\lambda_{Plan} = 0.0001$, $a = 1$ and $1 - \gamma = 0.95$ gives $N = 29,958$. Thus with 30,000 subjects he could detect one or more adverse reactions with a probability of success of 0.95. Alternatively, the entry with $\lambda_{Plan} = 0.0001$, $a = 2$, $1 - \gamma = 0.80$ gives $N = 29,944$ and allows the detection of two or more reactions with probability of 0.80. The corresponding calculations using $^{S}S_{S}$ confirm these sample sizes.

Table 6.1 and Equations 6.6 and 6.7

Example 6.5 Single group - Prescription monitoring - Safety of pioglitazone
The prescription-event monitoring study of pioglitazone, an antidiabetic drug, conducted by Kasliwal, Wilton and Shakir (2008) identified 34,151 patients who had commenced treatment with pioglitazone from which useful information was available for 12,772. One event monitored was 'death attributed to pioglitazone' by the reporting General Practitioner (GP).

The statistical methods in the paper specified: "A cohort of at least 10,000 would allow with 95% certainty that events not observed in the cohort occurred less frequently than one in 3,333 cases."

This calculation implies $\lambda_{Plan} = 1/3,333 = 0.0003$ and $1 - \gamma = 0.95$, hence equation (6.7) gives $N = -log0.05/0.0003 = 9,986$, which the authors sensibly round to 10,000.

The statistical methods in the paper also specified "… a cohort of 10 000 should allow for the detection of at least three cases of an event with 85% power, if the event occurs at a rate of at least one in 2000 patients (assuming the background rate is zero)."

This calculation implies $\lambda_{Plan} = 1/2{,}000 = 0.0005$, $a = 3$ and $1 - \gamma = 0.85$, then **Table 6.1** implies the sample size required is between 8,559 and 10,645. A more precise solution of equation (6.6) using $^S S_S$ gives $N = 9{,}447$.

The eventual study of 12,772 patients reported no 'deaths attributed to pioglitazone'.

Table 6.2 and Equation 6.8

Example 6.6 Background rate known – Several event types - Gastric cancer
Suppose that a possible side effect of a new drug, D, when given to patients with a particular condition is an increased incidence of gastric cancer. In an elderly population, it is presumed that the annual incidence of gastric cancer is 1%, and D will be deemed unacceptable if this increases to 1.5%. What size of study is required? Also of concern is a possible increase in cardiovascular events of much the same magnitude as the possible increased incidence of gastric cancer. How would this affect the sample size?

If the investigators are prepared to discount any result that states that D actually prevents gastric cancer, then this is a 1-sided test at, say, $\alpha = 0.05$. Furthermore, if the required power to detect this increase is $1 - \beta = 0.9$, then with $\lambda_{Back} = 0.01$ and $\varepsilon_{Plan} = 0.005$ equation (6.8) gives

$$N = \frac{\left[1.6449\sqrt{0.01} + 1.2816\sqrt{0.01 + 0.005} \right]^2}{0.005^2} = 4{,}133.3.$$ Thus the study requires approximately 4,200

subjects who are taking D. The calculations using $^S S_S$ give $N = 4{,}134$ as does **Table 6.2**.

If cardiovascular events were also to be monitored, then $s = 2$ and the study team might set $\alpha/2 = 0.025$, in place of 0.05 in the above calculations. Calculations using $^S S_S$ then give $N = 4{,}984$, which is an increase of 850 subjects so clearly a larger study is suggested. Similarly, if $s = 3$ event types were to be monitored then $\alpha/3 = 0.0167$ and $N = 5{,}467$.

Equations 6.2 and 6.9

Example 6.7 Background rate unknown - Very low rates – Osteoarthritis and rheumatoid arthritis
In a randomised trial conducted by Silverstein, Faich, Goldstein, *et al* (2000) celecoxib (C) was compared with non-steroidal anti-inflammatory drugs ($NSAID$) for osteoarthritis and rheumatoid arthritis. The annualised incidence rates of upper GI ulcer complications alone and combined with symptomatic ulcers were 0.76% with C and 1.45% with $NSAID$. If this comparison is to be repeated in a prospective but non-randomised post-marketing surveillance study, what size of study might be contemplated?

Assuming a 1-sided $\alpha = 0.05$, as one would only wish to show that upper GI complications are reduced with C, and power $1 - \beta = 0.8$, then with planning values $\lambda_C = 0.0076$ and $\lambda_{NSAID} = 0.0145$, equation (6.2) gives $PU = 5{,}740$ or a post-marketing study of approximately $N = 6{,}000$ patients, with 3,000 in each study arm.

Since the rates λ_C and λ_{NSAID} are relatively small, hence $\varepsilon_{Plan} = 0.0069$ is also small, it may be prudent for the investigators to use the more precise methods of sample size calculation given by equation (6.9) with $k = 1$, in which case $^S S_S$ gives $N = 5{,}676$, although this too suggests recruiting approximately 6,000 patients.

Table 6.3 and Equations 6.9 and 6.10

Example 6.8 Background rate unknown - Gastric cancer

If the investigators of *Example 6.6* did not know the annual incidence of gastric cancer with D but were prepared also to monitor for gastric cancer incidence a comparable control population (C) of equal size but who have not been prescribed the drug in question, how many subjects should be monitored in each group?

With $\lambda_C = 0.01$ and $\varepsilon_{Plan} = 0.005$, equation (6.10) gives $\bar{\lambda} = \dfrac{\left[0.01 + 1 \times (0.01 + 0.005)\right]}{1+1} = 0.0125$. For $k = 1$, 1-sided $\alpha = 0.05$, $1 - \beta = 0.9$, equation (6.9) gives the number of units required as $n_T =$

$$\left(\frac{1+1}{1}\right) \frac{\left\{1.6449\sqrt{(1+1)\times 0.0125 \times 0.9875} + 1.2816\sqrt{1 \times 0.01 \times 0.99 + (0.01 + 0.005)(1 - 0.01 - 0.005)}\right\}^2}{0.005^2}$$

$= 8{,}455.5$ or $8{,}456$. This is close to the corresponding entry in **Table 6.3** and $_SS_S$ of $n_T = 8{,}455$. As equal numbers per group are anticipated, $n_C = n_T = 8{,}455$ and the total number of subjects required is $N \approx 17{,}000$.

It should be emphasised that, although the actual incidence for C is unknown, the planning team has to provide its anticipated value in order to estimate the required number of patients. Patient numbers are quite sensitive to this value. Thus, if $\lambda_C = 0.005$ replaces 0.01, the number of subjects in each group for the same test size and power is substantially lowered to $n_C = n_T = 5{,}098$ or approximately $N = 10{,}000$ subjects in total.

Suppose the investigators planning this study have access to an appropriate cancer registry as a source for controls who are not receiving the drug under investigation. This would enable many more controls than patients receiving the drug of interest to be monitored for gastric cancer. What effect does this have on the number of patients required?

Again with 1-sided $\alpha = 0.05$, $1 - \beta = 0.90$, $\lambda_{CPlan} = 0.01$ and $\varepsilon_{Plan} = 0.005$, but now $k = 5$, **Table 6.3** suggests recruiting $n_T = 4{,}968$ patients to receive the drug and $n_C = 5 \times 4{,}968 = 24{,}840$ controls to be obtained from the registry. Thus, this suggests a study of $N = 4{,}968 + 24{,}840 = 29{,}808$ or approximately $30{,}000$ individuals.

Table 6.4 and Equations 6.11 and 6.12

Example 6.9 Matched-case-control - New analgesic

It is postulated that a relatively new analgesic (A) may be associated with a particular type of adverse reaction. To investigate if indeed this is so, a matched-case-control study is planned in which it is important to detect a possible relative risk of 1.2 by the use of A as compared to those that have been in current use (C). It is anticipated that the adverse event has a prevalence of 0.05 amongst users of C. How many cases, that is, those receiving A, experiencing the adverse reaction ought the investigators to recruit?

Here $\lambda_C = 0.05$ and the relative risk, $RR_{Plan} = \lambda_A / \lambda_C = 1.2$, then the anticipated prevalence with A is $\lambda_A = 1.2 \times 0.05 = 0.06$. From this we have $\varepsilon_{Plan} = \lambda_A - \lambda_C = 0.01$. If $m = 1$ is assumed, then each unit comprises two matched individuals—one A and one C.

With the planning values specified, equation (6.12) gives $\Omega = \dfrac{0.05 + 0.01}{1 + 0.01} = 0.0594$ and

$\Pi = \dfrac{0.05}{1+1}\left(1 + \dfrac{0.0594}{0.05}\right) = 0.0547$. Then with $m = 1$, 1-sided $\alpha = 0.05$ and $1 - \beta = 0.8$, equation (6.11) gives

$$U = \frac{1}{1 \times (0.05 - 0.0594)^2} \left\{ 1.6449 \sqrt{(1+1) \times 0.0547 \times 0.9453} + 0.8416 \sqrt{(0.05 \times 0.95) + (1 \times 0.0594 \times 0.9406)} \right\}^2$$

$= 7{,}235.9$ matched pairs.

As $m = 1$, the $n_A = 7{,}236$ individuals using A are pair-matched with $n_C = 1 \times 7{,}236$ individuals using C. This implies a total study size of $N = 15{,}000$ subjects. **Table 6.4** and $^S\!S_S$ with $m = 1$ give a similar value of $U = 7{,}227$.

On the other hand, if $m = 5$, then each unit comprises one A individual matched to five having used C. In this situation, $^S\!S_S$ gives $U = 4{,}257$ and therefore implies fewer subjects receiving A need to be included. However, although n_A ($= 4{,}257$) is now reduced, a far larger C group is required as $n_C = 5 \times 4{,}257 = 21{,}285$. Such a study would involve $N = 4{,}257 + 21{,}285 = 25{,}542$ individuals.

References

Technical

Brooker S, Bethony J, Rodrigues L, Alexander N, Geiger S and Hotez P (2005). Epidemiological, immunological and practical considerations in developing and evaluating a human hookworm vaccine. *Expert Review of Vaccines*, **4**, 35–50.

Edwardes MD (2001). Sample size requirements for case-control study designs. *BMC Medical Research Methodology*, **1**, 11.

Hanley JA and Lippman-Hand A (1983). If nothing goes wrong, is everything alright? *Journal of the American Medical Association*, **259**, 1743–1745.

Keene ON, Jones MRK, Lane PW and Anderson J (2007). Analysis of exacerbation rates in asthma and chronic obstructive pulmonary disease: example from the TRISTAN study. *Pharmaceutical Statistics*, **6**, 89–97.

Lewis JA (1981). Post-marketing surveillance: how many patients? *Trends in Pharmacological Sciences*, **2**, 93–94.

Lewis JA (1983). Clinical trials: statistical developments of practical benefit to the Pharmaceutical Industry. *Journal of the Royal Statistical Society* (A), **146**, 362–393.

Pandis N and Machin D (2012). Sample calculations for comparing rates. *American Journal of Orthodontics and Dentofacial Orthopedics*, **142**, 565–567.

Smith PG and Morrow R (1996). *Field Trials of Health Interventions in Developing Countries: A Toolbox.* Macmillan, London

Strom BL (2013). Sample size considerations for pharmacoepidemiology studies. In Strom BL, Kimmel SE and Hennessy S (eds) *Pharmacoepidemiology*, (5th edn) Wiley, Chichester.

Tubert-Bitter P, Begaud B, Moride Y and Abenhaim L (1994). Sample size calculations for single group post-marketing cohort studies. *Journal of Clinical Epidemiology*, **47**, 435–439.

Zu H and Lakkis H (2014). Sample size calculation for comparing two negative binomial rates. *Statistics in Medicine*, **33**, 376–387.

Examples

Baron-Cohen S, Scott FJ, Allison C, Williams J, Bolton P, Matthews FE and Brayne C (2009). Prevalence of autism-spectrum conditions: UK school-based population study. *British Journal of Psychiatry*, **194**, 500–509.

Chong S-A, Tay JAM, Subramaniam M, Pek E and Machin D (2009). Mortality rates among patients with schizophrenia and tardive dyskinesia. *Journal of Clinical Psychopharmacology*, **29**, 5–8.

Kasliwal R, Wilton LV and Shakir SAW (2008). Monitoring the safety of pioglitazone. *Drug Safety*, **31**, 839–850.

Lie S-FDJ, Ozcam M, Verkerke GJ, Sandham A and Dijkstra PU (2008). Survival of flexible, braided, bonded stainless steel retainers: a historic cohort study. *American Journal of Orthodontics and Dentofacial Orthopedics*, **30**, 199–204.

Silverstein FE, Faich G, Goldstein JL, Simon LS, Piincus T, Whelton A, Makuch R, Eisen G, Agrawal NM, Stenson WF, Burr AM, Zhao WW, Kent JD, Lefkowith JB, Verburg KM and Geis GS (2000). Gastrointestinal toxicity with celecoxib vs nonsteroidal anti-inflammatory drugs for osteoarthritis and rheumatoid arthritis. *Journal of the American Medical Association*, **284**, 1247–1255.

Table 6.1 Sample size, *N*, required to observe a total of *a* or more adverse events with a given probability $1 - \gamma$ and anticipated incidence λ_{Plan} [Equation 6.6].

λ_{Plan}	*a*	Probability $1 - \gamma$				
		0.5	0.8	0.9	0.95	0.99
0.0001	1	6,932	16,095	23,026	29,958	46,052
	2	16,784	29,944	38,898	47,439	66,384
	3	26,741	42,791	53,224	62,958	84,060
	4	36,721	55,151	66,808	77,537	100,452
	5	46,710	67,210	79,936	91,536	116,047
0.0005	1	1,387	3,219	4,606	5,992	9,211
	2	3,357	5,989	7,780	9,488	13,277
	3	5,349	8,559	10,645	12,592	16,812
	4	7,345	11,031	13,362	15,508	20,091
	5	9,342	13,442	15,988	18,308	23,210
0.001	1	694	1,610	2,303	2,996	4,606
	2	1,679	2,995	3,890	4,744	6,639
	3	2,675	4,280	5,323	6,296	8,406
	4	3,673	5,516	6,681	7,754	10,046
	5	4,671	6,721	7,994	9,154	11,605
0.005	1	139	322	461	600	922
	2	336	599	778	949	1,328
	3	535	856	1,065	1,260	1,682
	4	735	1,104	1,337	1,551	2,010
	5	935	1,345	1,599	1,831	2,321
0.01	1	70	161	231	300	461
	2	168	300	389	475	664
	3	268	428	533	630	841
	4	368	552	669	776	1,005
	5	468	673	800	916	1,161

Table 6.2 Sample size, *N*, required for detection of a specific increase in adverse reactions, ε_{Plan}, with background incidence, λ_{Back}, known [Equation 6.8].

λ_{Back}	1-sided $\alpha = 0.05$; Power $1 - \beta = 0.8$							
	Additional incidence, ε_{Plan}							
	0.001	0.0025	0.005	0.01	0.025	0.05	0.075	0.1
0.0025	17,433	3,216	963	311	79	31	18	13
0.005	32,943	5,728	1,608	482	110	40	23	16
0.0075	48,419	8,217	2,239	645	139	48	27	18
0.01	63,886	10,699	2,864	804	166	55	30	20
0.025	156,644	25,555	6,589	1,744	322	97	50	32
0.05	311,214	50,291	12,778	3,295	573	161	79	49
0.075	311,214	75,024	18,962	4,842	822	224	108	65
0.1	620,345	99,755	25,146	6,389	1.070	287	136	81

λ_{Back}	1-sided $\alpha = 0.05$; Power $1 - \beta = 0.9$							
	Additional incidence, ε_{Plan}							
	0.001	0.0025	0.005	0.01	0.025	0.05	0.075	0.1
0.0025	24,984	4,782	1,494	509	140	57	35	25
0.005	46,474	8,267	2,391	747	184	70	41	29
0.0075	67,914	11,717	3,266	974	224	81	47	32
0.01	89,339	15,156	4,134	1,196	262	92	52	35
0.025	217,826	35,736	9,295	2,499	479	150	79	51
0.05	431,933	70,001	17,868	4,648	827	240	120	75
0.075	646,032	104,260	26,435	6,792	1,172	327	160	98
0.1	860,130	138,517	35,001	8,934	1,516	414	199	120

Table 6.3 Sample size, n_T, required for the *Test* group to detect a specific additional adverse reaction rate, ε_{Plan}, over an unknown background incidence, λ_{PlanC}, for the *Control* group [Equation 6.9]. Each cell gives the number of subjects required in the *Test* group, n_T. Hence, the total sample size for the study is $N = (k+1)n_T$.

| | | 1-sided $\alpha=0.05$; Power $1-\beta=0.8$ | | | | |
| | | Planned Ratio $k=n_C/n_T$ | | | | |
λ_{CPlan}	ε_{Plan}	1	2	3	4	5
0.005	0.001	67634	50221	44,410	41,502	39,757
0.01	0.001	128,470	95,858	84,984	79,546	76,282
	0.005	6,105	4,477	3,931	3,657	3,492
0.05	0.005	24,603	18,362	16,281	15,240	14,615
	0.01	6,426	4,774	4,223	3,947	3,781
0.1	0.005	45,500	34,045	30,227	28,317	27,171
	0.01	11,620	8,675	7,693	7,202	6,907
	0.05	540	398	350	325	311
0.15	0.005	63,924	47,873	42,523	39,848	38,242
	0.01	16,195	12,111	10,750	10,069	9,661
	0.05	714	528	467	436	417
	0.1	197	145	127	118	113

| | | 1-sided $\alpha=0.05$; Power $1-\beta=0.9$ | | | | |
| | | Planned Ratio $k=n_C/n_T$ | | | | |
λ_{CPlan}	ε_{Plan}	1	2	3	4	5
0.005	0.001	93,683	69,983	62,073	58,115	55,738
0.01	0.001	177,951	133,195	118,271	110,807	106,328
	0.005	8,455	6,283	5,554	5,188	4,968
0.05	0.005	34,078	25,510	22,652	21,224	20,366
	0.01	8,901	6,651	5,899	5,524	5,298
0.1	0.005	63,024	47,225	41,958	39,325	37,745
	0.01	16,094	12,049	10,700	10,026	9,621
	0.05	748	556	492	460	441
0.15	0.005	88,545	66,371	58,980	55,284	53,066
	0.01	22,432	16,805	14,929	13,991	13,428
	0.05	988	737	653	611	586
	0.1	273	203	179	167	160

Table 6.4 Number of units, U, comprising 1 case to m controls, to be observed in a matched-case-control study [Equation 6.11].
Each cell gives the number of units required, U. Hence, the number of cases, $n_{Cases} = U$ while the number of controls, $n_{Controls} = mU$. The total sample size for the study is $N = n_{Cases} + n_{Controls}$.

$\lambda_{Control}$	ε_{Plan}	1-sided $\alpha = 0.05$; Power $1 - \beta = 0.80$				
		Number of controls per case, m				
		1	2	3	4	5
0.005	0.001	68,415	50,804	44,927	41,986	40,220
0.01	0.001	131,273	97,955	86,845	81,289	77,955
	0.005	6,273	4,601	4,041	3,760	3,591
0.05	0.005	27,466	20,504	18,183	17,022	16,325
	0.01	7,227	5,372	4,753	4,443	4,257
0.1	0.005	56,608	42,367	37,619	35,246	33,821
	0.01	14,567	10,880	9,651	9,036	8,667
	0.05	718	529	466	434	415
0.15	0.005	89,178	66,801	59,342	55,612	53,374
	0.01	22,770	17,036	15,125	14,169	13,595
	0.05	1,066	791	699	653	625
	0.1	316	233	205	191	183

$\lambda_{Control}$	ε_{Plan}	1-sided $\alpha = 0.05$; Power $1 - \beta = 0.90$				
		Number of controls per case, m				
		1	2	3	4	5
0.005	0.001	94,765	70,793	62,792	58,788	56,385
0.01	0.001	181,833	136,104	120,855	113,229	108,653
	0.005	8,688	6,457	5,708	5,332	5,106
0.05	0.005	38,045	28,482	25,293	23,698	22,741
	0.01	10,010	7,481	6,637	6,214	5,961
0.1	0.005	78,411	58,760	52,209	48,934	46,968
	0.01	20,176	15,108	13,418	12,573	12,066
	0.05	993	740	655	612	587
0.15	0.005	123,525	92,600	82,291	77,136	74,044
	0.01	31,540	23,632	20,996	19,678	18,887
	0.05	1,475	1,102	977	915	877
	0.1	438	326	288	269	258

7

Survival Time Outcomes

SUMMARY

This chapter describes methods for calculating sample sizes for studies in which the outcome of primary concern is assessed by the period between a specific time-point and the subsequent occurrence of a particular event. In general the time-interval to the event is termed the 'survival time'. For example, in a study of post-operative wound healing, the time-point would be the 'date of the operation' while the event would be the 'healed' wound and the period between them is the 'healing time'. When comparing groups, the ratio of the instantaneous event rates in the two groups, termed the hazard ratio (*HR*), is used to describe the relative outcome measure. The null hypothesis of *HR* = 1 is often tested by the Logrank test or using Cox proportional hazards regression.

In some situations such as, for example, when death is the 'event', then a death, when it occurs, may be attributed to one of many possible causes. Thus all the potential causes of death 'compete' with each to be the actual cause of the eventual fatality. Competing risks studies seek to quantify the contributions of the 'specific' causes to the overall mortality. Sample size methods for comparative studies concerned with competing risks' endpoints are also included in this chapter.

7.1   Introduction

There are many investigations in which individual subjects from two particular groups are identified for a clinical study and, once included, are then followed over time until they experience a predefined critical event. The length of this period for each subject is then used to compare the two interventions.

If the endpoint of interest is a death, then the 'survival time' may be the actual duration of time from the date of recruitment to a clinical trial until the date of death of a cancer patient, or, if the occurrence of any Methicillin-resistant *Staphylococcus aureus* (MRSA) infections is being monitored in a hospital, then the time from hospital admission to contracting the infection will be recorded as the 'infection-free survival time'. However, in this latter example, events are expected to be rare and most patients are likely to be discharged without experiencing the 'event'.

For subjects in whom the single 'event-of-interest' occurs while the study is in progress, their actual survival time, t, is observed. In those for whom the event has not (yet) occurred, their duration in the study is noted and recorded. However as the event has not occurred, these duration times are termed 'censored' and denoted as, t^+.

It should be emphasised that it is not essential in survival time studies that all patients are followed until the critical event occurs. For example, in many cancer clinical trials with time to death as the endpoint, some patients will live for many years post randomisation. Thus observation of their deaths

Sample Sizes for Clinical, Laboratory and Epidemiology Studies, Fourth Edition. David Machin, Michael J. Campbell, Say Beng Tan and Sze Huey Tan.
© 2018 John Wiley & Sons Ltd. Published 2018 by John Wiley & Sons Ltd.

and hence recording of the corresponding dates would not be possible in a reasonable time-frame. One option in such circumstances is for the investigators to fix a (calendar) date beyond which no further information is to be collected so that all patients surviving beyond this date will provide censored survival times. Similarly, only those patients who contract MRSA infection will have an actual infection-free survival time while for the remainder the time from hospital admission to discharge will provide a censored observation.

The consequence of having such censored observations is that the focus is to determine the necessary number of subjects, N, in order to guarantee that the requisite number of events, E, are observed. This in turn implies that a study might, instead of fixing a date for closure, recruit the N subjects and then wait until the required E events are observed before conducting the analysis and reporting of the results. In a study without censored survival times, N will equal E but such a situation will not often arise.

The eventual analysis of these data, which involves either t or t^+ for every subject, will involve calculating the Kaplan-Meier (K-M) estimates of the survival curves for each group. Statistical comparisons between the groups can be made using the Logrank test or, now more commonly, Cox proportional hazards regression. These essentially test the null hypothesis of equal death (often from any cause) rates in, for example, two interventions *Standard* (*S*) and *Test* (*T*) that are to be compared in a randomised controlled trial. The corresponding summary statistic used is the hazard ratio (*HR*).

In other situations, there may be several types of events to consider. Perhaps, rather than death from any cause being the (compound) event, the individual causes of death are of interest. In which case, each cause will compete with every other possible cause to be the one that ultimately brings about the demise. The individual possible causes are termed the competing risks (CR). In comparative studies, methods for accounting for CRs use either the cause-specific hazard ratio (*csHR*) associated with the K-M approach or the sub-distribution hazard ratio (*subHR*) which is associated with the *CuMulative Incidence method* (*CMI*).

7.2   Events of a Single Type

Exponential Survival Times

Suppose the single event of interest is death from any cause and that two interventions, S and T, give rise to survival distributions with constant but possibly different instantaneous death rates, λ_S and λ_T. The instantaneous death rate is the probability of death in a unit of time, and is often called the hazard. In certain situations, it is possible to postulate an Exponential distribution for the distribution of survival times. In which case, from equation (1.15), the survivor function for the intervention S with a hazard rate, λ_S, at time, t, is

$$S_S(t) = exp(-\lambda_S t),$$

(7.1)

with $\lambda_S > 0$ and $t \geq 0$.

The relationships between the hazard rate, λ_S, the proportion alive, $\pi_S(\tau)$, at a fixed point of time, τ, and the median survival time, M_S, can be summarised by

$$\lambda_S = \frac{-log\pi_S(\tau)}{\tau} = \frac{-log0.5}{M_S}.$$

(7.2)

There are analogous expressions for the intervention group T.

Hazard ratio

The ratio of the risks in the S and T groups is the HR with possible values ranging from 0 to ∞ and which can be expressed in the following ways:

$$HR = \frac{\lambda_T}{\lambda_S} = \frac{log\pi_T}{log\pi_S} = \frac{M_S}{M_T}. \tag{7.3}$$

As we are concerned with the Exponential distribution of survival times, the value of the ratio $log\pi_T/log\pi_S$ remains the same irrespective of the time chosen so that component '(τ)' of equation (7.2) is omitted from this expression. Note also that it is M_S (not M_T) which is in the numerator of equation (7.3).

When $\lambda_S > \lambda_T$ then $HR < 1$, and when $\lambda_S < \lambda_T$ then $HR > 1$. The test of the null hypothesis of equality of event rates for the interventions with respect to the endpoint concerned is expressed by H_0: $HR = 1$.

In planning a comparative study, the investigators will need to provide planning values of λ_S and λ_T, or π_S and π_T, or M_S and M_T and then use (7.3) to obtain an anticipated HR_{Plan}. However, equation (7.3) can be rearranged to give, for example,

$$\pi_T = exp\left(HR \times log\pi_S\right), \tag{7.4}$$

so that if planning values for π_S and HR are provided, then the corresponding planning value of π_T can be determined.

Proportional Hazards

As we have shown in equation (7.3), when comparing two interventions in which the corresponding survival times have Exponential distributions with different but constant hazards, the HR remains the same at whatever point in time, τ, is considered. This property is termed Proportional Hazards (PH).

PH can apply even if the respective death rates in the two groups fluctuate over time, provided their ratio remains unchanged. In which case

$$HR = \frac{\lambda_T(t)}{\lambda_S(t)}. \tag{7.5}$$

Thus, although the respective hazards in the numerator and denominator may change with time, their ratio and hence the HR itself does not.

Number of Events

When comparing two interventions with a survival-time endpoint, the results are usually summarised graphically by the K-M survival curves and the corresponding HR quoted. As we have indicated, one statistical test used to compare the groups is the Logrank test.

If we assume that patients are to be entered into a clinical trial and randomised to receive one of two interventions in the ratio 1:φ with anticipated HR_{Plan}, 2-sided test size α, and power $1 - \beta$ then two approximations have been derived for the total number of events, E, to be observed. These are

$$E_{Sch} = \frac{\left(1+\varphi\right)^2}{\varphi} \frac{\left(z_{1-\alpha/2} + z_{1-\beta}\right)^2}{\left(logHR_{Plan}\right)^2}, \tag{7.6}$$

and

$$E_F = \left(\frac{1}{\varphi}\right)\left[\frac{1+\varphi HR_{Plan}}{1-HR_{Plan}}\right]^2 \left(z_{1-\alpha/2} + z_{1-\beta}\right)^2. \tag{7.7}$$

Values for $z_{1-\alpha/2}$ and $z_{1-\beta}$ can be obtained from **Table 1.2**.

Table 7.1 compares E_{Sch} of equation (7.6) with E_F of (7.7) and shows that the latter method requires more events to be observed. Consequently **Table 7.2** uses equation (7.7) to give the number of events required for combinations of the anticipated proportions surviving at a given time point in the two groups.

Number of Subjects

Equations (7.6) and (7.7) contain the 'effect size' as expressed by the single summary HR_{Plan} and these lead directly to the total number of events required, E. However, in order to calculate the number of subjects needed, it is necessary to specify anticipated values for π_S and π_T. As these will in general both change with time, the values selected for planning will be chosen at a convenient follow-up time by the investigators. For example, for the S intervention the published literature may provide information on the median survival time, M_S, from which automatically $\pi_S(M_S) = 0.5$. Since HR_{Plan} has previously been specified when calculating E, use of equation (7.4) leads to a corresponding planning value for π_T.

The total number of subjects required is

$$N = \frac{E}{\Psi_{Plan}} \text{ where } \Psi_{Plan} = \frac{(1-\pi_S)+\varphi(1-\pi_T)}{1+\varphi}. \tag{7.8}$$

Here Ψ_{Plan} is the anticipated proportion of subjects likely to experience the failure event in the trial. The corresponding number of subjects in each intervention are then $n_S = N/(1+\varphi)$ and $n_T = N\varphi/(1+\varphi)$ respectively.

Table 7.3 gives the corresponding numbers of subjects required with the number of events, E, first having been calculated using equation (7.7). Both **Table 7.2** and **7.3** indicate how sensitive E, and consequently the number of subjects required, N, are to the planning values set by the investigating team.

Study Duration

The reliability of a 'time-to-event' study depends on the total number of events, E, that are eventually observed. For these studies there is clearly a period of accrual, a, during which subjects are recruited and some events will occur. Once recruitment is closed there is usually a further period of follow-up, f, in which time more events are accumulated. The duration of the trial is therefore, $D = a + f$. It is implicit in these studies that all who are recruited will eventually fail although the study team may not observe some of the failures as the trial will need to be reported before they all occur. For example, in many cancer clinical trials, 'death' may be the failure of concern but the investigators will wish to report their results before the demise of the longer-term survivors.

In order to observe the pre-specified number of events, E, the investigating team has a number of options to consider which will include the availability of patients and the anticipated (median) time to failure. They can, for example, plan to make (i) a as short as possible but have an extensive f, or (ii) have longer a to allow more recruits but short f, or (iii) achieve a balance between a and f to minimise the total duration, D.

The approach taken depends on the availability of subjects for the study, the event rate in the control arm and practical considerations, such as the costs of accrual and follow-up. For example, in rare diseases N will clearly be small so extending f is likely to be desirable. However, the shortest duration of a study occurs when all patients are entered for the period 0 to a after which time there is no further follow-up accumulated hence $f = 0$. In which case $D = a$.

7.3 Competing Risks

In certain types of study, there may be many alternative causes leading to the event of concern. For example, suppose a study is conducted of workers at a nuclear installation who are exposed to the risk of dying from leukaemia, which is the *main* risk. However, they may also die from *competing risks (CR)* such as a different cancer, accident, cardiovascular disease, diabetes, and so on and therefore cannot die from leukaemia. These causes can be regarded as all competing within each individual to be responsible for the ultimate death. Thus, in a sense, we can think of these causes all racing to be the first and hence to be '*the*' cause of the actual death and thereby preventing the '*other*' causes from being responsible. This implies that if the death is caused by a cardiovascular accident (*CVA*), then t_{CVA} is observed while, for example, $t_{Leukaemia}$, $t_{OtherCancer}$, $t_{Accident}$ and $t_{Diabetes}$ will never be observed but have the corresponding censored survival times $t_{Leukaemia}^+$, $t_{OtherCancer}^+$, $t_{Accident}^+$, and $t_{Diabetes}^+$ that are all censored at a time equal to t_{CVA}.

Once a study is concluded there are two approaches to the summary. One uses the K-M approach to estimate the survival curves, the other the *CuMulative Incidence (CMI)* method. Details are given by, for example, Tai and Machin (2014, Chapters 6 and 10).

In the following description we generally assume that events of only two types, A and B, are competing.

Cause-Specific

Cause-specific hazard ratio (*csHR*)
For a *specific* cause of death, say A, the K-M estimate of the proportion alive at a convenient time can be used to derive the associated hazard, λ^A. Essentially this regards a death from the *other* cause B at t_B, as providing a censored survival time for A as $t_A^+ = t_B$. It then views these B events in the same way as censored observations of A which arise if patients are still alive or are lost to follow-up at the time of analysis. When comparing S and T with respect to the event A, the corresponding hazard ratio (now denoted *csHR*) is

$$csHR_A = \frac{\lambda_T^A}{\lambda_S^A} \tag{7.9}$$

If published values for CMI_S^A and CMI_S^B are available at a *given* time-point, a planning value for the rate with S may be derived from

$$\lambda_S^A = CMI_S^A \times \frac{-log\left[1 - CMI_S^A - CMI_S^B\right]}{t\left[CMI_S^A + CMI_S^B\right]}, \tag{7.10}$$

and similarly for T. Should a third event, C, be of interest, then the term CMI_S^C will be subtracted within [.] in the numerator and added to the denominator.

Here $csHR_A$ of equation (7.9) is assumed to remain constant over time corresponding to a PH situation and further the rather stringent assumption is made that the interventions S and T have no effect on the competing risk, B.

Sample-size

When considering the number of events required when using $csHR_A$ as the effect size, equation (7.7) can be used directly to obtain csE^A. However, to obtain the total sample size for events of type A to be anticipated now includes considerations of the competing event, B. This implies modifying the expression Ψ_{Plan} of equation (7.8). First considering intervention S, we define

$$\Psi_{Plan,S}^A = \frac{\lambda_S^A}{\left(\lambda_S^A + \lambda_S^B\right)} \times \left\{1 - \frac{exp\left[-\left(\lambda_S^A + \lambda_S^B\right)f\right] - exp\left[-\left(\lambda_S^A + \lambda_S^B\right)\times(f+a)\right]}{\left(\lambda_S^A + \lambda_S^B\right)a}\right\}, \tag{7.11}$$

where λ_S^A and λ_S^B denote the respective anticipated hazards of events A and B within intervention S. There is a corresponding expression for $\Psi_{Plan,T}^A$. As defined earlier, a is the planned recruitment duration, and f is a further period of follow-up. Combining the results from equation (7.11) for S and T, we have

$$\Psi_{Plan}^A = \frac{\Psi_{Plan,S}^A + \varphi\Psi_{Plan,T}^A}{1+\varphi}. \tag{7.12}$$

Finally, the total number of subjects to be recruited is given by

$$csN^A = \frac{csE^A}{\Psi_{Plan}^A}. \tag{7.13}$$

The corresponding number of subjects in each intervention is then $csn_S^A = csN^A/(1+\varphi)$ and $csn_T^A = csN^A\varphi/(1+\varphi)$ respectively.

Sub-Distribution

Sub-distribution Hazard Ratio (*subHR*)

In the presence of *CRs*, the *CuMulative Incidence* (*CMI*) method estimates the cumulative probability for each cause of failure, in the presence of all risks acting on the subjects concerned. Then if A, as opposed to the competing event B, is the main event of concern, the sub-distribution *HR* for comparing S and T is defined as

$$subHR_A = \frac{log\left[1-CMI_T^A\right]}{log\left[1-CMI_S^A\right]}, \tag{7.14}$$

when values for CMI_T^A and CMI_S^A are available at a *given* time-point. Alternatively when a planning value of CMI_T^A is not available but λ_S^A is, then assuming Exponential distributions for the event times,

$$CMI_S^A(t) = 1 - exp\left(-\lambda_S^A t\right). \tag{7.15}$$

In a similar way, a planning value for $CMI_T^A(t)$ can be obtained if λ_T^A is provided.

Sample size

To calculate the sample size required, the number of events, $subE_A$, is obtained from equation (7.7) but now using the planning value $subHR_{Plan}$. Before equation (7.13) can then be used to obtain the total sample size, $subN^A$, it is first necessary to provide a value for Ψ_{Plan}^A.

If the anticipated proportion of censored observations in the respective intervention groups at a *given* time-point, say c_S and c_T, are provided then

$$\Psi_{Plan,S}^A = \left(1-c_S\right)CMI_S^A \text{ and } \Psi_{Plan,T}^A = \left(1-c_T\right)CMI_T^A. \tag{7.16}$$

Alternatively if a study is planned to have a patient accrual period extending over a units of time with a follow-up of f further units then, provided appropriate values of CMI_S^A are available at key times, the proportion of A failures in intervention S can be estimated by

$$\Psi_{Plan,S}^A = \frac{1}{6}\left[CMI_S^A(f) + 4CMI_S^A(0.5a+f) + CMI_S^A(a+f)\right], \tag{7.17}$$

with a similar expression for $\Psi_{Plan,T}^A$. This implies that the investigators need to first specify a and f for the study as a whole and then provide planning values for CMI for each intervention group at three time points.

In circumstances when one value of $CMI(t)$ is known then, assuming an Exponential distribution of survival times, the corresponding λ can be estimated by solving equation (7.15). Once obtained then, for given a and f, values of $CMI(f)$, $CMI(0.5a+f)$ and $CMI(a+f)$ can be obtained from the same equation.

Once $\Psi_{Plan,S}^A$ and $\Psi_{Plan,T}^A$ are calculated, equation (7.12) is used to obtain the pooled value, Ψ_{Plan}^A. Finally, Ψ_{Plan}^A and $subE^A$ are used in equation (7.13) to obtain $subN^A$.

7.4 Subject Withdrawals

One aspect of a survival time study that will affect the number of subjects recruited is the anticipated proportion of those who are subsequently lost to follow-up. Since these subjects are lost, we will never observe and record the date of the critical event, even though it may have occurred. These subjects have censored observations in the same way as those for whom the event of interest has still not occurred by the time of analysis of the study. Such lost subjects however do not, and will never, contribute events for the analysis and, therefore, we need to compensate for their loss.

If the anticipated loss or withdrawal proportion is w ($100w\%$), then the required number of patients, N, derived from any of the preceding situations should be increased to

$$N_{Adjusted} = \frac{N}{1-w} \text{ or } N(1+w). \qquad (7.18)$$

Note that two options for $N_{Adjusted}$ are given here but, provided w is not too large, they are numerically similar. However, this is only a guideline so either option can be used but the one chosen should be specified in the study protocol and in the final report.

An appropriate value for w can often be obtained from reports of previous studies conducted by others. If there is no such information at hand, then a pragmatic value may be to take $w = 0.1$. We are assuming that the loss to follow-up is occurring at random and is not related to the current (perhaps health) status of the subject concerned.

7.5 Bibliography

Theory, formula and tables corresponding to equation (7.6) when $\varphi = 1$ are given by George and Desu (1974) while Schoenfeld (1983) modifies the formula to account for unequal allocation. Equation (7.7) was derived by Freedman (1982). In general, this latter expression leads to slightly larger sample sizes and so is recommended. George and Desu (1974) show that the shortest duration of a study occurs when all patients are entered for a fixed period after which time no further follow-up is accumulated.

When considering CRs, Latouche, Porcher and Chevret (2004) define the *subHR* of equation (7.14) while Pintilie (2002) gives equations (7.10) and (7.11). The method of accounting for patient recruitment rates and follow-up of equations (7.16) and (7.17) are given by Latouche and Porcher (2007). Wolbers, Koller, Stel, *et al* (2014) give, in the context of cardiology studies, a tutorial contrasting the respective roles of the cause-specific and the *CMI* functions while Tai, Chen and Machin (2015) describe their particular impact on the estimation of sample sizes.

7.6 Examples

Table 1.2
For two-sided test size, $\alpha = 0.05$, $z_{0.975} = 1.96$. For one-sided $1 - \beta = 0.8$ and 0.9, $z_{0.8} = 0.8416$ and $z_{0.9} = 1.2816$.

Table 7.1 and Equations 7.3 and 7.7

Example 7.1 Equal allocation - Number of events required – Advanced renal carcinoma
The randomised, double-blind, Placebo (P) controlled trial of Everolimus (EV) conducted by Motzer, Escudier, Oudard, *et al* (2008) in patients with advanced renal carcinoma assumed a planning value for the median progression-free survival with P as $M_P = 3.0$ months. They anticipated that a clinically meaningful improvement with EV would be $M_{EV} = 4.5$ months. How many events would be required if equal allocation is anticipated, the power is set at 90%, and with a 5% 2-sided test size?

From (7.3), $HR_{Plan} = M_P/M_{EV} = 3.0/4.5 = 0.6667$. In addition, with 2-sided $\alpha = 0.05$, power $1 - \beta = 0.9$ and $\varphi = 1$, equation (7.7) gives $E_F = \left(\dfrac{1}{1}\right)\left[\dfrac{1 + (1 \times 0.6667)}{1 - 0.6667}\right]^2 (1.96 + 1.2816)^2 = 262.76$ or 263. This can be implemented in $^S\!S_S$ by setting the proportion progression-free with P at the median as $\pi_P = 0.5$. **Table 7.1** with Δ set as $1/HR_{Plan} = 1/0.6667 \approx 1.5$ gives the same number of events.

Tables 7.1, 7.2 and 7.3 and Equations 7.4, 7.7 and 7.8

Example 7.2   Equal allocation - Type 2 diabetes mellitus
Zinman, Harris, Neuman, *et al* (2010) conducted a double-blind randomised trial comparing a combination of Rosiglitazone and Metformin (*RM*) with Placebo (*P*) in patients with impaired glucose tolerance with the objective of prevention of subsequent type 2 diabetes mellitus. In planning their trial, they postulated that the median time to develop diabetes in the control group would be $M_P = 6.25$ years and the extra delay with *RM* would result in a $HR_{Plan} = 0.545$. They further assumed a 2-sided $\alpha = 0.05$ and $1 - \beta = 0.8$.

Use of equation (7.7), with $\varphi = 1$, gives $E_F = \dfrac{1}{1}\left[\dfrac{1 + 0.545}{1 - 0.545}\right]^2 (1.96 + 0.8416)^2 = 90.50$ or 91 patients to be observed who develop diabetes. Further $\pi_P = 0.5$ implies from equation (7.4) that $\pi_{RM} = \exp(0.545 \times \log 0.5) = 0.685$. Hence, from equation (7.8) the anticipated trial size is

$$N = \dfrac{(1+1) \times 91}{[(1 - 0.5) + (1 - 0.685)]} = 223.42 \text{ or } 224 \quad \text{patients with impaired glucose tolerance. Thus}$$

$n_P = n_{EM} = 224/2 = 112$ would be randomised to each intervention.

The eventual trial results of Zinman, Harris, Neuman, *et al* (2010, Figure 2) concerned 207 patients, in whom 41 developed diabetes with *P* and 14 with *RM*, and yielded a $HR = 0.31$. The observed median time to develop diabetes in those receiving *P* was approximately 4 years, which was quite different from the value assumed at the planning stage. Had these values been used at the planning stage, then while $\pi_P = 0.5$ we have $\pi_{RM} = \exp(0.31 \times \log 0.5) = 0.807$. Using 2-sided $\alpha = 0.05$ and $1 - \beta = 0.8$, $^S\!S_S$ gives $E_F = 30$ events and $N = 88$ patients, suggesting that a much smaller trial would have been initiated.

These results can be essentially verified using **Table 7.1** with $HR = 1/0.31 = 3.22$, which is midway between the tabular entries of 3.0 and 3.5. Hence, using the Freedman column with a power of 80%, $E_F = (32 + 26)/2 = 29$. The Schoenfeld column entries all suggest fewer events are required. Here $E_{Sch} = (27 + 21)/2 = 24$. As a consequence, we have adopted a conservative approach in **Tables 7.2** and **7.3** and use equation (7.7) for their construction. The number of events required is confirmed by **Table 7.2** with $\pi_1 = 0.5$ and $\pi_2 = 0.8$. Hence $E_F = 30$ while **Table 7.3** suggests $N = 86$ subjects are recruited in order to observe these.

Equations 7.3, 7.4, 7.7 and 7.8

Example 7.3   Unequal allocation – Colorectal surgery
Fiore, Faragher, Bialocerkowski, *et al* (2013) conducted a randomised trial comparing Open (*O*) and Laparoscopic (*L*) colorectal surgery with respect to patient Time for Readiness to be Discharged (TRD). The median TRD for 24 patients with *O* was 6.0 days while for 30 receiving *L* it was 5.0 days. The patients were randomised on a 1:1.25 basis.

How many patients should be recruited to a confirmatory trial assuming $\varphi = 1.25$, 2-sided test 5% and power 90%?

Here $M_O = 6$, $M_L = 5$ and from equation (7.3) $HR_{Plan} = 6/5 = 1.2$, with 2-sided $\alpha = 0.05$, $1 - \beta = 0.9$ and $\varphi = 1.25$, and equation (7.7) gives $E_F = \frac{1}{1.25} \times \left[\frac{1 + (1.25 \times 1.2)}{1 - 1.2} \right]^2 \times (1.96 + 1.2816)^2 = 1,313.50$ or $1,314$.

To obtain the sample size, the corresponding proportions π_O and π_L have to be provided. The median time of 6 days for the control group corresponds to $\pi_O = 0.5$. Thus, from equation (7.4), $\pi_L = \exp(1.2 \times log0.5) = 0.4353$ and use of equation (7.8) with these values gives

$$\Psi_{Plan} = \frac{(1 - 0.5) + 1.25 \times (1 - 0.4353)}{1 + 1.25} = 0.5359, \text{ and } N_F = \frac{1,314}{0.5359} = 2,451.95 \text{ or } 2,452.$$

In order to be randomised in the ratio 1:1.25, the final sample size needs to be divisible by 9 and since $N_F/9 = 2,452/9 = 272.44$, this needs to be increased to 273. Thus $n_O = 273 \times 4 = 1,092$ and $n_L = 273 \times 5 = 1,365$ patients so that the final sample size chosen $N = 1,092 + 1,365 = 2,457$.

Equations 7.3, 7.4, 7.7, 7.8 and 7.18

Example 7.4   Accounting for withdrawals - Advanced squamous cell carcinoma of the lung
Soria, Felip, Cobo, *et al* (2015) conducted an international randomised trial in which 795 adults with stage IIIB or IV squamous cell carcinoma of the lung, who had progressed after at least four cycles of platinum-based chemotherapy, were randomised with 398 to Afatinib (AF) and 397 to Erlotinib (ER). The planning values used for the median overall survivals were $M_{AF} = 8.8$ and $M_{ER} = 7.0$ months respectively. Further, $\varphi = 1$, a 2-sided test of 5% and a power of 80% were stipulated. If it is assumed that there will be a 10% withdrawal of patients beyond the control of the investigator, how does this affect the planned trial size?

Use of equation (7.3) gives $HR_{Plan} = \frac{7.0}{8.8} = 0.7955$. Hence the number of events (here deaths) required to be observed is given from equation (7.7) with $\varphi = 1$, 2-sided $\alpha = 0.05$ and $\beta = 0.2$ as

$$E = \left(\frac{1}{1} \right) \left[\frac{1 + (1 \times 0.7955)}{1 - 0.7955} \right]^2 (1.96 + 0.8416)^2 = 605.06 \text{ or } 606.$$

In order to calculate the required number of patients to observe these events, planning values for the proportion of patients anticipated to be alive at $M_{ER} = 7.0$ months are required. For ER this is $\pi_{ER} = 0.5$, and from equation (7.4), $\pi_{AF} = \exp(0.7955 \times log0.5) = 0.5761$. Hence, from equation (7.8),

the proportion of patients likely to die is $\Psi_{Plan} = \frac{(1 - 0.5) + 1(1 - 0.5761)}{1 + 1} = 0.4620$. The number of

patients required is therefore $N = \frac{606}{0.4620} = 1311.68$ or approximately 1,300 patients with 650 assigned to each intervention.

Allowing for a withdrawal rate of 10% or $w = 0.1$ and using the first expression in (7.18), we obtain $N_{Adjusted} = 1,300/0.9 = 1,444$. The second expression suggests the smaller number $N_{Adjusted} = 1,300 \times (1 + 0.1) = 1,430$. However, these are only suggestions and both recommend an increase to about 1,400 subjects for this proposed trial.

After the trial was conducted, the observed median survival rates of $M_{AF} = 7.9$ and $M_{ER} = 6.8$ months reported by Soria, Felip, Cobo, *et al* (2015) were lower, in each group, than had been anticipated.

Were these to be used as planning values for a confirmatory trial, $HR_{Plan} = \dfrac{6.8}{7.9} = 0.8608$. Then, with the same test size and power, the number of deaths required $\boxed{^SS_S}$ is, $E = 1,404$. Further with $\pi_{ER} = 0.5$ but now $\pi_{AF} = exp(0.8608 \times log0.5) = 0.5506$, the number of patients required becomes $N = 2,958$ or 3,000.

Equations 7.3, 7.7 and 7.8

Example 7.5   Unequal allocation - Stroke

Chen, Venketasubramanian, Lee, *et al* (2013) reported the number of vascular events (a composite of several event types including non-fatal recurrent stroke and death as two of these) occurring in 1,099 stroke patients in the first 90 days following a double-blind randomisation to Placebo (*P*) or a traditional Chinese medicine (*MLC601*). The individual times to the vascular events were recorded should they occur within the 90 days. For those who did not experience an event, their survival was censored at that time-point. A $HR = 0.51$ (95% CI 0.28 to 0.93) in favour of *MLC601* was reported. The K-M estimates of the event-free survival at 90 days were approximately 95% and 97.5% respectively (see their figure, page 3581). As can be confirmed using this sample size and result, this is consistent with setting a 2-sided $\alpha = 0.05, \beta = 0.2, \varphi = 1$ assuming $\pi_P = 0.94, \pi_{MLC601} = 0.975$ and $\delta_{Plan} = 0.975 - 0.94 = 0.035$ or 3.5%. The corresponding number of events anticipated with this plan is $E = 45$ and the investigators' report is based on 47.

Suppose a repeat trial is planned in patients with more advanced disease who are likely to experience more vascular events and so only 90% are now anticipated to be event free over the 90 days. Also, it is planned to allocate patients on a 2:3 basis in favour of *MLC601*. If we again assume 2-sided $\alpha = 0.05, \beta = 0.2$ and $\delta_{Plan} = 0.035$ but a reduced $\pi_P = 0.90$, then with these planning values and $\varphi = 1.5$, use of equations (7.3), (7.7) and (7.8) or $\boxed{^SS_S}$ gives $E = 154, N = 1,950$ and consequently $n_P = 780$ and $n_{MLC601} = 1,179$. Compared to $\varphi = 1$, when $E = 162$ and $N = 1,964$, the unequal allocation design results in a very similar sized trial. Both options suggest a trial about twice the size of that conducted by Chen, Venketasubramanian, Lee, *et al* (2013) would be required.

Equations 7.6, 7.10, 7.11, 7.12, 7.13, 7.15 and 7.17

Example 7.6   Competing risks – Infants with brain tumours

In a study described by Grundy, Wilne, Weston, *et al* (2007), the primary objective of giving chemotherapy to infants younger than 3 years with intracranial ependymoma was to avoid or delay the use of radiotherapy (RT) at such a young age. Following treatment, the infants were subsequently classified into one of four groups: (*A*) receive RT following progression; (*B*) have a progression but no RT, or die without documentation of progression; (*C*) receive (elective) RT without documentation of progression; and (*D*) continue to be alive without progression and without RT. *A*, *B* and *C* represent competing events, whereas the patient 'survival times' within group *D* are censored for all events. Some results of this study are presented by Tai, Grundy and Machin (2011) and are summarised in **Figure 7.1**.

Suppose a randomised trial is planned comparing surgical resection with adjuvant chemotherapy (*S-C*) and surgery alone (*S*) for infants with brain tumours with the purpose to determine which best delays or avoids RT. The design team uses the information of **Figure 7.1** for planning purposes and assumes a 1:1 allocation, a 2-sided test size of 5% and a power of 80%. They also specify that the

Competing event	Number of infants	CMI (5)	Histology Ependymoma (89) v Other (90)	
			csHR	subHR
A: Recurrence, hence RT	69	40%	0.63	1.21
B: Recurrence, no RT	60	30%	0.26	0.44
C: Elective RT	9	5%	0.14	0.20
D: No recurrence and alive	41	$c = 25\%$		
All events	179	100%		

Figure 7.1 Infants receiving chemotherapy for their brain tumour: Number experiencing differing events, with the corresponding 5-year *CMI* rates, and competing risk hazard ratios, *csHR* and *subHR*, comparing those with Ependymoma histology with those of Other malignant brain tumours (after Tai, Grundy and Machin, 2011).

event B is of major concern, and wish to compare the sub-distribution and cause-specific approaches to estimating the HR for comparing the treatment groups.

Subdistribution Approach

The investigators assume for event B that $CMI_B(5) = 0.3$, $c = 0.25$ and that use of S-C, as opposed to S, leads to the $subHR_{Plan} = 0.44$ of **Figure 7.1**. They then use equation (7.6) with $\varphi = 1$, 2-sided $\alpha = 0.05$ and $1 - \beta = 0.8$, to obtain the number of events required as $E^B_{sub} = \dfrac{(1+1)^2}{1} \dfrac{(1.96 + 0.8416)^2}{(log 0.44)^2} = 46.58$ or 47.

If $CMI_B(5) = 0.3$ is assumed as the average value for both S and C-S then, using one component of equation (7.16), $\Psi^B_{Plan} \sim (1-c) \times CMI_B(5) = 0.75 \times 0.3 = 0.225$. Hence, from (7.13), the number of infants required is $SubN^B = \dfrac{E^B_{sub}}{\Psi^B_{Plan}} = \dfrac{47}{0.225} = 209$ or $n_S = n_{S-C} = 105$ per treatment group.

Alternatively, if recruitment is planned to be for $a = 2$ years with $f = 3$ subsequent years of follow-up, then equation (7.15) can be solved with $a + f = 5$ to obtain an average value for $\lambda^B = -log\left[1 - CMI_B(5)\right]/5 = 0.0713$. Hence equation (7.15) can be used again to provide estimates of $CMI_B(f) = 0.1927$ and $CMI_B(0.5a + f) = 0.2482$. The with $CMI_B(5) = 0.3$, use of equation (7.17) gives $\Psi^B_{Plan} = [0.1927 + (4 \times 0.2482) + 0.3]/6 = 0.2476$. Finally from (7.13), the number of infants required is $SubN^B = \dfrac{E^B_{sub}}{\Psi^B_{Plan}} = \dfrac{47}{0.2476} = 189.82 \approx 190$ which is quite close to the 209 obtained earlier.

Cause-specific approach

The investigators now assume that use of C-S, as opposed to S, leads to the $csHR_{Plan} = 0.26$ of **Figure 7.1**. Equation (7.6) now gives $E^B_{cs} = \dfrac{(1+1)^2}{1} \dfrac{(1.96 + 0.8416)^2}{(log 0.26)^2} = 17.30$ or 18. Further, the investigators also specify $a = 2$ and $f = 3$, giving $D = 5$ years. The planning value for the cause-specific hazard is obtained from an extension of equation (7.10) to allow for the three CRs A, B and C and uses the *CMI* values of **Figure 7.1**. Hence

$$\lambda^B_S = CMI^B_S \times \frac{-log\left[1 - CMI^A_S - CMI^B_S - CMI^C_S\right]}{t\left[CMI^A_S + CMI^B_S + CMI^C_S\right]} = 0.3 \times \frac{-log\left[1 - 0.4 - 0.3 - 0.05\right]}{5\left[0.4 + 0.3 + 0.05\right]} = 0.3 \times 0.3697 = 0.1109.$$

Similarly, $\lambda_S^A = 0.4 \times 0.3697 = 0.1479$ and $\lambda_S^C = 0.05 \times 0.3697 = 0.0185$. These are summed to give $\lambda S = 0.1479 + 0.1109 + 0.0185 = 0.2773$. Thus, the anticipated proportion of events of type B is, from equation (7.11), $\Psi_{Plan,S}^B = \dfrac{0.1109}{0.2773} \times \left\{ 1 - \dfrac{exp[-0.2773 \times 3] - exp[-0.2773 \times 5]}{0.2773 \times 2} \right\} = 0.2664$. If the same value is assumed for $\Psi_{Plan,C-S}^B$ then equation (7.12) implies $\Psi_{Plan}^B = 0.2664$ also. This is then used in equation (7.13) to give $N_{cs}^B = \dfrac{E_{cs}^B}{\Psi_{Plan}^B} = \dfrac{18}{0.2664} = 67.58$ or $n_S = n_{S-C} = 34$ per treatment group. Alternatively, direct use of $\boxed{{}^S S_S}$ gives $N_{cs}^B = 68$.

Equations 7.6, 7.8, 7.10. 7.11, 7.12 and 7.16

Example 7.7   Competing risks – Advanced non-metastatic nasopharyngeal cancer
Tai, Wee and Machin (2011) present in **Figure 7.2** *csHR* and *subHR*, and the corresponding 95% CIs obtained from a trial of patients with advanced non-metastatic nasopharyngeal cancer randomised to receive either radiotherapy alone (*RT*) or RT with adjuvant chemotherapy (*ChemoRT*). When the competing event considered is distant metastases (*M*), there is a strong indication of a benefit for the use of *ChemoRT*. The estimated $csHR^M$ and $subHR^M$ both equal 0.43 with the corresponding CIs excluding the null hypothesis value $HR_0 = 1$. In contrast, for loco-regional recurrence (*R*) the $csHR^R = 0.84$ and $subHR^R = 0.91$ differ. However, neither CI excludes the possibility of $HR_0 = 1$.

Suppose a confirmatory randomised trial is planned and the design team uses the information of **Figure 7.2** but chooses a 1:1.5 allocation in favour of *ChemoRT*, a 2-sided test size of 5% and a power of 90%.

Subdistribution approach
The investigators assume event M is of principal importance and set a planning value from **Figure 7.2** of $subHR_{Plan}^M = 0.43$. They then use equation (7.6) with $\varphi = 1.5$, 2-sided $\alpha = 0.05$ and $1 - \beta = 0.9$, to obtain the number of events required as $E_{sub}^M = \dfrac{(1+1.5)^2}{1.5} \dfrac{(1.96+1.2816)^2}{(log\,0.43)^2} = 61.46$ or 62.

Competing event	CMI(5)				
	RT	ChemoRT		Cause-Specific	Sub-distribution
M: Distant metastases	0.45	0.20	HR	0.43	0.43
			95% CI	0.24 – 0.75	0.25 – 0.76
R: Loco-regional recurrence	0.12	0.12	HR	0.84	0.91
			95% CI	0.34 – 2.08	0.37 – 2.24
Censored rates	0.43	0.68			
Total	1.00	1.00			

Figure 7.2 Cause-specific and subdistribution *HRs* for the competing risks of distant metastases and local recurrence in patients with advanced non-metastatic nasopharyngeal cancer from a randomised trial comparing radiotherapy alone (*RT*) and RT with adjuvant chemotherapy (*ChemoRT*) (after Tai, Wee, Machin, 2011, Table 3).

If, from **Figure 7.2**, the censoring proportions for *RT* and *ChemoRT* are set as $c_{RT} = 0.43$ and $c_{ChemoRT} = 0.68$ and $CMI_{RT}^{M}(5) = 0.45$ and $CMI_{ChemoRT}^{M}(5) = 0.20$, then equation (7.16) gives $\Psi_{RT}^{M} = (1 - c_{RT})CMI_{S}^{M}(5) = 0.57 \times 0.45 = 0.2565$. Similarly, $\Psi_{ChemoRT}^{M} = 0.32 \times 0.20 = 0.064$. Combining these as in equation (7.12) gives $\Psi_{Plan}^{M} = \dfrac{0.2565 + (1.5 \times 0.064)}{1 + 1.5} = 0.1410$. Then from equa-

tion (7.8) the total number of patients required is $N_{sub}^{M} = \dfrac{E_{sub}^{M}}{\Psi_{Plan}^{M}} = 62/0.1410 = 439.72$ or 440. As $\varphi = 1.5$ the required numbers in each group becomes $n_{RT} = 176$ and $n_{ChemoRT} = 264$ respectively.

In contrast, if event *R* is considered as the main event, then with $subHR_{Plan}^{R} = 0.91$ equation (7.7) now gives $E_{sub}^{R} = \dfrac{(1+1.5)^{2}}{1.5} \dfrac{(1.96 + 1.2816)^{2}}{(log0.91)^{2}} = 4{,}922.57$, which would imply a prohibitively large trial.

Cause-specific approach

The investigators again assume that use of *ChemoRT*, as opposed to *RT*, leads to the $csHR^{M} = 0.43$ of **Figure 7.2**, which is the same magnitude as $subHR^{M}$ and hence leads to the same number of events required, namely $E_{cs}^{M} = 62$.

Further, the investigators specify an accrual duration, $a = 4$, and additional follow-up, $f = 1$, giving a total duration $D = 5$ years. The planning value for the cause-specific hazard is obtained from equation (7.10) and uses the *CMI* values at $t = 5$ years of **Figure 7.2**. Hence

$$\lambda_{RT}^{M} = CMI_{RT}^{M} \times \frac{-log\left[1 - CMI_{RT}^{M} - CMI_{RT}^{R}\right]}{t\left[CMI_{RT}^{M} + CMI_{RT}^{R}\right]} = 0.45 \times \frac{-log\left[1 - 0.45 - 0.12\right]}{5\left[0.45 + 0.12\right]} = 0.45 \times 0.2961 = 0.1333 \cdot$$

Similarly, $\lambda_{RT}^{R} = 0.12 \times 0.2961 = 0.0355$. These are summed to give $\lambda_{RT} = 0.1333 + 0.0355 = 0.1688$. Thus, the anticipated proportion of events of type *M* is, from equation (7.11),

$$\Psi_{Plan,RT}^{M} = \frac{0.1333}{0.1688} \times \left\{1 - \frac{exp[-0.1688 \times 1] - exp[-0.1688 \times 5]}{0.1688 \times 4}\right\} = 0.3046.$$ The corresponding values for

ChemoRT are $\lambda_{ChemoRT}^{M} = 0.0482$, $\lambda_{ChemoRT}^{R} = 0.0289$, $\lambda_{ChemoRT} = 0.0771$ and $\Psi_{Plan,ChemoRT}^{M} = 0.1271$. Thus, from equation (7.12), $\Psi_{Plan}^{M} = [0.3046 + (1.5 \times 0.1271)]/(1 + 1.5) = 0.1981$.

The final sample size is from equation (7.8), $N_{cs}^{M} = \dfrac{E_{sc}^{M}}{\Psi_{Plan}^{M}} = 62/0.1981 = 312.97$. As $\varphi = 1.5$ then, if

312.97 is rounded up to 315, the required numbers in each group are $n_{RT} = 126$ and $n_{ChemoRT} = 189$.

In this example, the subdistribution approach leads to a larger sample size than that for the cause-specific approach.

References

Technical

Freedman LS (1982). Tables of the number of patients required in clinical trials using the logrank test. *Statistics in Medicine*, **1**, 121–129.

George SL and Desu MM (1974). Planning the size and duration of a clinical trial studying the time to some critical event. *Journal of Chronic Diseases*, **27**, 15–24.

Latouche A, Porcher R and Chevret S (2004). Sample size formula for proportional hazards modelling of competing risks. *Statistics in Medicine*, **23**, 3263–3274.

Latouche A and Porcher R (2007). Sample size calculations in the presence of competing risks. *Statistics in Medicine*, **26**, 5370–5380.

Pintilie M (2002). Dealing with competing risks: testing covariates and calculating sample size. *Statistics in Medicine*, **21**, 3317–3324.

Schoenfeld DA (1983). Sample-size formula for the proportional hazards regression model. *Biometrics*, **39**, 499–503.

Tai BC, Chen ZJ and Machin D (2018). Estimating sample size in the presence of competing risks – Cause-specific hazard or cumulative incidence approach? *Statistical Methods in Medical Research*, **27**, 114–125.

Tai BC, Grundy R and Machin D (2011). On the importance of accounting for competing risks in paediatric brain cancer: II. Regression modeling and sample size. *International Journal of Radiation Oncology, Biology and Physics*, **79**, 1139–1146.

Tai B-C and Machin D (2014). *Regression Methods for Medical Research*. Wiley Blackwell, Chichester.

Wolbers M, Koller MT, Stel VS, Schaer B, Jager KJ, Leffondré K and Heinze G (2014). Competing risks analyses: objectives and approaches. *European Heart Journal*, **35**, 2936–2941.

Examples

Chen CLH, Venketasubramanian N, Lee C-F, Wong L and Bousser M-G (2013). Effects of ML601 on early vascular events in patients after stroke: The CHIMES study. *Stroke*, **44**, 3580–3583.

Fiore JF, Faragher IG, Bialocerkowski A, Browning L and Denchy L (2013). Time for readiness for discharge is a valid and reliable measure of short-term recovery after colorectal surgery. *World Journal of Surgery*, **37**, 2927–2934.

Grundy RG, Wilne SA, Weston CL, Robinson K, Lashford LS, Ironside J, Cox T, Chong WK, Campbell RHA, Bailey CC, Gattamaneni R, Picton S, Thorpe N, Mallucci C, English MW, Punt JAG, Walker DA, Ellison DW and Machin D (2007). Primary postoperative chemotherapy without radiotherapy for intracranial ependymoma in children: the UKCCSG / SIOP prospective study. *Lancet Oncology*, **8**, 696–705.

Motzer RJ, Escudier B, Oudard S, Hutson TE, Porta C, Bracardo S, Grünwald V, Thompson JA, Figlin RA, Hollaender N, Urbanowitz G, Berg WJ, Kay A, Lebwohl D and Ravaud A (2008). Efficacy of everolimus in advanced renal cell carcinoma: a double-blind, randomised, placebo-controlled phase III trial. *Lancet*, **372**, 449–456.

Soria J-C, Felip E, Cobo M, Lu S, Syrigos K, Lee KH, Goker E, Georgoulias V, Li W, Isla D, Guclu SZ, Morabito A, Min YJ, Ardizonni A, Gadgeel SM, Wang B, Chand VK, and Goss GD (2015). Afatinib versus erlotinib as second-line treatment of patients with advanced squamous cell carcinoma of the lung (LUX-Lung 8): an open-label randomised controlled phase 3 trial. *Lancet Oncology*, **16**, 897–907.

Tai B-C, Wee J and Machin D (2011). Analysis and design of randomised clinical trials involving competing risks endpoints. *Trials*, **12**, 127.

Zinman B, Harris SB, Neuman J, Gerstein HC, Retnakaran RR, Raboubd J, Qi Y and Hanley AJG (2010). Low-dose combination therapy with rosiglitazone and metformin to prevent type 2 diabetes mellitus (CANOE trial): a double-blind randomised controlled study. *Lancet*, **376**, 103–111.

Table 7.1 Number of critical events for comparison of two survival distributions compared when the hazards remain proportional (PH) over time [Equations 7.6 and 7.7]. Each cell gives the total number of events for the comparison of two interventions. If $HR_{Plan} < 1$ enter the table using the reciprocal, $1/HR_{Plan}$.

	2-sided $\alpha = 0.05$			
	Power $1 - \beta$			
	0.8		0.9	
HR	Schoenfeld Equation (7.6)	Freedman Equation (7.7)	Schoenfeld Equation (7.6)	Freedman Equation (7.7)
1.1	3,457	3,462	4,627	4,634
1.2	945	950	1,265	1,272
1.3	457	462	611	618
1.4	278	283	372	379
1.5	191	197	256	263
1.6	143	148	191	198
1.7	112	117	150	157
1.8	91	97	122	129
1.9	77	82	103	110
2.0	66	71	88	95
2.1	58	63	77	84
2.2	51	56	68	75
2.3	46	51	61	68
2.4	41	47	55	62
2.5	38	43	51	58
2.6	35	40	47	54
2.7	32	38	43	50
2.8	30	35	40	47
2.9	28	34	38	45
3.0	27	32	35	43
3.5	21	26	27	35
4.0	17	22	22	30
4.5	14	20	19	26
5.0	13	18	17	24

Table 7.2 Total number of critical events, E, required with subjects allocated equally to the two intervention groups [Equation 7.7].

π_2	2-sided $\alpha=0.05$; Power $1-\beta=0.8$							
	π_1							
	0.1	0.2	0.3	0.4	0.5	0.6	0.7	0.8
0.15	843	–	–	–	–	–	–	–
0.2	251	–	–	–	–	–	–	–
0.25	128	1,415	–	–	–	–	–	–
0.3	80	378	–	–	–	–	–	–
0.35	57	178	1,678	–	–	–	–	–
0.4	43	105	427	–	–	–	–	–
0.45	34	70	192	1,664	–	–	–	–
0.5	28	50	109	409	–	–	–	–
0.55	23	38	70	178	1,441			
0.6	20	30	49	98	343	–	–	–
0.65	17	24	36	61	145	1,087	–	–
0.7	15	20	27	41	77	249	–	–
0.75	13	17	21	29	46	101	685	–
0.8	12	14	17	22	30	52	148	–
0.85	12	12	14	17	21	30	57	318
0.9	10	11	12	13	15	27	27	62

π_2	2-sided $\alpha=0.05$; Power $1-\beta=0.9$							
	π_1							
	0.1	0.2	0.3	0.4	0.5	0.6	0.7	0.8
0.15	1,128	–	–	–	–	–	–	–
0.2	335	–	–	–	–	–	–	–
0.25	171	1,894	–	–	–	–	–	–
0.3	108	506	–	–	–	–	–	–
0.35	76	238	2,247	–	–	–	–	–
0.4	57	140	571	–	–	–	–	–
0.45	45	93	257	2,228	–	–	–	–
0.5	37	67	145	547	–	–	–	–
0.55	31	51	93	238	1,928	–	–	–
0.6	26	40	65	131	459	–	–	–
0.65	23	32	47	81	193	1,455	–	–
0.7	20	26	36	55	103	333	–	–
0.75	18	22	28	39	62	135	917	
0.8	16	19	23	29	40	69	199	–
0.85	14	16	19	22	28	40	76	426
0.9	13	14	15	17	20	25	36	82

Table 7.3 Total number of subjects, *N*, required with subjects allocated equally to the two intervention groups [Equations 7.7, 7.8 and combined].

π_2	2-sided $\alpha=0.05$; Power $1-\beta=0.8$							
	π_1							
	0.1	0.2	0.3	0.4	0.5	0.6	0.7	0.8
0.15	964	–	–	–	–	–	–	–
0.2	296	–	–	–	–	–	–	–
0.25	156	1,826	–	–	–	–	–	–
0.3	102	506	–	–	–	–	–	–
0.35	74	246	2,486	–	–	–	–	–
0.4	58	152	658	–	–	–	–	–
0.45	48	104	308	2,894	–	–	–	–
0.5	42	78	182	744	–	–	–	–
0.55	36	62	122	340	3,034	–	–	–
0.6	32	52	90	198	764	–	–	–
0.65	28	42	70	130	342	2,900	–	–
0.7	26	38	54	92	194	712	–	–
0.75	24	34	38	70	124	312	2,492	–
0.8	22	30	38	56	86	174	592	–
0.85	22	26	34	46	66	110	254	1,818
0.9	20	26	30	38	50	136	136	414

π_2	2-sided $\alpha=0.05$; Power $1-\beta=0.9$							
	π_1							
	0.1	0.2	0.3	0.4	0.5	0.6	0.7	0.8
0.15	1,290	–	–	–	–	–	–	–
0.2	396	–	–	–	–	–	–	–
0.25	208	2,444	–	–	–	–	–	–
0.3	136	676	–	–	–	–	–	–
0.35	100	330	3,330	–	–	–	–	–
0.4	78	202	880	–	–	–	–	–
0.45	64	138	412	3,876	–	–	–	–
0.5	54	104	242	996	–	–	–	–
0.55	46	82	162	454	4,060	–	–	–
0.6	42	68	120	264	1,022	–	–	–
0.65	38	56	90	172	456	3,880	–	–
0.7	34	48	72	124	258	952	–	–
0.75	32	42	60	92	166	416	3,336	–
0.8	30	40	52	74	116	232	796	–
0.85	28	34	46	60	88	146	338	2,436
0.9	26	32	38	50	68	100	180	548

8

Paired Binary, Ordered Categorical and Continuous Outcomes

SUMMARY
The purpose of this chapter is to describe methods for calculating sample sizes for studies which yield paired data for the situations where the outcomes are binary, ordered categorical or continuous. Common designs include: comparisons using paired organs, such as eyes of the same individual; before-and-after studies in which a subject may be assessed both before and after an intervention is given; case-control designs in which an individual with a particular disease may be matched to one or more individuals without the disease; randomised, two-period, two-treatment cross-over trials in which each treatment is given in sequential order to every patient; and split-mouth designs in which a tooth in one part of the mouth is compared to one from a different location in the same oral cavity.

8.1 Introduction

Chapters 4, **5** and **6** describe sample-size calculations for the comparison of two groups under the assumption that the data for one group are independent of that of the other. Thus, whatever the results in one group, they would not influence the results obtained from the other and vice-versa. However, a common situation is when the data in the two groups are linked in some way and so the assumption of independence no longer holds. Linked data arise in a number of ways. In a two-treatment, two-period, cross-over trial, both treatments are evaluated in every patient. Thus, two endpoint observations are made for each individual (one following each treatment) to form a pair. In a case-control study design, each case with the disease in question may be matched, for example by age and gender, with a disease-free control to form a pair. In other situations, the same patient may be assessed before and after receiving a particular intervention, while in dental applications two teeth within the same patient may be compared. In these instances, the basic endpoint unit for analysis is a measure of difference between the observations made on the two components of each pair however so defined.

Here, we describe sample-size calculations for the comparison of paired data when these differences have a binary, ordered categorical or continuous form.

8.2 Within and Between Subject Variation

If only one measurement is made per individual, it is then impossible to separate the *within* subject and *between* subjects sources of variation. The *within*-subject variance, σ^2_{Within}, quantifies the anticipated variation among repeated measurements on the *same* individual. It is a compound of the true

Sample Sizes for Clinical, Laboratory and Epidemiology Studies, Fourth Edition. David Machin, Michael J. Campbell, Say Beng Tan and Sze Huey Tan.
© 2018 John Wiley & Sons Ltd. Published 2018 by John Wiley & Sons Ltd.

variation in the individual and any measurement error. The *between*-subject variance, $\sigma^2_{Between}$, quantifies the anticipated variation *between* subjects. In such cases the variance formula summarises a composite of both the *within* and *between* subject sources so that the total variation comprises $\sigma^2_{Total} = \sigma^2_{Between} + \sigma^2_{Within}$. However, use of a paired design eliminates the between subject variation from the comparison so that effectively $\sigma^2_{Total} = \sigma^2_{Within}$ and the total variance is thus reduced. This leads to a more sensitive comparison between groups and hence lower sample sizes than the independent groups (unpaired) designs of **Chapters 3, 4 and 5**.

8.3 Designs

Cross-over Trial

Suppose a cross-over trial is planned in which patients are to be asked whether they obtain relief of symptoms on each of two medications, *Standard* (*S*) and *Test*(*T*). In such a trial half the patients would receive *S* in the first period of the design followed by *T* in the second period (denoted by the sequence *ST*), and the other half would receive the sequence *TS*. In practice the two sequences would be assigned at random to the patients on a 1:1 basis. For expository purposes, we summarise the results of such a trial in the format of **Figure 8.1** and indicate 'Yes' as implying a response or success and 'No' a lack of response or failure.

In **Figure 8.1**, *r* is the number of patients whose response was 'No' with both treatments and *u* is the number whose response is 'Yes' with both treatments. Thus, for example, r/N_{Pairs} estimates π_{00}. In contrast, *s* patients fail to respond to *S* but respond to *T* while *t* patients respond to *S* but fail on *T*. The anticipated proportions of patients who will respond on *S* is π_S, on *T* is π_T, and the anticipated proportion of discordant outcomes is $\pi_{Dis} = \pi_{01} + \pi_{10}$.

Matched Case-control Study

Figure 8.2 illustrates the situation for a paired Case-Control study in which each index *Case* with the disease of interest is matched to a single *Control* of someone without that disease. In this setting the matching variables chosen are potential covariates which, unless accounted for in some way, may

Response to S	Response to T — No	Response to T — Yes	Total	Anticipated proportions
No	$r\ (\pi_{00})$	$s\ (\pi_{10})$	$r + s$	$[1 - \pi_S]$
Yes	$t\ (\pi_{01})$	$u\ (\pi_{11})$	$t + u$	$[\pi_S]$
Total	$r + t$	$s + t$	N_{Pairs}	
Anticipated proportions	$[1 - \pi_T]$	$[\pi_T]$		[1]

Figure 8.1 Notation for a 2 × 2 cross-over trial comparing treatments *S* and *T* for a binary endpoint with associated parameters.

	Control		
Case	Not exposed	Exposed	Total
Not exposed	r	s	$r + s$
Exposed	t	u	$t + u$
Total	$r + t$	$s + t$	N_{Pairs}

Figure 8.2 Notation for a 1 to 1 matched Case-Control study with a binary endpoint.

obscure the true difference between *Case* and *Control*. Once the matching is made, the relevant exposure history to the risk of concern is ascertained so that each Case-Control pair can then be assigned to one of the four categories of **Figure 8.2**.

Before-and-After Design

In a typical 'before-and-after' design, one intervention is under study and an observation is made on each subject *Before* (at baseline, *B*) the intervention is received, and a second observation is recorded *After* (*A*) the intervention is completed. These provide the paired data items. The corresponding difference in these observations measures the effect of the intervention within the individual participants. For a binary endpoint, the results would be summarised in a similar format to **Figure 8.2** but, for example, 'Baseline' measures replacing 'Controls'.

Paired Organs Design

If the organ concerned is the eye, then studies may be concerned with observations taken from each eye. For example, if both eyes have the same condition that requires therapy then a trial may be designed to give intervention (say) *S* to one eye chosen at random and the other then receives *T*. The paired data are then summarised as a difference between the respective assessments of the two eyes post-intervention. Such designs may also be used, for example, to investigate alternative approaches to treating severe burns in different locations on the same patient.

Split-mouth Design

One design used in dental studies is to identify two eligible (perhaps) carious teeth, one on each side of the oral cavity, and consider such studies in a similar manner to the paired-organ situation except that there is the strong likelihood of cross-contamination of the two interventions concerned.

8.4   Binary Data

Mcnemar Test

The binary data arising from the designs of either **Figures 8.1** or **8.2** are often summarised using the odds ratio, $\psi = \pi_{10}/\pi_{01}$, while the corresponding test of significance is McNemar's test.

For illustration we focus on a cross-over trial, where $\psi = s/t$ is a measure of how much more likely it is that a patient will respond 'Yes' with T and 'No' with S as opposed to 'Yes' with S and 'No' with T. We note that the $(r + u)$ patients who respond to both S and T in the same way (that is, they either fail on both treatments or respond to both treatments) do not enter this calculation. This odds-ratio, and the corresponding McNemar test, are termed 'conditional' as they are calculated using only the discordant proportion which is comprised of $\pi_{Dis} = \pi_{10} + \pi_{01}$. Thus, they are 'conditional' on the discordance.

Sample size

For a two-period, two-treatment, cross-over trial, a 1:1 matched case-control study, a before-and-after design and other types of paired design, the number of pairs required, with 2-sided test size α and power $1 - \beta$, is

$$N_{Pairs} = \frac{\left[z_{1-\alpha/2}\left(\psi + 1\right) + z_{1-\beta}\sqrt{\left[\left(\psi + 1\right)^2 - \left(\psi - 1\right)^2 \pi_{Dis}\right]} \right]^2}{\left(\psi - 1\right)^2 \pi_{Dis}}. \tag{8.1}$$

Some sample sizes for this situation are given in **Table 8.1** for a range of values of ψ and π_{Dis}, for a 2-sided $\alpha = 0.05$ and $1 - \beta = 0\,8$ and 0.9.

An alternative approach is to first calculate the number of discordant pairs required by

$$m_{Dis} = \frac{\left[z_{1-\alpha/2}\left(\psi + 1\right) + 2z_{1-\beta}\sqrt{\psi} \right]^2}{\left(\psi - 1\right)^2}. \tag{8.2}$$

When designing a study one could therefore use equation (8.2) to estimate the discordant sample size and then recruit subject-by-subject until m_{Dis} paired observations are made, at which point recruitment stops. The attraction of this method is that the investigator only has to provide a planning value of the effect size, ψ_{Plan}, of interest.

Unfortunately, this strategy implies that the total number of subjects to be recruited is not known in advance. So even though we can base enrolment into a study on the discordant sample size, there still has to be some estimate of the total sample size for planning and budgetary purposes.

Then, with anticipated values of any two of π_{Dis}, π_{01} and ψ, since

$$\pi_{Dis} = \pi_{01}\left(1 + \psi\right), \tag{8.3}$$

the total sample size required is obtained from

$$N_{Pairs} = \frac{m_{Dis}}{\pi_{Dis}}. \tag{8.4}$$

Thus, a combination of equations (8.2) with (8.4) provides an alternative means of determining the number of pairs required. This enables the consequences of changes in planning values for ψ to be directly examined through equation (8.2) and those of changing π_{Dis} with equation (8.4).

Effect size

When designing a study, as $\psi = \pi_{10}/\pi_{01}$, an investigator has to provide planning values for two of ψ, π_{01} and π_{10}.

Alternatively, an investigator may be able to specify planning values for the marginal probabilities of response to S and T, that is π_S and π_T. If they assume that the response to S is *independent* of the response to T in each subject then, from **Figure 8.1**, $\pi_T(1-\pi_S)$ and $\pi_S(1-\pi_T)$ provide estimates for π_{10} and π_{01} respectively. Further, as $\pi_{Dis} = \pi_{10} + \pi_{01}$, this can be estimated by $\pi_T(1-\pi_S) + \pi_S(1-\pi_T)$.

Finally, since $\psi = \pi_{10}/\pi_{01}$, the associated anticipated value is then $\psi_{Marginal} = \dfrac{\pi_T(1-\pi_S)}{\pi_S(1-\pi_T)}$.

Although the independence assumption may not be very likely, $\psi_{Marginal}$ may provide a reasonable basis for ψ_{Plan} in the initial stages of establishing an appropriate sample size.

Cross-over trial

In a two-period, two-treatment cross-over design, it is usual to randomly allocate the sequences ST and TS equally between the participants in the trial. Thus once N_{Pairs} is obtained, it will be rounded up to the nearest even number so that $n_{ST} = n_{TS} = N_{Pairs}/2$ can be allocated to each sequence.

1:C matched case-control design

In some circumstances the number of *Cases* (perhaps of a rare disease) available may be limited to a small number so that, for a given test-size, α, sufficient power cannot be attained with a 1:1 matching. This difficulty may be overcome by the use of multiple *Controls* per *Case*. In this situation, the number of *Cases* is *fixed* but the number of *Controls* per case is *increased* as necessary to achieve the desired power. In practice, there is little statistical benefit in having more than $C = 4$ controls for each case as the *gain* in power diminishes rapidly with each extra control included.

The matched unit, U, comprises a single case together with the corresponding C controls and so consists of $U = (1+C)$ individuals. To determine the number of units required, the study size is first calculated from equations (8.1), or (8.2) with (8.4), which assume one control for each case, to obtain N_{Equal}. The number of units required in a 1:C matching is then given by

$$N_{Units} = \frac{N_{Equal}(1+C)}{2C}. \tag{8.5}$$

Thus, the number of cases required is $n_{Cases} = N_{Units}$ and the number of controls required is $n_{Controls} = Cn_{Cases}$. Finally, the total number of subjects recruited to the study will be $N_{Subjects} = n_{Cases} + n_{Controls}$.

8.5 Ordered Categorical Data

Wilcoxon Signed Rank Test

Ordered categorical data that are paired arise in a number of clinical situations, such as in trials that compare a scored symptom or component of quality of life before and after treatment or a study to compare visual acuity measured before and after surgery. Alternatively, we may have continuous data for which the assumption of a Normal distribution does not hold and so we then regard it as categorical data but with many categories. In either case, the Wilcoxon signed rank test would be the most appropriate statistical test for analysis.

The format of data resulting from such studies extends the number of rows (and columns) of **Figure 8.1** from 2 to κ, where κ represents the number of ordered categories. Observations which then lie along the diagonal of such a $(\kappa \times \kappa)$ contingency table correspond to those whose category has not changed following the intervention, and these do not contribute information for the comparison.

Effect size

To calculate the sample size, it is necessary to specify the distribution of differences, that is, the proportion of subjects that are likely to agree in their own responses or differ (positively and negatively) by one, two and so on categories up to the greatest disagreements (negative and positive) of $\kappa - 1$ categories.

For example, with a 3-point scale the design team may suspect that the new treatment will be an improvement over the control so the difference in pairs will tend to be positive. They then anticipate that, conditional on the overall difference being positive, proportions ξ_2 and ξ_1 of the subjects will improve by $c_2 = +2$ and $c_1 = +1$ categories respectively. Similarly, they anticipate the proportions for $c_0 = 0$, $c_{-1} = -1$ and $c_{-2} = -2$ as ξ_0, ξ_{-1} and ξ_{-2}.

In general, once the $2(\kappa - 1) + 1$ anticipated probabilities ξ_j have been specified, the next step is to calculate the anticipated proportions in each of the $2(\kappa - 1)$ non-zero difference groups, that is, $v_j = \xi_j / (1 - \xi_0)$. From these the planning effect size is

$$\eta_{Plan} = \sum_{j=-(k-1)}^{k-1} v_j c_j \tag{8.6}$$

and the corresponding SD is

$$\sigma_{Dis} = \sqrt{\sum_{j=-(k-1)}^{k-1} v_j c_j^2 - \eta_{Plan}^2} . \tag{8.7}$$

The standardised difference for comparing groups is then defined by

$$\Delta_{Cat} = \frac{\eta_{Plan}}{\sigma_{Dis}} \tag{8.8}$$

Sample size

If the Wilcoxon signed rank sum test is to be used, then the required number of pairs for a 2-sided test size α and power $1 - \beta$, is

$$N_{Pairs} = \frac{2\left(z_{1-\alpha/2} + z_{1-\beta}\right)^2}{\Delta_{Cat}^2} + \frac{z_{1-\alpha/2}^2}{2} . \tag{8.9}$$

Practical note

In practice, if there are too many possible categories, there may be little information on which to base the anticipated values of ξ_j. Nevertheless, published data, collective views of the design team or a pilot study may provide some indications. In such instances a pragmatic approach is to reduce the individual scores in the discordant categories (for a 3 point scales these are −2, −1, 1 and 2) by ignoring their magnitude and merely anticipate a planning value for the likely odds ratio ψ of positives over negatives. In effect, this is returning to the binary situation of **Figure 8.1**.

Once ψ is provided it can be used in equation (8.2) to calculate the discordant sample size, m_{Dis}, and then with a corresponding π_{Dis}, equation (8.4) is used to estimate the total sample size, N_{Pairs}^{Binary}, for this 'binary' variable. However, having in reality several (>2) categories implies a greater potential to have discordance in the two observations made from a single individual. Thus the N_{Pairs}^{Binary} calculated as just described is likely to be a larger sample size than is necessary and so an averaged sample size of $N_{\kappa} = (m_{Dis} + N_{Pairs}^{Binary})/2$ may be a practical compromise.

8.6 Continuous Data

For binary and ordered categorical data, the components required for sample size determination comprise a measure related to the odds ratio and information on the number of discordant observations anticipated. For continuous data the measures to be estimated are the anticipated difference between two means, δ_{Diff}, and the associated SD of that difference, σ_{Diff}. For the design types we consider, the planning value for δ_{Diff} takes the same form. However, although the measures taken from the individuals in the case-control units (although matched) are independent, the two measures in a before-and-after design and a cross-over trial are taken from the same individual and hence cannot be regarded as independent. In these latter situations, the anticipated correlation between two observations needs to be taken into account in the planning value for σ_{Diff}.

When the units of observation are paired, the endpoint observations from the elements x_i and y_i from each unit are linked and the difference between them, $d_i = (x_i - y_i)$, is used as the endpoint for analysis. However, here in the case of a continuous variable, the tabulations similar to **Figures 8.1** and **8.2** cannot be constructed except in the unusual situation when many of the observed differences are tied and there are few such tied values. Tied observations are those that take exactly the same numerical value. Also with a continuous endpoint, although dependent on how accurately the data are recorded, there may be no pairs for which $x_i = y_i$ precisely. In which case, all pairs will be discordant.

Paired *t*-Test

Suppose in a case-control study, cases with a particular disease are matched, perhaps by age and gender, to healthy controls. The endpoint for analysis for pair i is then $d_i = (x_i - y_i)$ where x_i is the continuous observation from the case and y_i is the continuous observation from the control and there are N_{Pairs}.

For the situation of C controls for every case in a matched case-control study, the unit for analysis becomes $d_i = (x_i - \bar{y}_i)$ where $\bar{y}_i$ is the mean of the C continuous observations from the controls of matched group i.

The analysis of such designs involves calculating the mean difference, $\bar{d} = \dfrac{\sum d_i}{N_{Pairs}}$, and the corresponding *SD* of the differences, $s = \sqrt{\dfrac{\sum (d_i - \bar{d})^2}{N_{Pairs} - 1}}$. These allow a paired *t*-test, with degrees of freedom $df = N_{Pairs} - 1$, or in larger studies a z-test, of the null hypothesis of no difference between cases and controls.

Similar considerations apply to other paired designs.

Analysis of Variance (ANOVA)

For a two-treatment, two-period, cross-over design, the paired t-test, with $df = N_{Pairs} - 1$, for comparing the two treatments may be used only if it can be assumed that there is no effect of the Period in which a particular treatment was given. For example, in such a cross-over trial comparing S and T, patients will be randomised in equal numbers, n ($= n_{ST} = n_{TS} = N_{Pairs}/2$), to each of the sequences ST and TS. If no Period effect is present, S given in Period-1 before T in Period-2 will have the same effect as if S is given in Period-2 preceded by T given in Period-1. This similarly applies if T is given first. These assumptions are usually justified by introducing a washout between the two periods of the design during which neither S nor T is given.

Further the treatment effect, δ_{Treat}, is then estimated by the difference, $\bar{d}$, of all observations made on T versus all those made on S, where

$$\bar{d} = \frac{\left(\bar{t}_1 + \bar{t}_2\right)}{2} - \frac{\left(\bar{s}_1 + \bar{s}_2\right)}{2}. \tag{8.10}$$

Here $\bar{t}_1$ and $\bar{t}_2$ are the mean values of those receiving treatment T in Period-1 and Period-2 respectively, each based on n values with similar definitions for $\bar{s}_1$ and $\bar{s}_2$ respectively.

On the other hand, although the effect of treatment is still estimated by equation (8.10), if a Period effect is present then the ANOVA approach to analysis is required to take account of this (see Senn, 2002). Essentially, ANOVA for a cross-over trial partitions the total variation into components due to treatment and period (each with 1 degree of freedom), as well as a within subjects' (residual) term with $df = (N_{Pairs} - 2)$. It is usual to be conservative and assume that a Period effect is present with the associated $df = N_{Pairs} - 2$.

Effect size

The effect size, δ_{Plan}, is the anticipated mean of the paired differences considered in the design.

Standard deviation of the difference (σ_{Diff})

If we consider one individual then, for example, their blood pressure (BP) will vary over time even if the underlying average value remains essentially unchanged over time. An individual measurement may depart from this 'average' level, but were we to take successive readings from the same individual we would hope that the mean of these would estimate the underlying mean level, μ_{BP}. Also their SD estimates the within-subject SD, σ_{Within}, which essentially quantifies the random variation. For design purposes it is assumed that that σ_{Within} will be the same for all subjects included in the corresponding study, although the format of σ_{Diff} will depend on the design chosen.

Sample size

For planning purposes, the anticipated planning values δ_{Plan} and σ_{Plan} are proposed for δ_{Diff} and σ_{Diff} from which the standardised effect size is

$$\Delta_{Cont} = \frac{\delta_{Plan}}{\sigma_{Plan}}. \tag{8.11}$$

The sample size required to detect an anticipated standardised difference Δ_{Cont}, for 2-sided significance level α and power $1 - \beta$, is

$$N_{Pairs} = \frac{2\left(z_{1-\alpha/2} + z_{1-\beta}\right)^2}{\Delta_{Cont}^2} + \frac{z_{1-\alpha/2}^2}{2}. \tag{8.12}$$

For a cross-over trial, if N_{Pairs} determined from (8.12) is an odd number then it will be increased to the next even integer so that equal subject numbers for each sequence are obtained.

For small sample size situations, the first term components $z_{1-\alpha/2}$ and $z_{1-\beta}$ of this expression would be replaced by $t_{df,1-\alpha/2}$ and $t_{df,1-\beta}$ respectively of the t-distribution and the last term omitted. However, this final term corrects for small sample settings and so equation (8.12) gives the required sample size in all situations. Some sample sizes are given in **Table 8.2** for a range of values of Δ and $1 - \beta$ for a 2-sided $\alpha = 0.05$.

Case-control

The subjects recruited to the units of a 1:C matched case-control design are usually assumed as independent of each other even though they are linked. In this case, the SD of a paired difference is

$$\sigma_{Diff} = SD(d_i) = SD\left(x_i - \bar{y}_i\right) = \sqrt{\sigma_{With}^2 + \frac{\sigma_{With}^2}{C}} = \sigma_{With}\sqrt{\left(1 + \frac{1}{C}\right)}. \tag{8.13}$$

In the situation of a 1:1 matched design, $C = 1$ and $\sigma_{Diff} = \sigma_{With}\sqrt{2}$.

Before-and-after, cross-over and other designs

In these situations it is the same individual who is assessed on the two separate occasions and so the resulting observations are not independent. Thus, they are associated to an extent determined by the magnitude of the Pearson correlation coefficient, ρ, between the values of the outcome measure obtained from the component pairs. In this case

$$\sigma_{Diff} = SD(d_i) = SD\left(b_i - a_i\right) = \sqrt{\sigma_{Within}^2 - 2\rho\sigma_{Within}^2 + \sigma_{Within}^2}$$
$$= \sigma_{Within}\sqrt{2(1-\rho)}. \tag{8.14}$$

The correlation could be estimated if, for example, a baseline value was collected and then correlated with the post-intervention values from one of the treatment groups. Thus, if a planning value of σ_{Within} is available and ρ can be anticipated, then together these can provide a planning value, σ_{Plan}, for σ_{Diff}.

Practice

Since σ_{Diff} depends on the choice of ρ in equation (8.14), an exploratory approach to determining the chosen sample size is to try out various values of ρ to see what influence this will have on the proposed sample size.

For example, it is unlikely that ρ would be negative since paired studies are designed to exploit the positive association within pairs. Consequently, if we set $\rho = 0$, then $\sigma_{Diff} = \sigma_{Within}\sqrt{2}$ takes its largest possible value and hence a conservative estimate of the required sample size is obtained. In this worst-case scenario, the sample size for the cross-over trial would be half that of the corresponding (independent) two-group trial obtained from equation (5.4) with $\varphi = 1$. On the other hand, if one could be sure of a positive correlation, then the sample size would be smaller than this.

8.7 Bibliography

Equation (8.1) was derived from Connett, Smith and McHugh (1987, Equation 6), which they compared with the discordant pairs approach of (8.2) and (8.4). They concluded that the approach of (8.1) is 'preferable overall' although the latter provides an adequate approximation provided the power is not too large or π_{Dis} is not close to 0 or 1. The latter approach was also advocated by Lachin (1992, p1250, Point 7). Julious and Campbell (1998, equation (1)) give equation (8.12), which was originally derived by Guenther (1981).

8.8 Examples and Use of the Tables

Table 1.2
For two-sided test size, $\alpha = 0.05$, $z_{0.975} = 1.96$. For one-sided $1 - \beta = 0.8$ and 0.9, $z_{0.80} = 0.8416$ and $z_{0.90} = 1.2816$ respectively.

Table 8.1 and Equation 8.1

Example 8.1 Split mouth - Binary data - Atraumatic dental restorative treatment
Lo, Luo, Fan and Wei (2001) compared in a split-mouth design the clinical performance of two glass-ionomer cements, ChemFlex (C) and Fuji IX GP (F), when used with atraumatic dental restorative

Fuji IX GP (F)	ChemFlex (C)			Total (%)
	Absent	Slight defect or wear	Present and sound	
Absent				8.0
Slight defect or wear		(r)	(s)	16.0
Present and sound		(t)	(u)	76.0
Total (%)	4.0	4.0	92.0	100

Figure 8.3 Results from the split-mouth trial of two glass-ionomer cements used in children with bilateral matched pairs of carious posterior primary teeth (after Lo, Luo, Fan and Wei, 2001, Table 1).

treatment (ART) in 26 children aged between 6 and 14 years with bilateral matched pairs of carious posterior primary teeth. Despite using a paired design, the 2-year follow-up assessments of the ART are presented as in the margins of **Figure 8.3**, although for our purpose, and to comply with the notation of **Figure 8.1**, the 'Absent' and 'Slight defect or wear' groups are merged.

Suppose a repeat trial is planned with the same split-mouth design. How many children with bilateral matched pairs of carious posterior primary teeth are required assuming 2-sided $\alpha = 0.05$, $1 - \beta = 0.80$?

Using the notation of **Figure 8.1**, we have $\pi_C = 0.92$ and $\pi_F = 0.76$. Under the assumption of independence of response for each subject, we therefore anticipate that $\dfrac{s}{N_{Pairs}}$ estimates $\pi_{10} = (1 - \pi_F)$ $\pi_C = 0.24 \times 0.92 = 0.2208$ and $\dfrac{t}{N_{Pairs}}$ estimates $\pi_{01} = (1 - \pi_C)\,\pi_F = 0.08 \times 0.76 = 0.0608$.

Together these give the anticipated $\pi_{Dis} = 0.2208 + 0.0608 = 0.2888$ and $\psi = \pi_{10}/\pi_{01} = 0.2208/0.0608 = 3.63$. Using either equation (8.1) or S_{Ss} with input values $\pi_{Dis} = 0.29$ and $\psi_{Plan} = 3.63$ suggests that $N_{Pairs} = 82$ children with suitable bilateral carious posterior primary teeth would be required.

More realistic planning values of (say) $\pi_{Dis} = 0.3$ and $\psi_{Plan} = 3$ give from **Table 8.1** $N_{Pairs} = 103$ or, if $1 - \beta$ is increased to 0.9, $N_{Pairs} = 136$.

Table 8.1 and Equations 8.1, 8.2 and 8.4

Example 8.2   Case-control - Binary data - Out-of-hours *General Practitioner* consultations
Using 40 case-control pairs, Morrison, Gilmour and Sullivan (1991) wished to identify the reasons why some children less than 10 years old received more out-of-hours visits by general practitioners (GP) than others. The cases were 'high out-of-hours' users and the controls 'not high out-of-hours users' who were matched by age and gender. It was postulated that the marital status (single/divorced or married/cohabiting) of the child's mother might be a determinant of referral. The associated data are summarized in **Figure 8.4**.

The estimated odds ratio of being married/cohabiting in those of 'Low out-of-hours attendance' compared to mothers who are 'High out-of-hours' is $\psi = s/t = 12/1 = 12$, $\pi_{01} = 1/40 = 0.025$, $\pi_{10} = 12/40 = 0.3$, hence $\pi_{Dis} = (12 + 1)/40 = 0.325$.

Suppose a similar study is planned but in GP practices from another geographical area. However, the effect size is anticipated to be close to $\psi = 3$, which is much less than experienced previously. In addition, the research team expects that π_{01} is likely to be larger than for the previous study and sets a planning value for $\pi_{01} = 0.125$. Together these suggest $\pi_{10} = 0.125 \times 3 = 0.375$ and $\pi_{Dis} = 0.5$.

Cases	Controls (Low out-of-hours attendance)		
(High out-of-hours)	Single/divorced	Married/cohabiting	Total
Single/divorced	3 (r)	12 (s)	15
Married/cohabiting	1 (t)	24 (u)	25
Total	4	36	40

Figure 8.4 Case-Control status by whether a child's mother was single/divorced or married/cohabiting (after Morrison, Gilmour and Sullivan, 1991).

From equation (8.1), assuming a 2-sided $\alpha = 0.05$, $1 - \beta = 0.9$ and $\psi_{Plan} = 3$, the number of pairs

$$N_{Pairs} = \frac{\left[1.96 \times (3+1) + 1.2816\sqrt{\left\{(3+1)^2 - (3-1)^2 \times 0.125\right\}}\right]^2}{(3-1)^2 \times 0.125} = 79.82 \text{ or approximately } 80.$$

required is

Utilising either **Table 8.1** with $\psi_{Plan} = 3$ and $\pi_{Dis} = 0.5$ or $\boxed{^{S}S_S}$ with the same input values gives $N_{Pairs} = 80$. The same results would be obtained if $\psi_{Plan} = 1/3$.

Alternatively from equation (8.2), we anticipate that $m_{Dis} = \dfrac{\left[1.96 \times (3+1) + (2 \times 1.2816 \times \sqrt{3})\right]^2}{(3-1)^2} =$

37.70 or 38 discordant pairs are required. The use of equation (8.4) then implies $N_{Pairs} = 38/0.5 = 76$.

Table 8.1 and Equation 8.1

Example 8.3 Case-control - Binary data - Anticipated marginal probabilities - Out-of-hours GP consultations

Suppose the investigators of *Example 8.2* did not have a very clear view of the proportion of discordant pairs but believed that about 90% of controls would be married/cohabiting mothers compared to 70% of cases. How many matched-pairs need to be recruited assuming again 2-sided $\alpha = 0.05$, $1 - \beta = 0.9$?

Using the notation of **Figure 8.1**, we have $\pi_T = 0.9$ and $\pi_S = 0.7$ where T and S now represent *Case* and *Control* respectively. Under the assumption of independence of response for each subject, we therefore anticipate that $\dfrac{s}{N_{Pairs}}$ estimates $\pi_{10} = (1 - \pi_T)\,\pi_S = 0.3 \times 0.9 = 0.27$. Similarly, $\dfrac{t}{N_{Pairs}}$ estimates $\pi_{01} = (1 - \pi_T)\,\pi_S = 0.1 \times 0.7 = 0.07$. Together these give the anticipated $\pi_{Dis} = 0.27 + 0.07 = 0.34$ and $\psi = \pi_{10}/\pi_{01} = 0.27/0.07 = 3.86$. Using either equation (8.1) or $\boxed{^{S}S_S}$ with input values $\pi_{Dis} = 0.34$ and $\psi = 3.86$ gives $N_{Pairs} = 86$.

However, a cautious investigator may also consider a reduced ψ of (say) 3.0 and values of π_{Dis} perhaps ranging from 0.15 to 0.35. These latter options suggest, with **Table 8.1** or $\boxed{^{S}S_S}$, the number of pairs varying from 277 down to 116. Thus, a sensible (compromise) sample size might be $N_{Pairs} = 150$.

Table 8.1 and Equations 8.1 and 8.5

Example 8.4 Multiple matched-controls - Binary data - Out-of-hours GP consultations

Suppose a researcher wished to repeat the results of Morrison, Gilmour and Sullivan (1991) and believed that he would be able to obtain four controls for every case in the study. How does this affect the sample size if we presume that $\pi_{Dis} = 0.5$ and $\psi = 3$?

In this case, use of equation (8.1), **Table 8.1** or $\boxed{^{S}S_S}$ gives $N_{Equal} = 80$ and so with $C = 4$, use of equation (8.5) estimates $N_{Units} = \dfrac{80 \times (1+4)}{2 \times 4} = 50$. This implies that $n_{Cases} = 50$ (1 per unit) and hence $n_{Controls} = C \times n_{Cases} = 4 \times 50 = 200$ (4 per unit). Thus the 50 units of size 5 imply $N_{Total} = 50 + 200 = 250$ children would be involved. If $C = 5$, then $n_{Cases} = 48$, and now $N_{Total} = 6 \times 48 = 288$ children. This implies 2 fewer Cases would need to be identified, but data from 38 more children would have to be obtained.

Table 8.2 and Equations 8.6, 8.7, 8.8 and 8.9

Example 8.5   Case-control - Ordered categorical data - Haemorrhagic stroke

Zodpey, Tiwari and Kulkarni (2000) conducted a case-control study investigating risk factors in 166 hospital based patients with haemorrhagic stroke. The corresponding age and gender matched controls were selected from patients who attended the study hospital for conditions other than cardiovascular and cerebrovascular diseases. Their results with respect to the levels of hypertension in the pairs are summarised in **Figure 8.5** with the numbers in parentheses indicating the score difference, $d = Case - Control$.

Assuming the 2-sided test size is 5% and the power 80%, how many case-control pairs would be required for a repeat of this study?

The calculations necessary to evaluate equations (8.6) and (8.7) are summarised in **Figure 8.6**, from which planning values of $\eta = 1.3550$, $\sum_{j=-3}^{j=+3} v_j c_j^2 = 5.1620$, hence $\sigma_{Dis} = \sqrt{5.1620 - 1.3550^2} = 1.8237$, are obtained. The corresponding standardised effect size of equation (8.8) is $\Delta_{Cat} = \dfrac{1.3550}{1.8237} = 0.7430$. Finally, use of equation (8.9) or $\boxed{S_{S}}$ gives $N_{pairs} = \dfrac{2(1.96 + 0.8416)^2}{0.7544^2} + \dfrac{1.96^2}{2} = 30.36$ or 31 pairs. However, in repeating such a study in practice, it may be prudent to double this number to allow a better possibility of obtaining at least one paired observation in each of the sixteen cells from which **Figure 8.6** is derived. This remains far fewer than the 166 case-control pairs of the initial study.

Alternatively, if we had ignored the ordinal nature of the data and simply taken the ratio of the number of positive differences over the number of negatives in **Figure 8.3**, we would have $\psi = \dfrac{14 + 26 + 32}{4 + 7 + 10} = \dfrac{72}{21} = 3.43$. If we then use this value in equation (8.2), we obtain

Case		Control				
		Normal	Mild	Moderate	Severe	
	Score	0	1	2	3	Total
Normal	0	65 (0)	2 (−1)	3 (−2)	4 (−3)	74
Mild	1	10 (+1)	1 (0)	5 (−1)	4 (−2)	20
Moderate	2	22 (+2)	1 (+1)	2 (0)	3 (−1)	28
Severe	3	32 (+3)	4 (+2)	3 (+1)	5 (0)	44
Total		129	8	13	16	166

Figure 8.5 Reported levels of hypertension present in 166 Case-Control pairs (after Zodpey, Tiwari and Kulkarni, 1999, Table 3).

	Difference in Score (Case – Control)							
c	−3	−2	−1	0	1	2	3	Total
Frequency	4	7	10	73	14	26	32	166
Observed proportions								
	0.0241	0.0422	0.0602	0.4398	0.0843	0.1566	0.1928	1.0000
Discordant proportions								
ξ	0.0430	0.0753	0.1075		0.1505	0.2795	0.3442	1.0000
$\xi \times c$	−0.1290	−0.1506	−0.1075		0.1505	0.5590	1.0326	$\eta = 1.3550$
$\xi \times c^2$	0.3870	0.3012	0.1075		0.1505	1.1180	3.0968	5.1620

Figure 8.6 Distribution of score differences between cases and controls (data from Zodpey, Tiwari and Kulkarni, 1999, Table 3).

$$m_{Dis} = \frac{\left[1.96 \times (3.43+1) + 2 \times 0.8416\sqrt{3.43}\right]^2}{(3.43-1)^2} = 23.58 \quad \text{or} \quad 24.$$ The proportion discordant is $\pi_{Dis} =$ $(72+21)/166 = 0.5602$ and so, from equation (8.4), $N_{Pairs} = 24/0.5602 = 42.84$ or 43. As might be expected, regarding the assessment as binary, rather than of four ordered levels, results in a loss of information and therefore requires a larger sample size for the study.

However, if we regard the 4-point scoring system as providing numerically continuous data and use **Table 8.2**, this gives, for 2-sided $\alpha = 0.05$, $1 - \beta = 0.8$ and $\Delta_{Cat} = 0.75$, $N_{Pairs} = 30$.

Equation 8.12

Example 8.6 Before-and-after design - Continuous date - Whole blood clotting time
Butenas, Cawthern, van't Meer, *et al* (2001) measured the effect of taking aspirin on whole blood clotting time in minutes in 3 subjects. The samples were taken before and after 3 days of aspirin (an anti-platelet drug) at 325 mg twice per day. *Before* aspirin the results were 4.2, 3.1 and 5.1 min and *After* aspirin 3.7, 4.1 and 3.6 min respectively.

The paired differences are 0.5, −1.0 and 1.5 min from which the mean value $\bar{d} = +0.33$ min and their $SD = 1.26$ min are calculated. This gives, using the t-statistic with 2 degrees of freedom, a very wide 95% CI of from −2.80 to +3.46 min. So, after completion of the study, there remains a great deal of uncertainty about the true direction and magnitude of this difference. In their design there are 3 'units', and each 'unit' is formed of the pair of measures from the same individual.

If we were to repeat this study using the values they obtained of $\bar{d} = +0.33$ and $SD = 1.26$ as planning values for δ_{Plan} and σ_{Plan} respectively, then these give $\Delta_{Plan} = 0.33/1.26 \approx 0.25$. Substituting this into equation (8.12) with a 2-sided test size $\alpha = 0.05$ and power $1 - \beta = 0.8$ gives

$$N_{Pairs} = \frac{2(1.96+0.8416)^2}{0.25^2} + \frac{1.96^2}{2} = 253.08 \quad \text{or} \quad 254 \text{ pairs.}$$

However, if we were only interested in establishing whether there is a major decrease in clotting times with the use of aspirin, we might set $\delta_{Plan} = 1$ min, then $\Delta_{Plan} = 1/1.26 \approx 0.8$ and the study size calculations using equation (8.12) lead to $N_{Pairs} = 27$. By any reasonable standards, the choice of only 3 subjects for the study conducted by Butenas, Cawthern, van't Meer, *et al* (2001) was far too small.

Table 8.2 and Equations 8.11, 8.12 and 8.14

Example 8.7   Cross-over trial - Continuous data -Refractory dyspnoea

Abernethy, Currow, Frith, *et al* (2003) conducted a cross-over trial of sustained release morphine (M) against placebo (P) for the management of 38 patients with refractory dyspnoea. They observed that use of M indicated a reduction of 6.6 units (95% CI 1.6 to 11.6) in morning dyspnoea scores as measured by a visual analogue scale. From these results it can be deduced that the SD of the paired differences between M and P scores was approximately 15.73 units. On the basis of these results, a repeat trial is planned and the investigators set $\delta_{Plan} = 6$ and $\sigma_{Plan} = \sigma_{Diff} = 16$ to give, from equation (8.11), $\Delta_{Plan} = 6/16 = 0.375$. Hence, from equation (8.12) with a 2-sided significance level of 5% and 90%

power, $N_{Pairs} = \dfrac{2(1.96 + 1.2816)^2}{(0.375)^2} + \dfrac{1.96^2}{2} = 151.36$. This implies 152 patients are needed as in a cross-

over trial it is presumed that equal numbers are allocated to each sequence. In this case the randomisation would ensure that 76 patients receive treatment in the sequence PM and the same number for MP. Use of **Table 8.2** or S_{Ss} with $\Delta_{Plan} = 0.35$ and 0.40 both give the sample sizes of 174 and 134 respectively.

If we assume that the correlation between successive observations from the same patient is $\rho = 0.7$, then

equation (8.14) implies $\sigma_{Within} = \dfrac{\sigma_{Diff}}{\sqrt{2(1 - \rho)}} = \dfrac{16}{\sqrt{2(1 - 0.7)}} \approx 20$. **Figure 8.7** shows how the value of σ_{Diff}

would change, and the consequent effect on the sample size required, with changing ρ assuming $\sigma_{Within} = 20$. For example, σ_{Diff} reduces dramatically as ρ increases, while N_{Pairs} decreases from more than 450 to less than 10, resulting in very different scenarios that the investigating team would need to consider.

Table 8.2 and Equations 8.11 and 8.12

Example 8.8   Before-and-after - Continuous data - Carnitine deficiency

Cruciani, Dvorkin, Homel, *et al* (2006) gave 27 patients with known carnitine deficiency a 1-week supplementation of L-Carnitine. They measured their baseline (pre-) and post-supplementation carnitine levels. Both measures were taken in all but one patient. On the basis of the difference between the logarithms of these paired measures, the mean log carnitine value was raised over the period by 0.4651 with a standard deviation of 0.4332.

If a repeat Before-and-After study is planned, how many patients would need to be recruited, assuming a 2-sided test size of 5% and a power of 80%?

From the above, the design standardised effect size of equation (8.11) is $\Delta_{Plan} = 0.4651/0.4332 = 1.074 \approx 1$. This is a large effect size by the standards set by Cohen (1988). Using equation (8.12)

directly we obtain $N_{Pairs} = \dfrac{2(1.96 + 0.8416)^2}{1.0^2} + \dfrac{1.96^2}{2} = 17.62$ or 18.

A more cautious investigator may question the magnitude of the assumptions or perhaps wish to recruit patients with less evidence of carnitine deficiency. In which case, scenarios for a range of values for Δ_{Plan} would be investigated.

(a)   (b)

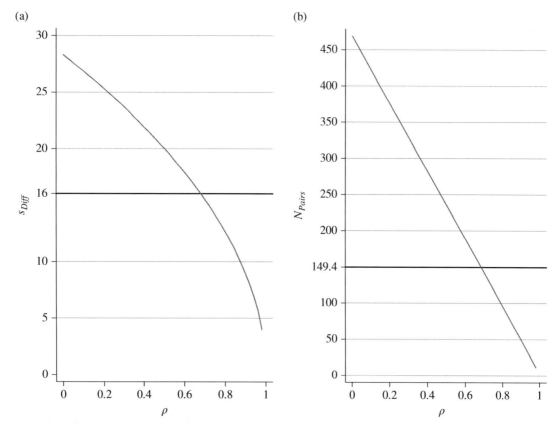

Figure 8.7 Influence of changing ρ on the planning values for (a) σ_{Diff} and hence (b) N_{Pairs} assuming $\sigma_{Within} = 20$. (*See insert for color representation of the figure.*)

Thus, for the above test size and power and Δ_{Plan} equal to 0.4, 0.6 and 0.8, the corresponding sample sizes from **Table 8.2** are $N_{Pairs} = 101$, 46 and 27. These can also be obtained from $^S S_S$ by setting $\delta = \Delta_{Plan}$ and $\sigma = 1$. With the original specification of $\Delta_{Plan} = 1.074$, $^S S_S$ gives $N_{Pairs} = 16$.

Table 8.2 and Equations 8.11, 8.12 and 8.14

Example 8.9 Cross-over trial - Continuous data - Intraocular pressure reduction
Realini (2009) reports a trial of 26 patients with ocular hypertension or open-angle glaucoma whose intraocular pressure (IOP) was currently controlled using a single IOP-lowering agent. As such they could safely undergo a 4-week washout before randomisation of one eye to apply Latanoprost (*L*) ophthalmic solution at night for 4 weeks while the other eye was left Untreated (*U*). At 4-weeks post-randomisation, the eyes receiving *L* had a mean IOP of 17.1 mmHg (SD = 3.1) and for *U* these were 20.3 (4.8) respectively. This represents a reduction in IOP by use of *L* of 3.2 mmHg.

If a repeat trial is planned, how many patients would need to be recruited, assuming a 2-sided test size of 5% and a power of 80%?

Following the results of Realini (2009), the investigators may set $\delta_{Plan} = 3$ mmHg. However, planning for a paired design requires the stipulation of σ_{Diff}, which can be obtained using equation

(8.14) if σ_{Within} and ρ can be specified. The trial data suggest $\sigma_{Within} \approx \sqrt{\dfrac{3.1^2 + 4.8^2}{2}} = 4.04$ and so $\sigma_{Diff} \approx 4.04\sqrt{2(1-\rho)} \approx 5.71\sqrt{1-\rho}$.

From the above, the standardised effect size of equation (8.11) is $\Delta_{Plan} = \dfrac{3}{5.71\sqrt{1-\rho}} = \dfrac{0.525}{\sqrt{1-\rho}}$.

If $\rho = 0.1$, $\Delta_{Plan} = 0.55$ and $\rho = 0.9$, $\Delta_{Plan} = 1.66$ then these two extremes give, from (8.12) or S_{Ss}, N_{Pairs} ranging from 54 to 8. As the original trial included 26 patients, it may be prudent for the new investigators to assume a low value for ρ and (perhaps) recruit 30 patients. Alternatively, they may think of using an intermediate value for $\rho = 0.5$, and hence $\Delta_{Plan} = 0.74$, but also increase the power to (say) 90%. Such a design would require $N_{Pairs} = 42$ with 21 patients receiving the sequences LU and UL respectively.

References

Technical

Cohen J (1988). *Statistical Power Analysis for the Behavioral Sciences*, (2nd edn) Lawrence Earlbaum, New Jersey.

Connett JE, Smith JA and McHugh RB (1987). Sample size and power for pair-matched case-control studies. *Statistics in Medicine*, **6**, 53–59.

Guenther WC (1981). Sample size formulas for normal theory *t* tests. *American Statistician*, **35**, 243–244.

Julious SA and Campbell MJ (1998). Sample sizes for paired or matched ordinal data. *Statistics in Medicine*, **17**, 1635–1642.

Lachin JM (1992). Power and sample size evaluation for the McNemar test with application to matched case-control studies. *Statistics in Medicine*, **11**, 1239–1251.

Examples

Abernethy AP, Currow DC, Frith P, Fazekas BS, McHugh A and Bui C (2003). Randomised, double blind, placebo controlled crossover trial of sustained release morphine for the management of refractory dyspnoea. *British Medical Journal*, **327**, 523–528.

Butenas S, Cawthern KM, van't Meer C, DiLorenzo ME, Lock JB and Mann KG (2001). Antiplatelet agents in tissue factor-induced blood coagulation. *Blood*, **97**, 2314–2322.

Cruciani RA, Dvorkin E, Homel P, Malamud S, Culliney B, Lapin J, Portenoy RK and Esteban-Cruciani N (2006). Safety, tolerability and symptom outcomes associated with L-carnitine supplementation in patients with cancer, fatigue, and carnitine deficiency: a phase I/II study. *Journal of Pain and Symptom Management*, **32**, 551–559.

Lo ECM, Luo Y, Fan MW and Wei SHY (2001). Clinical investigation of two glass-ionomer restoratives used with the atraumatic restorative treatment approach in China: Two-years results. *Caries Research*, **35**, 458–463.

Morrison JM, Gilmour H and Sullivan F (1991). Children seen frequently out of hours in one general practice. *British Medical Journal*, **303**, 1111–1114.

Realini TD (2009). A prospective, randomized, investigator-masked evaluation of the monocular trial in ocular hypertension or open-angle glaucoma. *Ophthalmology*, **116**, 1237–1242.

Zodpey SZ, Tiwari RR and Kulkarni HR (2000). Risk factors for haemorrhagic stroke: a case-control study. *Public Health*, **114**, 177–182.

Table 8.1 Sample sizes for paired binary data [Equation 8.1].
Each cell gives the number of pairs of subjects, N_{Pairs}, that should be entered into the study.

Odds Ratio ψ	2-sided $\alpha=0.05$; Power $1-\beta=0.8$									
	Proportion of Discordant Pairs, π_{Dis}									
	0.1	0.2	0.3	0.4	0.5	0.6	0.7	0.8	0.9	1
1.5	1960	979	652	489	391	325	278	243	216	194
1.6	1472	735	489	367	293	244	209	182	162	146
1.7	1166	582	387	290	232	193	165	144	128	115
1.8	960	479	319	239	190	158	135	118	105	94
1.9	813	406	270	202	161	134	115	100	89	80
2.0	705	351	234	175	139	116	99	86	77	69
2.1	622	310	206	154	123	102	87	76	67	60
2.2	556	277	184	138	110	91	78	68	60	54
2.3	504	251	167	125	99	82	70	61	54	49
2.4	461	230	152	114	91	75	64	56	50	44
2.5	425	212	141	105	84	69	59	51	46	41
3	312	155	103	77	61	50	43	37	33	29
4	216	107	71	53	42	34	29	25	22	20
5	175	86	57	42	33	27	23	20	18	16

Odds Ratio ψ	2-sided $\alpha=0.05$; Power $1-\beta=0.9$									
	Proportion of Discordant Pairs, π_{Dis}									
	0.1	0.2	0.3	0.4	0.5	0.6	0.7	0.8	0.9	1
1.5	2623	1310	872	653	522	434	372	325	288	259
1.6	1969	983	654	490	391	325	278	243	216	194
1.7	1560	778	517	387	309	257	220	192	170	153
1.8	1284	640	425	318	254	211	180	157	139	125
1.9	1087	542	360	269	215	178	152	133	118	105
2.0	942	469	312	233	185	154	131	114	101	91
2.1	831	414	274	205	163	135	116	101	89	80
2.2	744	370	245	183	146	121	103	90	79	71
2.3	673	335	222	166	132	109	93	81	71	64
2.4	616	306	203	151	120	100	85	74	65	58
2.5	568	282	187	139	111	92	78	68	60	53
3	417	206	136	101	80	66	56	49	43	38
4	288	142	94	69	55	45	38	33	29	25
5	233	114	75	55	43	36	30	26	22	20

Table 8.2 Sample Sizes for paired continuous data with 2-sided $\alpha = 0.05$ [Equation 8.12].

Each cell gives the number of pairs of subjects, N_{Pairs}, that should be entered into the study. If a cross-over trial is planned then any *odd* number tabular entries should be increased to the next *even* number above.

Standardised Effect size	Power: $1 - \beta$			
Δ	0.8	0.85	0.9	0.95
0.05	6,282	7,185	8,408	10,398
0.1	1,5721	1,798	2,104	2,601
0.15	700	801	936	1,158
0.2	395	451	528	652
0.25	254	290	339	418
0.3	177	202	236	291
0.35	131	149	174	215
0.4	101	115	134	165
0.45	80	91	106	1310
0.5	65	74	86	106
0.55	54	62	72	88
0.6	46	521	61	75
0.65	40	45	52	64
0.7	34	39	45	55
0.75	30	34	40	49
0.8	27	30	35	43
0.85	24	27	32	38
0.9	22	25	28	35
0.95	20	22	26	31
1	18	20	23	28
1.1	15	17	20	24
1.2	13	15	17	20
1.3	12	13	15	18
1.4	10	12	13	16
1.5	9	10	12	14

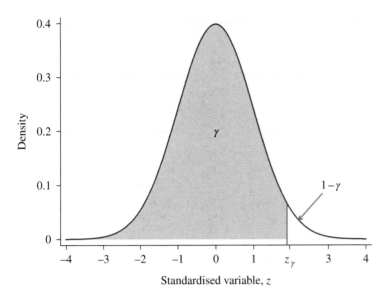

Figure 1.1 The probability density function of a standardised Normal distribution.

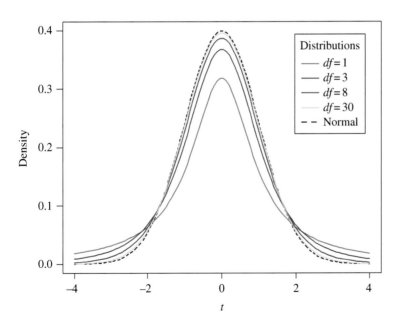

Figure 1.3 Central *t*-distributions with different degrees of freedom (*df*) and the corresponding Normal distribution.

Sample Sizes for Clinical, Laboratory and Epidemiology Studies, Fourth Edition. David Machin, Michael J. Campbell, Say Beng Tan and Sze Huey Tan.
© 2018 John Wiley & Sons Ltd. Published 2018 by John Wiley & Sons Ltd.

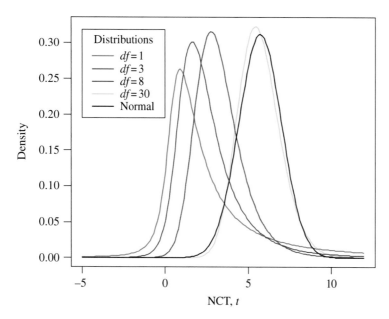

Figure 1.4 Non-central t-distributions with $\mu=\sigma=1$, hence non-centrality parameters $\psi=\sqrt{n}$, with increasing $df=n-1$ with n equal to 2, 4, 9 and 31. For $n=31$ the corresponding Normal distribution with mean $\sqrt{31}=5.57$ is added.

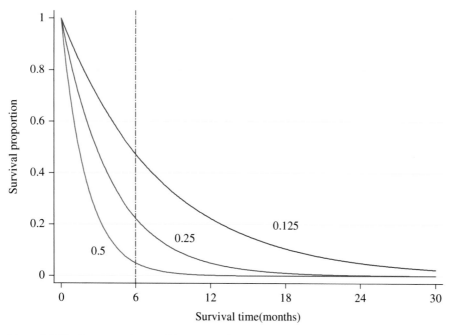

Figure 1.7 The Exponential survival function with constant hazards of $\theta=0.125$, 0.25 and 0.5.

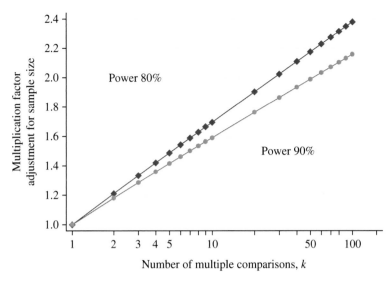

Figure 2.1 Sample size multiplication factors to compensate for k multiple comparisons when applying a Bonferroni correction with two-sided $\alpha = 0.05$ (after Fayers and Machin, 2016, Figure 11.3).

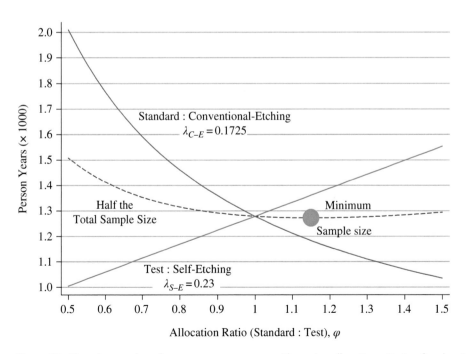

Figure 6.1 Changing number of person-years per group with varying allocation ratio 1: φ for planning values $\lambda_{C-E} = 0.23$ and $\lambda_{S-E} = 0.1725$, for a 2-sided $\alpha = 0.05$ and $1 - \beta = 0.90$ [Equation 6.2].

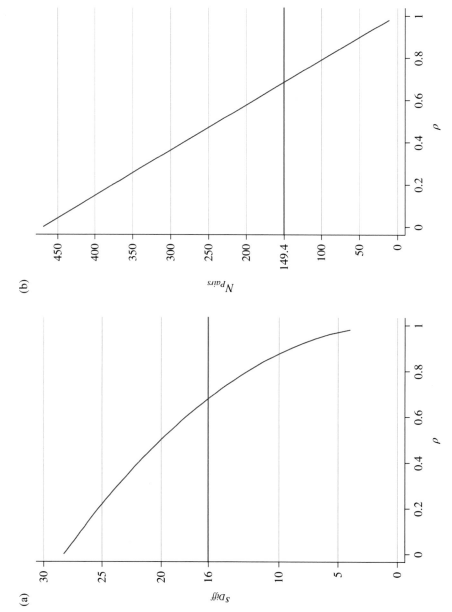

Figure 8.7 Influence of changing ρ on the planning values for (a) σ_{Diff} and hence (b) N_{Pairs} assuming $\sigma_{Within} = 20$.

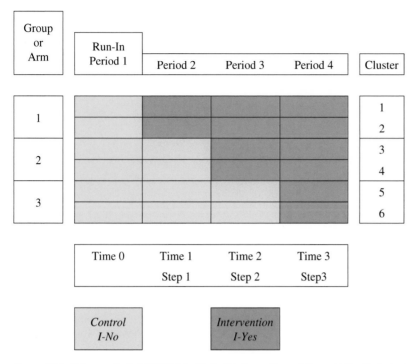

Figure 13.1 Schema of a full SWD trial with $\lambda = 2$ interventions, *I-No* and *I-Yes*, $K = 6$ clusters with $P = 4$ periods, $A = 3$ arms with $g = 2$ clusters randomised at each of $S = 3$ steps.

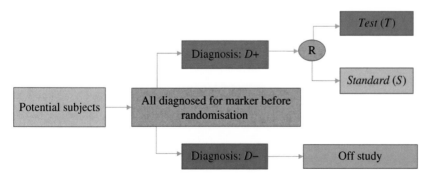

Figure 15.2 An Enrichment Design in which subjects are selected for randomisation provided they are diagnosis positive ($D+$) for a specific molecular target.

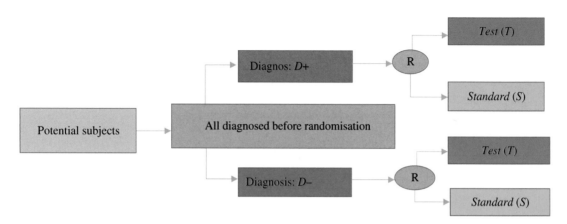

Figure 15.3 Biomarker stratified design (after Simon, 2008a, b).

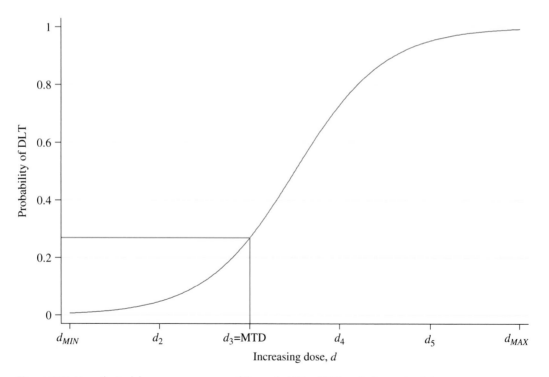

Figure 15.7 Hypothetical dose-response curve of the probability of DLT against a received dose.

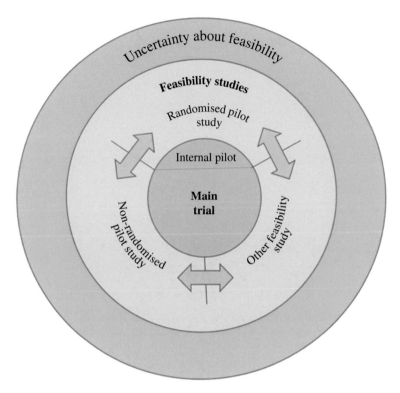

Figure 16.1 Conceptual framework for feasibility and pilot studies (from Eldridge, Lancaster, Campbell, *et al*, 2016, Figure 7).

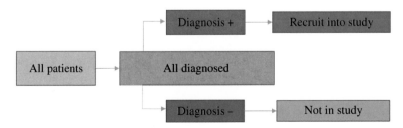

Figure 18.1 Enrichment Design for a TE Trial.

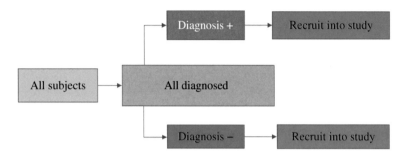

Figure 18.2 Biomarker stratified design for TE trials.

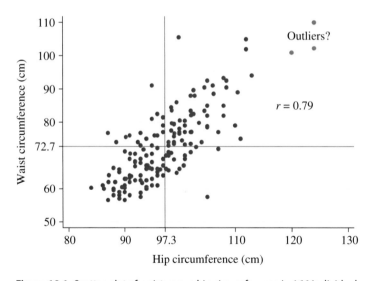

Figure 19.1 Scatter plot of waist versus hip circumference in 166 individuals.

9

Confidence Intervals

SUMMARY

This chapter describes how sample sizes may be derived by pre-specifying the width or relative width of the confidence interval the investigator wishes to obtain at the end of the study. Formulae are given for both binary and continuous outcome measures for a single group, for the comparison between two independent groups and for paired or matched groups.

9.1   Introduction

A sample size calculation is required for all clinical investigations whether concerned with a single group or for comparative studies.

If a single group study is envisaged, such as an epidemiological survey with the objective to determine the prevalence of asthma in young children in a particular locality, then an unbiased estimate of the prevalence can be obtained from a simple random sample of the target population. In designing such a survey, the investigators are likely to ask 'How many subjects do I need to examine in order to assess prevalence with a reasonable degree of accuracy?' This uncertainty can be expressed by the width of the corresponding confidence interval (CI) for the prevalence concerned. This implies that, if a large number of surveys all of the same size is conducted and 95% CIs calculated for each, then 95% of these intervals would contain the true prevalence, π_{Pop}, and 5% would not. Therefore it is *possible* that the CI, calculated after a single sample is taken, does *not* contain the true population prevalence.

In comparative studies and clinical trials, a pilot investigation (see **Chapter 16**) may be conducted with the objective of obtaining a preliminary idea of the magnitude of the difference between groups with a view to doing a later definitive study should this difference appear to be of clinical relevance. For such *learning* studies, the sample size can be selected in order to ensure a given level of precision is obtained, rather than consider the power in the traditional fashion, for a clinically relevant and pre-specified difference of interest. Thus, the estimation approach through the provision of CIs for the true difference replaces testing a formal null hypothesis to obtain a *p*-value.

In these situations, the sample size chosen is determined by two factors. First, how precise should the estimate be? If the investigator can allow only a small margin of uncertainty, then a large sample will be needed. The second is whether, for example, a 90% or 95% CI is to be planned for.

Sample Sizes for Clinical, Laboratory and Epidemiology Studies, Fourth Edition. David Machin, Michael J. Campbell, Say Beng Tan and Sze Huey Tan.
© 2018 John Wiley & Sons Ltd. Published 2018 by John Wiley & Sons Ltd.

Power Implications

For comparative studies, there is a relationship between conventional significance testing and *CI*s. Thus, for example, if zero lies outside the 95% *CI* for the difference of two means, a significance test would generally yield a result significant at 5%. Hence, one might question the disappearance of $z_{1-\beta}$ of equation (1.7) from the sample-size equations below. However, the methods we describe are equivalent to assuming a power of 50% or $1 - \beta = 0.5$, and thereby setting $z_{1-\beta} = 0$. Further, as neither a null nor an alternative hypothesis has been postulated, one cannot, for example, declare the null hypothesis to be rejected if *a priori* it was not set. The comparative studies envisaged in this chapter are exploratory in nature and so, although the results of a particular study may suggest a range of plausible differences between groups that exclude the null hypothesis, a subsequent definitive and formally powered study is likely to be required to get the necessary level of proof for any difference indicated.

Nevertheless, conventional equations or tables for power calculations of significance tests can be used to estimate the equivalent sample size for a specified width of *CI*s simply by setting the power as 50%.

9.2   Single Proportion

Large Populations - Response Rate not too Close to 0 or 1

Suppose a study for which the underlying population prevalence of the disease of interest, π_{Pop}, is to be designed. If N subjects are involved, then $p = r/N$, where r is the number of individuals observed to have the disease, estimates π_{Pop}. Provided that both Np and $N(1 - p)$ are not too small (a good guide is that they are both greater than 10), then we can use the Normal approximation to the Binomial distribution and obtain from these data an estimated $100(1 - \alpha)\%$ *CI* for π_{Pop} as

$$p - z_{1-\alpha/2}\sqrt{\frac{p(1-p)}{N}} \text{ to } p + z_{1-\alpha/2}\sqrt{\frac{p(1-p)}{N}}. \tag{9.1}$$

This is the same expression as equation (1.18).

At the design stage of the prevalence study, we have not yet observed p, and so we can only suggest the anticipated value of equation (9.1) by replacing p by π_{Plan}. This then represents the target *CI* for the study we have in mind. The width of this *CI*, for a specific choice of α, will depend on π_{Plan} and critically on the ultimate sample size, N chosen.

Using (9.1), $\omega_{Plan} = 2z_{1-\alpha/2}\sqrt{\dfrac{\pi_{Plan}(1-\pi_{Plan})}{N}}$ can be set as the pre-specified width of the desired *CI*.

Rearranging this expression, the corresponding sample size is given by

$$N = 4\left[\frac{\pi_{Plan}(1-\pi_{Plan})}{\omega_{Plan}^2}\right]z_{1-\alpha/2}^2 = 4\Omega_{Plan}z_{1-\alpha/2}^2, \tag{9.2}$$

where $\Omega_{Plan} = \dfrac{\pi_{Plan}(1-\pi_{Plan})}{\omega_{Plan}^2}$.

Alternatively, instead of pre-specifying the width, ω_{Plan}, of the *CI*, the investigators may wish to estimate π_{Pop} to within a certain percentage of its value, say $100\varepsilon\%$. So the anticipated *CI* is now envisaged as $\pi_{Plan} - (\pi_{Plan} \times \varepsilon_{Plan})$ to $\pi_{Plan} + (\pi_{Plan} \times \varepsilon_{Plan})$. This is equivalent to specifying that the *CI* should be no wider than $\omega_{Plan} = 2\pi_{Plan}\varepsilon_{Plan}$. To obtain the sample size we substitute this value for ω in equation (9.2) to obtain:

$$N = \left[\frac{1 - \pi_{Plan}}{\pi_{Plan}\varepsilon_{Plan}^2} \right] z_{1-\alpha/2}^2. \tag{9.3}$$

Expressions (9.2) and (9.3) will not be useful if the anticipated value of π_{Plan} is either 0 or 1 or close to these values. In which case, equation (9.5) below would be used in their place. Indeed, prudence suggests that this latter equation should always be used whatever the value of π_{Plan} and therefore this forms the basis of **Table 9.1**.

High or Low Anticipated Response Rate

As we have noted previously, if the sample size is not large or π_{Pop} is assumed close to 0 or 1, then the '*traditional*' method, which is the large sample approximation of equation (9.1) for calculating a *CI*, should not be used. Further we should note that although (9.1) is symmetric about the estimate p, strictly this symmetry only applies if $p = 0.5$; otherwise the true *CI* is not symmetric. Despite this we can still plan a study on the basis of the width of the interval, ω, even though the centre of the interval may not be p. In so doing we use the '*recommended*' method of equation (1.19) which we reproduce here with some small notational changes, including replacing r by $N\pi_{Plan}$, as we are now at the planning (rather than the analysis) stage of study development.

First, defining $A = 2N\pi_{Plan} + z_{1-\alpha/2}^2$, $B = z_{1-\alpha/2}\sqrt{z_{1-\alpha/2}^2 + 4N\pi_{Plan}(1-\pi_{Plan})}$, and $C = 2(N + z_{1-\alpha/2}^2)$, then the corresponding $100(1-\alpha)\%$ *CI* is given by

$$(A - B)/C \text{ to } (A + B)/C. \tag{9.4}$$

From this the width of the *CI* is $\omega = \dfrac{2B}{C}$ which after some algebra leads to a planning sample size of

$$N = \left[(2\Omega_{Plan} - 1) + \sqrt{(2\Omega_{Plan} - 1)^2 + \frac{1}{\omega_{Plan}^2} - 1} \right] z_{1-\alpha/2}^2. \tag{9.5}$$

Finite Populations

In some cases, the size of the population, N_{Pop}, from which a sample is to be taken is known precisely and may be of limited size. For example, the aim of the study may be to determine the prevalence of impotence amongst male patients on a diabetic register. The investigator could assess everyone on the register and thereby obtain the 'truth'. However, instead of assessing everyone, a sample from the register could be taken to estimate the prevalence and the corresponding *CI*.

It is clear that if one sampled 60 out of a total register of 100 subjects one would have a more accurate assessment of the prevalence than if one took a sample of 60 from a register of size 1000. In these circumstances, if p is estimated by the ratio of r cases from a sample of N diabetic patients from a register of size N_{Pop}, then equation (9.1) is modified somewhat to give an approximate $100(1-\alpha)\%$ *CI* for the true prevalence π_{Pop} as

$$p - z_{1-\alpha/2}\sqrt{\frac{p(1-p)}{N} \cdot \frac{N_{Pop} - N}{N_{Pop}}} \text{ to } p + z_{1-\alpha/2}\sqrt{\frac{p(1-p)}{N} \cdot \frac{N_{Pop} - N}{N_{Pop}}}. \tag{9.6}$$

Given that N is the sample size obtained from either equation (9.2), (9.3) or (9.5) for an (effectively) *infinite* population, then the sample size required for a population that is *finite* is:

$$N_{Finite} = \left(\frac{N_{Pop}}{N + N_{Pop}}\right) N. \tag{9.7}$$

The purpose of sampling is to reduce the number of observations to be made by the investigator. However, if the required sample size is a major proportion of the total population, say 80% or more, then it may be sensible to examine the whole population, N_{Pop}, rather than a sample from it.

9.3 Proportions from Two Groups

Independent Groups

Difference in proportions

The $100(1-\alpha)$% *CI* for a true difference in proportions between a *Standard* (S) and a *Test* (T) group, $\delta = \pi_T - \pi_S$, takes a form similar to (9.1) but now concerns $p_T - p_S$ and the corresponding $SE(p_T - p_S)$. It is estimated by

$$\left(p_T - p_S\right) - z_{1-\alpha/2}\sqrt{\frac{p_T\left(1-p_{T1}\right)}{n_T} + \frac{p_S\left(1-p_S\right)}{n_S}} \text{ to } \left(p_T - p_S\right) + z_{1-\alpha/2}\sqrt{\frac{p_T\left(1-p_{T1}\right)}{n_T} + \frac{p_S\left(1-p_S\right)}{n_S}}, \tag{9.8}$$

where p_T and p_S are the corresponding observed proportions in each of the two groups of size n_T and n_S respectively.

Thus, one may wish to calculate the number of subjects required to be able to obtain a *CI* of a specified width,

$$\omega_{Plan} = 2z_{1-\alpha/2}\sqrt{\frac{\pi_T\left(1-\pi_T\right)}{n_T} + \frac{\pi_S\left(1-\pi_S\right)}{n_S}}, \tag{9.9}$$

where, for ease of presentation, π_T and π_S, rather than π_{PlanT} and π_{PlanS}, denote the planning proportions considered by the design team. In which case, and first specifying $n_T = \varphi n_S$, and hence $N = n_S + n_T = (1 + \varphi)n_S$, the corresponding total sample size required is given by

$$N = 4\left(\frac{1+\varphi}{\varphi}\right)\left[\frac{\varphi\pi_S\left(1-\pi_S\right) + \pi_T\left(1-\pi_T\right)}{\omega_{Plan}^2}\right]z_{1-\alpha/2}^2. \tag{9.10}$$

This expression also gives a convenient check of the more complex calculations arising from equation (9.11) below.

Recommended method

An extension of the methodology of equation (9.4) allows a '*recommended*' method for calculating the *CI* for the difference between two proportions. This leads to the width of the $100(1-\alpha)$% *CI* as

$$\omega = \sqrt{\left(\pi_S - L_S\right)^2 + \left(U_T - \pi_T\right)^2} + \sqrt{\left(\pi_T - L_T\right)^2 + \left(U_S - \pi_S\right)^2}. \tag{9.11}$$

Here, $L_S = (A_S - B_S)/C_S$ and $U_S = (A_S + B_S)/C_S$, where $A_S = 2n_S\pi_S + z_{1-\alpha/2}^2$, $B_S = z_{1-\alpha/2}\sqrt{z_{1-\alpha/2}^2 + 4n_S\pi_S(1-\pi_S)}$, and $C_S = 2(n_S + z_{1-\alpha/2}^2)$.

There are similar expressions for L_T, U_T, A_T, B_T and C_T but with π_S and n_S replaced by π_T and n_T respectively.

Although details are omitted, once planning values for 2-sided α, φ, π_S, π_T are given, and ω_{Plan} is specified, equation (9.11) can be solved for N using an iterative procedure after first replacing n_S by $N/(1+\varphi)$ and n_T by $N_\varphi/(1+\varphi)$.

Since equation (9.11) can be used for all situations, it is used in place of equation (9.10) to calculate the sample sizes given in **Table 9.2** and those obtained from $^S S_S$.

Odds ratio

The comparison between two proportions can also be expressed through the odds ratio, *OR*, where

$$OR = \frac{p_T/(1-p_T)}{p_S/(1-p_S)} = \frac{p_T(1-p_S)}{p_S(1-p_T)}. \tag{9.12}$$

The corresponding estimated $100(1-\alpha)\%$ *CI* is

$$exp\left[logOR - z_{1-\alpha/2}SE(logOR)\right] \text{ to } exp\left[logOR + z_{1-\alpha/2}SE(logOR)\right], \tag{9.13}$$

where

$$SE(logOR) \approx \sqrt{\frac{1}{n_S\pi_S(1-\pi_S)} + \frac{1}{n_T\pi_T(1-\pi_T)}}. \tag{9.14}$$

As the *OR* is a ratio, rather than difference, it is usual to specify the requirement for the *CI* as a proportion of the *OR* itself, rather than by the width of the interval, ω_{Plan}. In which case, to estimate an *OR* to within $100\varepsilon_{Plan}\%$ of the true value, the sample size required is

$$N = \frac{(1+\varphi)\left[\dfrac{1}{\pi_S(1-\pi_S)} + \dfrac{1}{\varphi\pi_T(1-\pi_T)}\right]}{\left[log(1-\varepsilon_{Plan})\right]^2}z_{1-\alpha/2}^2, \tag{9.15}$$

and hence $n_S = N/(1+\varphi)$ and $n_T = \varphi n_S$. Sample sizes are given in **Table 9.3** for the situation of equal numbers of subjects in each group.

However, this requires two of the planning values of OR_{Plan}, π_S and π_T to be specified. If, for example, OR_{Plan} and π_S are given then π_T can be obtained from equation (9.12). Also, since equation (9.14) is an approximation, so too is (9.15). It is therefore suitable only when π_S and π_T do not take extreme values close to 0 or 1. So, if possible, formulating the study in terms of a difference in proportions to enable the corresponding *recommended* procedure implemented in $^S S_S$ is strongly advised.

Paired Groups

Difference in proportions

When the two proportions to be compared are from matched or paired data, the corresponding estimates are correlated. Thus when using the *recommended* procedure, this leads to the following rather complex expression for the width of the $100(1-\alpha)\%$ *CI*:

$$\omega = \sqrt{(\pi_S - L_S)^2 - 2\rho(\pi_S - L_S)(U_T - \pi_T) + (U_T - \pi_T)^2} \\ + \sqrt{(\pi_T - L_T)^2 - 2\rho(\pi_T - L_T)(U_S - \pi_S) + (U_S - \pi_S)^2}, \tag{9.16}$$

where $L_S = (A_S - B_S)/C_S$, $U_S = (A_S + B_S)/C_S$, $A_S = 2N_{Pairs}\pi_S + z_{1-\alpha/2}^2$, $B_S = z_{1-\alpha/2}$; $\sqrt{z_{1-\alpha/2}^2 + 4N_{Pairs}\pi_S(1-\pi_S)}$ and $C_S = 2(N_{Pairs} + z_{1-\alpha/2}^2)$, with similar expressions for L_T, U_T, A_T, B_T and C_T. Finally, ρ corrects for the fact that p_S and p_T are now correlated. For given planning values for 2-sided α, φ, π_S, π_T, ρ_{Plan} and ω_{Plan}, the entries of **Table 9.4** and $\boxed{^S\!S_S}$ use an iterative procedure to calculate the number of matched pairs required, N_{Pairs}.

9.4 Single Mean

For a single population mean μ_{Pop} of continuous data assumed to have a Normal distribution, the corresponding sample mean from N observations is $\bar{x}$ with SD, s. The estimate of the corresponding $100(1 - \alpha)\%$ CI for μ_{Pop} is

$$\bar{x} - t_{N-1,1-\alpha/2}\frac{s}{\sqrt{N}} \text{ to } \bar{x} + t_{N-1,1-\alpha/2}\frac{s}{\sqrt{N}}. \tag{9.17}$$

With some more detail given, this is the same expression as equation (1.17) with $df = N - 1$. If N is large then Student's $t_{N-1,1-\alpha/2}$, which depends on N as well as α, can be replaced by $z_{1-\alpha/2}$ from the Normal distribution.

In the same way as equation (9.2) is derived, to estimate μ_{Pop} with a pre-specified CI width ω_{Plan}, and a planning value for the standard deviation, s, as σ_{Plan}, the corresponding sample size is

$$N = 4\left[\frac{t_{N-1,1-\alpha/2}^2}{\Lambda_{Plan}^2}\right] \approx 4\left[\frac{z_{1-\alpha/2}^2}{\Lambda_{Plan}^2}\right], \tag{9.18}$$

where $\Lambda_{Plan} = \omega_{Plan}/\sigma_{Plan}$.

To estimate N, the right hand expression of equation (9.18) is first applied to obtain an initial sample size, say N_0, and if this is large (≥ 40) then this is taken as the sample size. If $N_0 < 40$, then $t_{N_0-1,1-\alpha/2}$ is obtained from **Table 1.3** and a revised sample size N_1 obtained using the corresponding part of equation (9.18). If this differs from N_0, repeat the process using $t_{N_1-1,1-\alpha/2}$ to obtain N_2 and so on. This iterative process usually terminates quite quickly (see *Example* 9.8).

If a proportionate target for the *CI* is set as $\mu_{Plan} - (\varepsilon_{Plan} \times \mu_{Plan})$ to $\mu_{Plan} + (\varepsilon_{Plan} \times \mu_{Plan})$ or μ_{Plan} $(1 - \varepsilon_{Plan})$ to $\mu_{Plan}(1 + \varepsilon_{Plan})$, then $\omega_{Plan} = 2\mu_{Plan}\varepsilon_{Plan}$. Substituting this in equation (9.18) gives

$$N = \frac{\sigma_{Plan}^2 t_{N-1,1-\alpha/2}^2}{\mu_{Plan}^2 \varepsilon_{Plan}^2} = \frac{t_{N-1,1-\alpha/2}^2}{\Theta_{Plan}^2 \varepsilon_{Plan}^2} \approx \frac{z_{1-\alpha/2}^2}{\Theta_{Plan}^2 \varepsilon_{Plan}^2}, \tag{9.19}$$

where $\Theta_{Plan} = \mu_{Plan}/\sigma_{Plan}$. As with equation (9.18) an iterative process may be required to obtain the sample size N.

It is important to note that, to calculate N from (9.18) or (9.19), an anticipated value of the population SD, σ, is required. In the absence of knowledge of this, a rough guide to σ_{Plan} is provided by the largest minus the smallest anticipated values of the measurement of concern divided by 4.

9.5   Difference Between Means

Independent Groups

If the SD can be assumed to be the same for both independent groups, then the estimated *CI* for the difference between them is

$$(\bar{x}_T - \bar{x}_S) - t_{df,1-\alpha/2}s_{Pool}\sqrt{\left[\frac{1}{n_T} + \frac{1}{n_S}\right]} \text{ to } (\bar{x}_T - \bar{x}_S) + t_{df,1-\alpha/2}s_{Pool}\sqrt{\left[\frac{1}{n_T} + \frac{1}{n_S}\right]}. \tag{9.20}$$

Here s_{Pool} is a combined estimate of σ_{Pop} obtained from the two samples weighted by their corresponding degrees of freedom, (*df*) $n_S - 1$ and $n_T - 1$.

Denoting the total sample size, $N = n_S + n_T$, with $n_T = \varphi n_S$, then the width of the anticipated *CI* can be expressed by

$$\omega_{Plan} = 2t_{df,1-\alpha/2}\sigma_{Plan}\sqrt{\left[\frac{1+\varphi}{N} + \frac{1+\varphi}{\varphi N}\right]}. \tag{9.21}$$

where $df = n_S + n_T - 2 = N - 2$. From this, the sample size required for a *CI* of width ω_{Plan} is

$$N = 4\frac{(1+\varphi)^2}{\varphi}\left[\frac{t_{df,1-\alpha/2}^2}{\Lambda_{Plan}^2}\right] \approx 4\frac{(1+\varphi)^2}{\varphi}\left[\frac{z_{1-\alpha/2}^2}{\Lambda_{Plan}^2}\right], \tag{9.22}$$

where $\Lambda_{Plan} = \omega_{Plan}/\sigma_{Plan}$.

As with equation (9.18) an iterative process may be required to obtain the final sample size N for smaller studies.

Paired or Matched Groups

When the units for observation are paired or matched, then the endpoint observations from the two members of each unit are linked. It is then the difference between these two measures from the N_{Pairs} units concerned that forms the endpoint for analysis. For example, if cases with a particular disease are matched, perhaps by age and gender to healthy controls, then the endpoint for pair *i* becomes $d_i = (x_i - y_i)$ where x_i is the observation from the case and y_i that of the same outcome measure from the control. The corresponding *CI* for a continuous variable is

$$\bar{d} - t_{df,1-\alpha/2}\frac{\sigma_{Pair}}{\sqrt{N_{Pair}}} \text{ to } \bar{d} + t_{df,1-\alpha/2}\frac{\sigma_{Pair}}{\sqrt{N_{Pair}}}. \tag{9.23}$$

By analogy with previous situations, an appropriate sample size for a given *CI* of width ω_{Plan} is

$$N_{Pair} = 4\left[\frac{\sigma_{Pair}^2}{\omega_{Plan}^2}\right]t_{df,1-\alpha/2}^2 = 4\frac{t_{df,1-\alpha/2}^2}{\Lambda_{Pair}^2} \approx 4\frac{z_{1-\alpha/2}^2}{\Lambda_{Pair}^2}. \tag{9.24}$$

where $\Lambda_{Pair} = \omega_{Plan}/\sigma_{Pair}$.

Note that (9.24) has a similar structure to equation (9.18) for the case of a single mean and to (9.22) for the difference of two means in independent groups. As a consequence **Table 9.5** can be used for the three situations.

9.6   Bibliography

Problems related to CIs for proportions and their differences are discussed by Newcombe and Altman (2000), who provide the '*recommended*' methods of equations (9.4) and (9.11) from which sample sizes can be deduced. Tan, Machin and Tan (2012) pointed out that an expression proposed by Bristol (1989) as an approximation to equation (9.10) when there is 1:1 allocation, and used in earlier editions of this book, appears to overestimate the required sample size obtained from the '*recommended*' method. The sample size formula (9.15), for use when differences are expressed by the odds ratio, is given by Lemeshow, Hosmer and Klar (1988). Newcombe and Altman (2000) also provide the basis for equation (9.16), which is used when calculating sample sizes for matched binary pairs.

9.7   Examples and Use of the Tables

Table 1.2

For a two-sided 90% CI, $\alpha = 0.1$ and $z_{0.9} = 1.6449$.
For two-sided 95% CI, $\alpha = 0.05$ and $z_{0.975} = 1.96$.

Table 9.1 and Equations 9.2 and 9.5

Example 9.1   Single group binary data - CI width specified - Disease prevalence
The prevalence of a disease among children in a particular area is unknown but is believed to be at a minimum of 5%. How many subjects are required if investigators wish to determine this prevalence with a 95% *CI* of width 10%?

They begin by considering $\pi_{Plan} = 0.05$ so that, using equation (9.2) with $\omega_{Plan} = 0.1$, the sample size obtained is $N = \dfrac{4 \times 0.05 \times (1 - 0.05) \times 1.96^2}{0.1^2} = 72.99$ or 73. However, they then check if this is regarded as a situation in which the method of calculation is sufficiently reliable. They obtain $N\pi_{Plan} = 3.65$, clearly < 10, and hence conclude that the recommended method of equation (9.5) should be used in this situation. Reference to **Table 9.1** or $^S\!S_S$ gives $N = 83$ children, which suggests a larger survey size would be necessary.

They further consider that the prevalence, although unlikely, could be as high as 20% and, as a matter of interest, calculate the potential survey size using both equation (9.2) and **Table 9.1** to obtain the same value of 245.

Finally, a compromise survey size of $N = 200$ is decided upon, which corresponds to the situation with $\pi_{Plan} \approx 0.15$.

Equation 9.3

Example 9.2   Single group binary data - Proportionate CI width specified - Disease prevalence
The prevalence rate of a disease among children in a particular area is believed to be about 30%. How many subjects are required if we wish to determine this prevalence to within about 4% of the true value, that is to have width of 8% for an anticipated *CI* of 26 to 34%?

Here, $\omega_{Plan} = 2 \times 0.3 \times \varepsilon_{Plan} = 0.08$, and therefore $\varepsilon_{Plan} = 0.08/0.6 = 0.1333$. Thus, from equation (9.3) and assuming a 95% CI is required, with $\pi_{Plan} = 0.3$ and $\varepsilon_{Plan} = 0.1333$, we obtain

$$N = \frac{(1-0.3) \times 1.96^2}{0.3 \times 0.1333^2} = 504.46 \text{ or } 505 \text{ children.}$$

Alternatively using the recommended method with $\boxed{^SS_S}$ and $\omega_{Plan} = 0.08$ gives $N = 502$, which agrees closely with the more approximate calculation. Should a 90%CI be required, then this sample size reduces to $N = 356$.

Equation 9.5

Example 9.3   Binary data - Low response rate - Autism-spectrum conditions
Baron-Cohen, Scott, Allison, *et al* (2009) conducted a survey of schools in Cambridgeshire, UK from which they estimated the prevalence of autism-spectrum conditions to be 94 per 10,000 of children aged 4 to 10 years with a 95% CI of 5 to 21 per 10,000. A repeat study is planned, but in an area in which the prevalence is anticipated to be higher, perhaps 150 per 10,000, but a narrower 95% CI close to a width of 11 per 10,000 is required. How large a study should be planned?

Here, the anticipated prevalence of $\pi_{Plan} = 150/10,000 = 0.015$ and $\omega_{Plan} = 11/10,000 = 0.0011$. Thus

$$\Omega_{Plan} = \frac{\pi_{Plan}(1 - \pi_{Plan})}{\omega_{Plan}^2} = \frac{0.015 \times (1 - 0.015)}{0.0011^2} = 12,210.74. \text{ As } \pi_{Plan} = 0.015 \text{ is close to zero, the recom-}$$

mended method of equation (9.5) is used for sample size purposes to give

$$N = \left[\{(2 \times 12,211) - 1\} + \sqrt{\{(2 \times 12,211) - 1\}^2 + \frac{1}{0.0011^2} - 1} \right] \times 1.96^2 = 187,696.$$

Alternatively using the recommended method with $\boxed{^SS_S}$ specifying $\omega_{Plan} = 0.0011$ gives $N = 187,686$, which agrees closely with the above calculation.

These calculations imply a study of approximately 200,000 children, which contrasts markedly with the study of Baron-Cohen, Scott, Allison, *et al* (2009), who attempted to deliver 11,635 questionnaire packets to participating schools.

Had the investigators set a larger $\omega_{Plan} = 16/10,000 = 0.0016$, as was obtained in the earlier study, then using $\boxed{^SS_S}$ results in a considerably reduced study size of $N = 88,741$ or approximately 90,000.

Equations 9.3 and 9.7

Example 9.4   Binary data - Finite population - Diabetes mellitus
Suppose that a register contains 1,000 male patients with diabetes mellitus but no clinical details are included with respect to whether they are impotent or not. If the estimated prevalence of impotence amongst these diabetics is assumed to be 20%, how many patients do we require in a survey to determine the prevalence of impotence if we are willing to allow a 95% CI of 4 percentage points on either side of the true prevalence?

Here, $\pi_{Plan} = 0.2$ and four percentage points of this prevalence implies that $\omega = 2\pi_{Plan}\varepsilon_{Plan} = 0.08$ so that $\varepsilon_{Plan} = 0.08/(2 \times 0.20) = 0.2$. From equation (9.3) or $\boxed{^SS_S}$ we would require about

$$N = \left[\frac{1-0.2}{0.2 \times 0.2^2} \right] 1.96^2 = 384.16 \text{ or } 385 \text{ subjects for a 95% } CI \text{ of the specified width. However, as the}$$

population is of a finite size, $N_{Pop} = 1,000$, this proposed sample size represents about 38% of the diabetics on the register. To adjust for the finite population, the ratio $\dfrac{N_{Pop}}{N+N_{Pop}} = \dfrac{1{,}000}{385+1{,}000} = 0.7220$

is required. As a consequence, the actual number of subjects to be sampled is reduced by equation

(9.7) to $N_{Finite} = 0.7220 \times 385 = 277.97$ or 280. This results in a considerable reduction in the anticipated study size.

Alternatively using $^{SS}_{S}$ with $\omega_{Plan} = 0.08$ gives $N = 383$, $\dfrac{N_{Pop}}{N+N_{Pop}} = \dfrac{1{,}000}{383+1{,}000} = 0.7231$ and

$N_{Finite} = 277$, which agrees closely with the earlier calculation.

Table 9.2 and Equations 9.10 and 9.11

Example 9.5 Binary data - Groups of equal and unequal sizes - Nausea after anaesthesia
In a study of two forms of anaesthesia, the respective nausea rates were anticipated to be 10% and 20%. How many patients are required if a width of 15% is set for the eventual 95% *CI* of the difference?

The planning values are $\pi_S = 0.1$, $\pi_T = 0.2$, and $\omega_{Plan} = 0.15$. Then, if equal numbers of subjects per anaesthesia group are required, $\varphi = 1$ and equation (9.10) gives

$$N = 4\left(\frac{1+1}{1}\right)\left[\frac{1\times 0.1\times(1-0.1)+0.2\times(1-0.2)}{0.15^2}\right]\times 1.96^2 = 341.46 \text{ or } 342. \text{ In which case, } n_S = n_T = 171$$

patients per intervention are required.

In some circumstances, an unequal allocation of subjects to the respective groups may be desired. If a 5:4 allocation is required, then $\varphi = 4/5 = 0.8$ and equation (9.10) leads to $N = 356.49$ with $n_S = 356.49/(1+0.8) = 198.05$ and $n_T = (0.8 \times 356.49)/(1+0.8) = 158.44$. Which, once conveniently rounded upwards to integers, become $n_S = 199$, $n_T = 159$ and hence $N = 358$. In contrast, if a 4:5 allocation is needed, then $\varphi = 5/4 = 1.25$ and it follows that $n_S = 149$, $n_T = 187$ and $N = 336$.

These sample sizes are somewhat different from those computed by $^{SS}_{S}$ which always defaults to the recommended method derived from (9.11). This gives for the 1:1 allocation, $N = 2n_S = 2 \times 175 = 350$ (as does **Table 9.2**); for the 5:4 allocation $n_S = 202$, $n_T = 162$, $N = 364$; and for the 4:5 allocation $n_S = 153$, $n_T = 192$, $N = 345$ subjects respectively.

However, if a 5:4 or 4:5 allocation ratio is required then it is best if the final total sample size derived is rounded upwards so as to be divisible by 9 (the block size). Thus in the preceding calculations for the 5:4 allocation using the recommended method, $N = 364$ would need to be increased to 369 to give $n_S = (5/9) \times 369 = 205$ and $n_T = (4/9) \times 369 = 164$. For the 4:5 allocation $N = 345$ would need to be increased to 351 to give $n_S = (4/9) \times 351 = 156$ and $n_T = (5/9) \times 351 = 195$.

Table 9.3 and Equations 9.12 and 9.15

Example 9.6 Odds ratio - Nausea after anaesthesia
In the study of nausea after anaesthesia of *Example 9.5*, what sample size would be required if the *OR* was to be determined to within 25% of its own value?

Here, from equation (9.12) the planning $OR_{Plan} = \dfrac{\pi_T/(1-\pi_T)}{\pi_S/(1-\pi_S)} = \dfrac{0.2/0.8}{0.1/0.9} = 2.25$. Then with $\varepsilon_{Plan} = 0.25$ this implies a desired *CI* of approximately $2.25 \times 0.75 = 1.69$ to $2.25 \times 1.25 = 2.81$. Use of equation

(9.15) with $\varphi = 1$ gives $N = \dfrac{(1+1)\left[\dfrac{1}{0.1\times 0.9} + \dfrac{1}{1\times 0.2\times 0.8}\right]}{\left[log(1-0.25)\right]^2} \times 1.96^2 = 1{,}611.68$ or 1,612. This suggests

$n_S = n_T = N/2 = 806$ patients per intervention.

	From Bidwell, *et al* (2005)				Planning		
	Blind				Blind		
Stroke	No	Yes	Total		No	Yes	Total
No	[95*]	[10*]	105		0.32	0.08	0.4
Yes	[229*]	[24*]	253		0.48	0.12	0.6
Total	324	34	358		0.8	0.2	1

* Not given by the authors but possible data consistent with the margins of the table.

Figure 9.1 Partial results from a survey of patients attending a hospital clinic (after Bidwell, Sahu, Edwards, *et al*, 2005).

The nearest tabular entries in **Table 9.3** are $\pi_1 = 0.1$, $OR = 2$ and $\pi_1 = 0.1$, $OR = 2.5$ which give, with $\varepsilon_{Plan} = 0.25$, the corresponding $N = 1,656$ and 1,578. The average of these is 1,617. This is quite close to the earlier 1,612.

Table 9.4 and Equation 9.16

Example 9.7 Paired binary data – Association of smoking with blindness and stroke
Bidwell, Sahu, Edwards, *et al* (2005) describe a survey of patients attending a hospital clinic on their awareness, and fear, of blindness (B) due to smoking, in comparison to stroke (S) and other smoking related diseases. A total of 358 patients responded to the survey, with only 34/358 (9.5%) believing that smoking caused blindness, as compared to 253/358 (70.6%) for stroke. This represents a $70.6 - 9.5 = 61.1\%$ difference. Although the authors do not provide full details, the results can be partially summarised as in the left panels of **Figure 9.1**.

The authors did not report any formal sample size calculations carried out before the start of the survey. Suppose however that they had wished to do this and had anticipated that 20% of patients believed smoking caused blindness while 60% believed smoking caused stroke. Moreover, they had planned to obtain a 95% *CI* of the difference in the proportions of width 10% and assumed a correlation coefficient of 0.6.

Since equation (9.16) must be solved iteratively for N, we use **Table 9.4** with $\pi_1 = 0.2$, $\pi_2 = 0.6$, $\omega_{Plan} = 0.1$ and $\rho_{Plan} = 0.6$ to obtain $N = 252$ patients for the survey. However, the final sample size is quite sensitive to the presumed value ρ_{Plan} so that if it takes the values 0.5 and 0.7, the corresponding sample sizes of 312 and 192 are obtained from $\boxed{S_{S}}$.

Tables 2.3 and 9.5 and Equations 9.18 and 9.19

Example 9.8 Continuous data - Small study - Cleft palate
As part of a larger study, Chapman, Hardin-Jones, Goldstein, *et al* (2008, Table 2) give the mean and SD of the number of stable consonants (SC) in 20 children with repaired cleft palate as 10.40 and 4.14 respectively. A repeat of the study is planned in a group of similar children from another location. How large should the study be to ensure that the width of the corresponding 95% *CI* is 3.6SC?

Here the anticipated values are $\sigma_{Plan} = 4.14$ and $\omega_{Plan} = 1.5$, hence $\Lambda_{Plan} = 1.5/4.14 = 0.3623$. For a 95% *CI*, the final term of equation (9.18) gives $N \approx 4 \times 1.96^2/0.3623^2 = 117.07$ or 118. As the $df = N - 1 = 117$ is large, $t_{117,0.975} \approx 1.96$ so that no refinement is required and the final sample size remains 118 or approximately 120 children. Use of $\boxed{^{SS}_S}$ with $\Lambda_{Plan} = 0.3623$ gives $N = 120$. Alternatively, direct entry with $\Lambda_{Plan} = 0.35$ (rather than 0.3623) in **Table 9.5** gives $N = 128$.

Had a larger $\Lambda_{Plan} = 0.7$ (implying $\omega_{Plan} = 3.0$) been anticipated, then the last expression in equation (9.18) gives an initial size of $N_0 \approx 4 \times 1.96^2/0.7^2 = 31.36$ or 32. However, since $N_0 < 40$ it may be regarded as small, so the first component of equation (9.18) is required. Thus with $N_0 = 32$, **Table 2.3** gives $t_{32-1, 0.975} = 2.0395$ leading to $N_1 = 4 \times 2.0395^2/0.7^2 = 33.96$ or 34. Again from **Table 2.3**, $t_{34-1, 0.975} = 2.0345$ resulting in $N_2 = 33.79$ or 34 once more. Thus the final sample size is $N = 34$ as given in **Table 9.5**.

Table 9.5 and Equation 9.22

Example 9.9 Continuous data - Large study - Epidural analgesia during labour and baby delivery
Sng, Woo, Leong, *et al* (2014, Table 2) reported the mean time-weighted local anaesthetic (LA) consumption for the mothers during labour and delivery receiving computer-integrated patient-controlled epidural analgesia (CIPCEA) was 8.9 mg/H (SD = 3.5) in those 76 women randomised to receive no initial basal infusion (CIPCEA0) and 9.9 (SD = 3.5) in the 76 women randomised to receive a 5 ml/H initial basal infusion (CIPCEA5). These results imply an observed difference of 1.0 mg/H with a 95%CI of –0.11 to 2.11 mg/H, which has a width of 2.22 mg/H. The CI covers the null hypothesis value of no difference between the CIPCEA0 and CIPCEA5 groups. What sample size would be required to reduce the 95% CI width to 1.5 mg/H?

Here $\sigma_{Plan} = 3.5$, $\omega_{Plan} = 1.5$ is required, hence $\Lambda_{Plan} = \omega_{Plan}/\sigma_{Plan} = 1.5/3.5 = 0.43$. The latter part of equation (9.22) with $\varphi = 1$ is used to obtain $N_0 = 4\dfrac{(1+1)^2}{1}\dfrac{1.96^2}{0.43^2} = 332.43$ or 334 patients with equal numbers per treatment group. The corresponding entries in **Table 9.5** for Λ_{Plan} equal to 0.40 and 0.45 are 388 and 306 respectively.

Table 9.5 and Equation 9.24

Example 9.10 Paired continuous data - Diastolic blood pressure
Suppose the study reported by Altman and Gardner (2000) in which systolic blood pressure levels in 16 middle-aged men before and after a standard exercise were to be repeated. In that study the mean 'After – Before' exercise difference was 6.6 mmHg, the standard deviation of this difference was 6.0 mmHg and the corresponding 95% CI was from 3.4 to 9.8 mmHg. The new investigators would like to reduce the width of the resulting CI to about 80% of that of the previous one.

The planning values are therefore $\omega_{Plan} = 0.8 \times (9.8 - 3.4) = 5.12$ and $\sigma_{Plan} = 6.0$, hence $\Lambda_{Plan} = 5.12/6.0 = 0.8533$. Using these values in the latter part of equation (9.24) for a 95% CI gives a sample size of $N_{Pairs} = \dfrac{4 \times 1.96^2}{0.8533^2} = 21.1$ or 22 middle-aged men. As $N_{Pairs} < 40$, an iteration is required. Thus from **Table 2.3**, $t_{22-1, 0.975} = 2.0796$, leading to $N_1 = 4 \times 2.0796^2/0.8533^2 = 23.76$ or 24, hence $t_{24-1, 0.975} = 2.0687$ and $N_2 = 4 \times 2.0796^2/0.8533^2 = 23.75$ or 24 once more. This is also given by $\boxed{^{SS}_S}$. Direct entry into **Table 9.5** with $\Lambda_{Plan} = 0.85$ also gives $N = 24$ men.

References

Technical

Altman DG and Gardner MJ (2000). Means and their differences. In Altman DG, Machin D, Bryant TN and Gardner MJ (eds). *Statistics with Confidence.* (2nd edn) British Medical Journal Books, London, 31–32.

Bristol DR (1989). Sample sizes for constructing confidence intervals and testing hypotheses. *Statistics in Medicine*, **8**, 803–811.

Lemeshow S, Hosmer DW and Klar J (1988). Sample size requirements for studies estimating odds ratios or relative risks. *Statistics in Medicine*, **7**, 759–764.

Newcombe RG and Altman DG (2000). Proportions and their differences. In Altman DG, Machin D, Bryant TN and Gardner MJ (eds). *Statistics with Confidence.* (2nd edn) British Medical Journal Books, London, 45–56.

Tan S-H, Machin D and Tan S-B (2012). Sample sizes for estimating differences in proportions – Can we keep things simple? *Journal of Biopharmaceutical Statistics*, **22**, 133–140.

Examples

Baron-Cohen S, Scott FJ, Allison C, Williams J, Bolton P, Matthews FE and Brayne C (2009). Prevalence of autism-spectrum conditions: UK school-based population survey. *The British Journal of Psychiatry*, **194**, 500–509.

Bidwell G, Sahu A, Edwards R, Harrison RA, Thornton J and Kelly SP (2005). Perceptions of blindness related to smoking: a hospital-based cross-sectional study. *Eye*, **19**, 945–948.

Chapman KL, Hardin-Jones MA, Goldstein JA, Halter KA, Havlik J and Schulte J (2008). Timing of palatal surgery and speech outcome. *Cleft Palate-Cranofacial Journal*, **45**, 297–308.

Sng BL, Woo D, Leong WL, Wang H, Assam PN and Sia ATH (2014). Comparison of computer-integrated patient-controlled epidural analgesia with no initial basal infusion versus moderate basal infusion for labor and delivery: A randomized controlled trial. *Journal of Anaesthesiology Clinical Pharmacology*, **30**, 496–501.

Table 9.1 Sample size, *N*, required to observe a pre-specified confidence interval width for an anticipated proportion [from equation (9.5)].

	Confidence Interval (*CI*)							
	90%				95%			
	Planned width of *CI*, ω_{Plan}				Planned width of *CI*, ω_{Plan}			
π_{Plan}	0.05	0.1	0.15	0.2	0.05	0.1	0.15	0.2
0.01	76	30	18	12	108	43	25	17
0.02	107	36	20	14	152	52	29	19
0.03	142	43	23	15	201	61	33	21
0.04	178	51	26	16	252	72	37	23
0.05	214	59	29	18	304	83	41	25
0.06	251	67	32	20	356	95	46	28
0.07	287	75	35	21	407	107	50	30
0.08	323	83	39	23	458	118	55	32
0.09	358	92	42	25	508	130	60	35
0.10	392	100	45	26	554	139	62	35
0.11	426	108	49	28	604	153	69	40
0.12	459	116	52	30	651	164	74	42
0.13	491	123	55	31	696	175	78	44
0.14	522	131	58	33	741	186	83	47
0.15	552	138	62	35	784	196	87	49
0.16	582	146	65	36	826	206	92	51
0.17	611	153	68	38	867	216	96	54
0.18	639	159	71	40	907	226	100	56
0.19	666	166	73	41	945	236	104	58
0.20	692	172	76	43	982	245	108	60
0.25	810	202	89	49	1150	286	126	70
0.30	907	226	99	55	1288	320	141	78
0.35	983	244	107	60	1395	347	152	84
0.40	1037	258	113	63	1472	366	161	89
0.45	1069	266	117	65	1518	377	166	92
0.50	1080	268	118	65	1533	381	167	93

Table 9.2 Sample sizes required to observe a given confidence interval width for the difference between proportions from two independent groups of equal size [derived iteratively from equation (9.11)].

Each cell gives the total number of subjects required, N. Hence, $n_S = n_T = N/2$ will be in each group.

Planning values		Confidence Intervals (CI)							
		90%				95%			
π_1	π_2	Planned width of CI, ω_{Plan}				Planned width of CI, ω_{Plan}			
		0.05	0.1	0.15	0.2	0.05	0.1	0.15	0.2
0.1	0.2	2170	548	246	140	3082	776	350	200
	0.3	2600	652	292	164	3692	926	414	234
	0.4	2858	716	318	180	4058	1014	452	254
	0.5	2944	736	328	184	4180	1044	464	260
	0.6	2856	714	318	178	4056	1014	450	252
	0.7	2598	650	288	162	3688	922	410	230
	0.8	2166	542	242	136	3074	770	342	194
	0.9	1564	394	178	102	2220	560	252	144
0.2	0.3	3202	800	356	200	4546	1136	504	282
	0.4	3462	864	382	214	4914	1226	544	304
	0.5	3548	884	392	220	5036	1256	556	312
	0.6	3460	864	382	214	4912	1226	542	304
	0.7	4332	798	354	198	4544	1134	502	280
	0.8	2770	692	306	172	3932	982	434	244
	0.9	2166	542	242	136	3074	770	342	194
0.3	0.4	3892	970	430	240	5526	1378	610	340
	0.5	3978	992	438	246	5648	1408	622	348
	0.6	3892	970	430	240	5526	1378	608	340
	0.7	3632	906	400	224	5158	1286	568	318
	0.8	4332	798	354	198	4544	1134	502	280
	0.9	2598	650	288	162	3688	922	410	230
0.4	0.5	4238	1056	468	260	6016	1500	662	370
	0.6	4152	1034	458	256	5894	1468	650	362
	0.7	3892	970	430	240	5526	1378	610	340
	0.8	3460	864	382	214	4912	1226	542	304
	0.9	2598	650	288	162	3688	922	410	230
0.5	0.6	4238	1056	468	260	6016	1500	662	370
	0.7	3978	992	438	246	5648	1408	622	348
	0.8	3548	884	392	220	5036	1256	556	312
	0.9	2944	736	328	184	4180	1044	464	260

Table 9.3 Total sample size required to observe a proportionate confidence interval width when comparing two independent groups of equal size expressed via their Odds Ratio (*OR*) [from equation (9.15)].

Each cell gives the total number of subjects required, *N*. Hence, the numbers per group are $n_S = n_T = N/2$.

Planning values		Confidence Intervals (*CI*)							
		90%				95%			
π_1	*OR*	Planning proportion of the *OR*, ε_{Plan}				Planning proportion of the *OR*, ε_{Plan}			
		0.1	0.15	0.2	0.25	0.1	0.15	0.2	0.25
0.1	1.25	9970	4190	2224	1338	14154	5950	3156	1900
	1.50	9398	3950	2096	1262	13344	5608	2976	1790
	1.75	8994	3780	2006	1208	12770	5368	2848	1714
	2.00	8694	3654	1938	1166	12344	5188	2752	1656
	2.50	8282	3482	1848	1112	11760	4942	2622	1578
0.2	1.25	5734	2410	1280	770	8142	3422	1816	1092
	1.50	5506	2314	1228	740	7816	3286	1744	1050
	1.75	5350	2250	1194	718	7596	3192	1694	1020
	2.00	5242	2204	1170	704	7442	3128	1660	998
	2.50	5108	2148	1140	686	7250	3048	1618	974
0.3	1.25	4468	1878	996	600	6344	2666	1416	852
	1.50	4368	1836	974	586	6202	2608	1384	832
	1.75	4312	1814	962	580	5122	2574	1366	822
	2.00	4284	1800	956	576	6082	2556	1356	816
	2.50	4274	1798	954	574	6068	2552	1354	814
0.4	1.25	3998	1680	892	538	5676	2386	1266	762
	1.50	3982	1674	888	534	5654	2376	1262	760
	1.75	3994	1678	892	536	5670	2384	1264	762
	2.00	4022	1692	898	540	5710	2400	1274	766
	2.50	4112	1728	918	552	5838	2454	1302	784
0.5	1.25	3924	1650	876	528	5572	2342	1244	748
	1.50	3982	1674	888	534	5654	2376	1262	760
	1.75	4058	1706	906	546	5760	2422	1284	774
	2.00	4144	1742	924	556	5884	2474	1312	790
	2.50	4340	1824	968	582	6160	2590	1374	828
0.6	1.25	4180	1758	932	562	5936	2496	1324	798
	1.50	4320	1816	964	580	6134	1289	684	824
	1.75	4472	1880	998	600	6350	5156	2832	852
	2.00	4632	1948	1034	622	6576	2764	1466	882
	2.50	4964	2088	1108	666	7048	2964	1572	946
0.7	1.25	4886	2054	1090	656	6936	2916	1548	932
	1.50	5142	2162	1148	990	7302	3070	1628	980
	1.75	5406	2274	1206	726	7676	3226	1712	1030
	2.00	5676	2386	1266	762	8060	3388	1798	1082
	2.50	6224	2616	1388	836	8836	3714	1970	1186
0.8	1.25	6558	2756	1462	880	9310	3914	2076	1250
	1.50	7028	2954	1568	944	9978	4194	2226	1340
	1.75	7370	3154	1674	1008	10654	4478	2376	1430
	2.00	7982	3356	1780	1074	11334	4764	2528	1522
	2.50	8946	3760	1996	1200	12702	5338	2832	1704

Table 9.4 Sample sizes required to observe a given confidence interval width for the difference between two paired or matched proportions [from equation (9.16)].

Each cell gives the number of pairs required, N_{Pairs}.

			Confidence Interval (CI)							
Planning values			**90% CI**				**95% CI**			
ρ	π_1	π_2	Planned width of CI, ω_{Plan}				Planned width of CI, ω_{Plan}			
			0.05	0.1	0.15	0.2	0.05	0.1	0.15	0.2
0.2	0.1	0.3	1063	267	120	68	1508	379	170	96
		0.4	1175	294	131	74	1668	418	186	105
		0.5	1212	303	135	76	1721	430	191	107
		0.6	1174	293	130	73	1667	416	185	104
	0.2	0.4	1392	347	154	86	1976	493	218	122
		0.5	1427	356	158	88	2026	505	224	125
		0.6	1391	347	153	86	1975	492	218	122
		0.7	1283	320	142	79	1822	454	201	112
	0.3	0.5	1593	397	175	98	2261	563	249	139
		0.6	1557	388	171	96	2211	551	243	136
		0.7	1453	362	160	89	2063	514	227	126
		0.8	1283	320	142	79	1822	454	201	112
	0.4	0.6	1660	413	183	102	2357	587	259	144
		0.7	1557	388	171	96	2211	551	243	136
		0.8	1391	347	153	86	1975	492	218	122
		0.9	1174	293	130	73	1667	416	185	104
	0.5	0.7	1593	397	175	98	2261	563	249	139
		0.8	1427	356	158	88	2026	505	224	125
		0.9	1212	303	135	76	1721	430	191	107
0.4	0.1	0.3	825	208	94	54	1172	296	133	76
		0.4	921	231	103	58	1307	328	146	83
		0.5	953	238	106	60	1352	338	150	85
		0.6	920	230	102	57	1305	326	145	81
	0.2	0.4	1053	263	117	65	1494	373	165	93
		0.5	1081	270	119	67	1535	383	169	95
		0.6	1052	262	116	65	1493	372	164	92
		0.7	966	241	106	59	1371	341	151	84
	0.3	0.6	1169	291	128	71	1659	413	182	101
		0.7	1089	271	120	66	1546	385	169	94
		0.8	966	241	106	59	1371	341	151	84
	0.4	0.6	1245	310	136	76	1767	439	194	107
		0.7	1169	291	128	71	1659	413	182	101
		0.8	1052	262	116	65	1493	372	164	92
		0.9	920	230	102	57	1305	326	145	81
	0.5	0.7	1196	298	131	73	1698	423	186	104
		0.8	1081	270	119	67	1535	383	169	95
		0.9	953	238	106	60	1352	338	150	85

(Continued)

Table 9.4 (Continued)

Planning values			Confidence Interval (CI)							
			90% CI				95% CI			
ρ	π_1	π_2	Planned width of CI, ω_{Plan}				Planned width of CI, ω_{Plan}			
			0.05	0.1	0.15	0.2	0.05	0.1	0.15	0.2
0.6	0.1	0.3	589	150	69	40	836	213	97	57
		0.4	667	168	75	43	946	238	107	61
		0.5	693	174	77	44	984	246	110	62
		0.6	665	166	74	41	944	236	105	59
	0.2	0.4	714	179	80	45	1014	254	113	64
		0.5	735	183	81	45	1044	260	115	64
		0.6	713	177	78	44	1012	252	111	62
		0.7	648	161	71	39	920	229	101	56
	0.3	0.5	800	199	88	49	1135	282	124	69
		0.6	780	194	85	47	1107	275	121	67
		0.7	726	180	79	44	1030	256	112	62
		0.8	648	161	71	39	920	229	101	56
	0.4	0.6	829	206	90	50	1177	292	128	71
		0.7	780	194	85	47	1107	275	121	67
		0.8	713	177	78	44	1012	252	111	62
		0.9	665	166	74	41	944	236	105	59
	0.5	0.7	800	199	88	49	1135	282	124	69
		0.8	735	183	81	45	1044	260	115	64
		0.9	693	174	77	44	984	246	110	62
0.8	0.1	0.3	353	93	44	27	500	131	62	38
		0.4	413	105	48	28	586	149	68	39
		0.5	433	109	48	27	615	154	69	39
		0.6	410	102	45	25	582	145	64	36
	0.2	0.4	377	96	44	25	535	136	62	36
		0.5	390	98	44	25	554	139	62	35
		0.6	374	93	41	23	530	132	58	32
		0.7	331	82	36	20	470	116	51	28
	0.3	0.5	403	100	44	24	572	142	62	34
		0.6	391	97	42	23	556	137	59	32
		0.7	362	89	39	21	514	126	55	30
		0.8	331	82	36	20	470	116	51	28
	0.4	0.6	413	102	44	24	587	144	62	34
		0.7	391	97	42	23	556	137	59	32
		0.8	374	93	41	23	530	132	58	32
		0.9	410	102	45	25	582	145	64	36
	0.5	0.7	403	100	44	24	572	142	62	34
		0.8	390	98	44	25	554	139	62	35
		0.9	433	109	48	27	615	154	69	39

Table 9.5 Sample sizes for a planned confidence interval width for (a) single mean, *N*, or a matched pair of means, N_{Pair}. [derived from equations (9.18) and (9.24)] and (b) the difference between two means from independent groups of equal size ($N=2n$) [from equation (9.22)].

	(a)		(b)	
	N: Equation (9.18) N_{Pairs}: Equation (9.24)		$N=2n$: Equation (9.22)	
Λ_{Plan}	*CI*: 90%	*CI*: 95%	*CI*: 90%	*CI*: 95%
0.05	4,331	6,149	17,318	24,588
0.10	1,085	1,540	4.332	6,150
0.15	483	686	1,926	2,736
0.20	273	387	1,086	1,540
0.25	176	249	696	986
0.30	123	174	484	686
0.35	91	128	356	506
0.40	70	99	274	388
0.45	56	79	216	306
0.50	46	64	176	250
0.55	38	54	146	206
0.60	32	46	124	174
0.65	28	39	106	148
0.70	24	34	92	128
0.75	22	30	80	112
0.80	19	27	70	100
0.85	17	24	62	88
0.90	16	22	56	80
0.95	14	20	50	72
1.0	13	18	46	64
1.1	11	16	38	54
1.2	10	14	34	46
1.3	9	12	28	40
1.4	8	11	26	34
1.5	7	10	22	30
1.6	7	9	20	28
1.7	6	8	18	24
1.8	6	8	16	22
1.9	6	7	16	20
2.0	5	7	14	18

10

Repeated Outcome Measures

SUMMARY
Sample size requirements for two group repeated measure designs from a continuous outcome measure are described. These designs may include repeated pre-intervention as well as repeated post-intervention assessments over time. The relevant measure of the difference between interventions may be, for example, the difference in means of all the post-assessment values in each group or the respective slopes of a linear regression obtained from these values. If baseline or additional pre-assessment measures are available, then any analysis will take these into account.
In some circumstances, particularly if a single specimen from an individual such as a histology slide is repeatedly assessed several times by the same individual (or possibly different individuals), the influence of the time element may be ignored and the mean of the various assessments is then taken as the outcome measure of interest. An example of this type of application is included.

10.1 Design Features

A common clinical trial design is one which measures the outcome variable of concern repeatedly over time. In some cases, the outcome is also measured at the baseline (immediately before allocation to the respective interventions is made), and in some situations also at times preceding the baseline.

Illustration

Consider the trial described by Levy, Milanowski, Chakrapani, *et al* (2007) where blood phenylalanine concentration was assessed in patients with phenylketonuria at 4 time points before and 4 time points after randomised assignment to Placebo (P) or Salpropterin (S). A summary of their results is given in **Figure 10.1**. They measured the blood phenylalanine concentrations at 2 weeks and 1 week before randomisation, at randomisation (week 0) and at 1, 2, 4 and 6 weeks afterwards. They were particularly interested in the 6-week outcome, and used earlier measurements to impute values that may have been missing at 6 weeks (using the last observation carried forward for the procedure).

However, the reasons for measuring the outcome repeatedly are not always made clear by investigators. Commonly, they might wish to investigate the time response of the intervention. For example, they might want to see whether the treatment increases response quite rapidly and then stays constant, or whether any benefit consistently accumulates. Often the main investigation is to look at the

Sample Sizes for Clinical, Laboratory and Epidemiology Studies, Fourth Edition. David Machin, Michael J. Campbell, Say Beng Tan and Sze Huey Tan.
© 2018 John Wiley & Sons Ltd. Published 2018 by John Wiley & Sons Ltd.

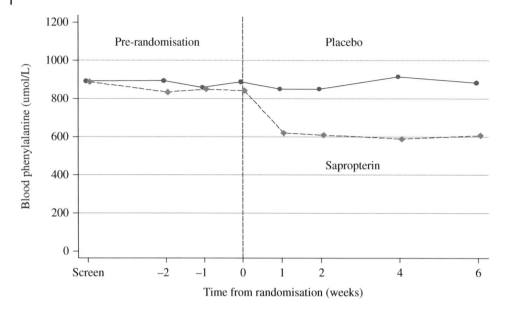

Figure 10.1 Mean blood phenylalanine concentration over time in patients with phenylketonuria pre-and post-randomisation to Placebo (*P*) or Salpropterin (*S*) (after Levy, Milanowski, Chakrapani, *et al*, 2007).

long-term benefit, so a study may consider the final measurement as the main endpoint. In any event, the sample size calculation requires a specific model for the analysis to be identified.

In general if there are a total of ν baseline and pre-baseline measures and w post-randomisation measures, then $t = -\nu + 1,\ -\nu + 2,\ ...,\ -1,\ 0,\ 1,\ 2,\ ...,\ w - 1,\ w$. For example, the study shown in **Figure 10.1** has 3 pre-baseline measures and a baseline, hence $\nu = 4$. Further, there are 4 post-randomisation measures so $w = 4$. Thus values for patient i are therefore denoted $y_{i,Screen},\ y_{i,-2},\ y_{i,-1},\ y_{i0},\ y_{i1},\ y_{i2},\ y_{i4},$ and y_{i6}.

Models and Intra-class Correlation

A simple model for these continuous data is

$$y_{it} = \alpha_0 + \beta x_{it} + \varepsilon_{it}, \tag{10.1}$$

where there are $i = 1,\ 2,\ ...,\ N = n_S + n_T$ subjects. This model implies that prior to randomisation, all subjects commence at the same underlying baseline value with a population mean of α_0, while at post-randomisation the two groups will differ by β in their population means. Randomisation occurs at the time $t = 0$, so n_T individuals are allocated the *Test* (*T*) intervention, which implies $x_{it} = 1$ once $t > 0$, and similarly $x_{it} = 0$ for the n_S assigned to *Standard* (*S*). This corresponds to the situation of **Figure 10.1** where one might anticipate values for α_0 and β close to 900 and 200 μmol/L respectively.

It is usual to assume the ε_{it} are Normally distributed with a constant variance σ^2. Nevertheless, given that the measures over time are repeated on a single individual, the ε_{it} are unlikely to be independent.

An extension of equation (10.1) is to assume that each individual i has their own baseline value, or intercept, α_{0i}^*. Assuming there are no pre-randomisation assessments, the model becomes

$$y_{it} = \alpha_{0i}^* + \beta x_{it} + \eta_{it}, \tag{10.2}$$

where $t = 1, 2, ..., w$. This is known as the *random intercepts* model. Here, the α_{0i}^* are assumed to follow an independent Normal distribution with mean α_0^* and variance, σ_α^2 while the η_{it} are also assumed to have an independent Normal distribution but with mean 0 and variance σ^2.

It follows that the correlation between any two measurements on the *same* individual is given by

$$\rho = \frac{\sigma_\alpha^2}{\sigma_\alpha^2 + \sigma^2}. \tag{10.3}$$

This is known as 'compound symmetry' or the 'exchangeable' assumption. It is the same assumption that is made in the analysis of cluster randomised trials of **Chapter 12** where ρ is termed the intra-class correlation coefficient (*ICC*).

Models (10.1) and (10.2) can be extended to allow for baseline and pre-baseline measures by allowing values of t to be zero and negative. Thus, as indicated above, the (final) baseline measure would be taken just prior to $t = 0$ and earlier baseline values will have an associated t which is negative. Thus with a single baseline measure at $t = 0$, we have

$$y_{it} = \gamma_0 y_{0i} + \alpha_{0i}^* + \beta x_{it} + \eta_{it}, \tag{10.4}$$

where γ_0 is the regression coefficient corresponding to the baseline measure and $t = 1, 2, ..., w$. Note that equation (10.1) estimates the common intercept using only post-randomisation observations whereas in equation (10.4) the actual baseline values are included in the model.

This model can be extended by adding additional pre-baseline covariates $y_{-1,i}, y_{-2,i}, ..., y_{-v+1,i}$ with corresponding regression coefficients $\gamma_{-1}, \gamma_{-2}, ..., \gamma_{-v+1}$, to give

$$y_{it} = \gamma_{-v+1} y_{i,-v+1} + ... + \gamma_{-2} y_{i,-2} + \gamma_{-1} y_{i,-1} + \gamma_0 y_{i0} + \alpha_{0i}^* + \beta x_{it} + \eta_{it}. \tag{10.5}$$

One method of analysis for such a situation is to compute for each individual the mean of their pre-randomisation observations, $\bar{y}_{Pre,i}$ and the mean of those post-randomisation, $\bar{y}_{Post,i}$. The corresponding model now becomes

$$\bar{y}_{post,i} = \gamma_0 \bar{y}_{pre,i} + \alpha_{0i}^* + \beta x_i + \varepsilon_i. \tag{10.6}$$

The suffix t is no longer present as the observations over the time points have been averaged and so there is no longer any time dependence. Such an analysis would imply obtaining the mean from Screen, -2, -1 and 0 week values and those from weeks 1, 2, 4 and 6 for each individual contributing to **Figure 10.1**.

10.2 Design Effects and Sample Size

Endpoint: Post-intervention Means

In this case, the two interventions are compared, using the difference in post-treatment means between the groups as the effect size and the pre-treatment means as a covariate. Then with the anticipated effect size, δ_{Plan}, and corresponding SD, σ_{Plan}, the total sample size for a 1: φ allocation, 2-sided test α and power $1 - \beta$ uses equation (5.4) to give

$$N = R \times \left[\frac{\left(1+\varphi\right)^2}{\varphi} \frac{\left(z_{1-\alpha/2} + z_{1-\beta}\right)^2}{\left(\delta_{Plan}/\sigma_{Plan}\right)^2} + \frac{z_{1-\alpha/2}^2}{2} \right], \tag{10.7}$$

where what is termed the design effect (*DE*) is

$$R = \left[\frac{1+\left(w-1\right)\rho}{w} - \frac{v\rho^2}{\left[1+\left(v-1\right)\rho\right]} \right]. \tag{10.8}$$

For the case of no pre-baseline or earlier observations, $v = 0$ and (10.8) becomes

$$R = \left[\frac{1+\left(w-1\right)\rho}{w} \right]. \tag{10.9}$$

This latter expression is very similar in form to **Chapter 12** equation (12.5) for the *DE* for a clustered data study except that w in the numerator is replaced by m to distinguish the two situations and there is no divisor.

Table 10.1 gives the value of R for differing v, w and ρ. It shows that R goes *up* with ρ when $v = 0$ and goes *down* with ρ when $v > 0$. This is because when $v = 0$ we are only considering the mean of the post-treatment measurements, and the variance of this mean increases as ρ increases. In general, as v increases, R decreases, as does its value as w increases. These decreases in R imply a reduction in required sample size for a given effect size, test size and power. In contrast, as ρ increases, R tends to first increase to a maximum and thereafter declines. When a baseline measurement is made, hence $v \geq 1$, then the effect is to reduce R and hence the sample size.

The treatment effect is now conditional on the alternative interventions having the same baseline value. This is always the case when the interventions are assigned at random. In the case of one baseline and one outcome measure, $v = w = 1$, and equation (10.8) implies $R = 1 - \rho^2$. This can have dramatic effects on the required sample size. Thus even under a relatively weak assumption that $\rho = 0.5$, the required sample size is reduced by 25%.

However, the assumption of equal baseline values for all subjects is not necessarily true for groups obtained from observational data where, for example, subjects with high values at baseline may be more likely to get the test intervention. An alternative in these circumstances is to look at the absolute change from the baseline for each subject, $y_{it} - y_{i0}$, although this may also be the relevant outcome measure in a clinical trial. Here we are treating the baseline as if it were an 'outcome' measure, and so essentially $v = 0$, $w = 2$ and hence from equation (10.9) $R = (1 + \rho)/2$. However, the analysis assumes the effect size is the average of the baseline measure and that taken at follow-up time, t. In which case, this average estimates half the slope of the regression model (10.2), namely $\beta/2$. Consequently, we need to multiply the design effect by 4 to get the adjustment for the sample size.

This leads to a modified $R = 4 \times [(1+\rho)/2] = 2(1+\rho)$. This shows that the analysis using absolute changes will always require a larger sample size than an analysis of the outcome measure, y_{it}, on its own. This is because the baseline is measured with the same error as the outcome, and this leads to an increased variance when it is used to establish the change. This contrasts to the situation when the analysis of covariance (effectively adjusting for baseline) is used, which will always lead to a reduction in the sample size required provided $\rho \neq 0$.

Endpoint: Post-intervention Slopes

If an investigator was interested in comparing two slopes, we need the time that each measurement was made, $t_1, t_2, \ldots, t_w$, to be recorded so that

$$D_t^2 = \sum_{j=1}^{w}\left(t_j - \bar{t}\right)^2 = \sum_{j=1}^{w} t_j^2 - \frac{\left(\sum_{j=1}^{w} t_j\right)^2}{w} \tag{10.10}$$

can be calculated. In which case, the DE of equation (10.8) is replaced by

$$R_{Slope} = \frac{1-\rho}{D_t^2}. \tag{10.11}$$

Then, for a random intercepts model with slopes considered fixed, SD of the intercepts σ_{Plan}, and assuming compound symmetry with fixed ρ, the total number of subjects required to detect a difference in slopes, δ_{Plan} uses equation (10.7) with R replaced by R_{Slope}.

Endpoint: Selected Post-intervention Assessements

In certain circumstances, a particular comparison of the repeated observations is of interest. For example, although post-randomisation observations may be taken on w occasions, only the mean value from the last two, when compared to a baseline assessment, may be of particular interest. For planning purposes, in this case, the investigators would have to specify an effect size δ_{Plan} as the anticipated difference between $\mu_{Plan} = \mu_{Baseline} - (\mu_{w-1} + \mu_w)/2$ for S and T, where $\mu_{Baseline}$, μ_{w-1} and μ_w are the anticipated mean values at the respective observation points. At the analysis stage, this would imply the calculation of the contrast $C = -1 \times y_0 + 0.5 \times y_{w-1} + 0.5 \times y_w$ for each subject, and then the mean of these values for each intervention group would be compared.

In general, the contrast for each group is defined by

$$C = \sum_{k} W_k \mu_k, \tag{10.12}$$

where the values taken for k will depend on the weights chosen for the $v + w$ observation points. The corresponding variance is given by

$$Var(C) = \sum_{l}\sum_{k} W_l W_k \theta_{lk}, \tag{10.13}$$

Weights	$W_0=-1$	$W_{w-1}=0.5$	$W_w=0.5$
$W_0=-1$	$W_0^2\sigma^2=\sigma^2$	$W_0W_{w-1}\rho\sigma^2=-0.5\rho\sigma^2$	$W_0W_w\rho\sigma^2=-0.5\rho\sigma^2$
$W_{w-1}=0.5$	$W_{w-1}W_0\rho\sigma^2=-0.5\rho\sigma^2$	$W_{w-1}^2\sigma^2=0.25\sigma^2$	$W_{w-1}W_w\rho\sigma^2=0.25\rho\sigma^2$
$W_w=0.5$	$W_wW_0\rho\sigma^2=-0.5\rho\sigma^2$	$W_wW_{w-1}\rho\sigma^2=0.25\rho\sigma^2$	$W_w^2\sigma^2=0.25\sigma^2$
$Var(C)=(1+0.25+0.25)\,\sigma^2+(-0.5-0.5-0.5+0.25-0.5+0.25)\rho\sigma^2=1.5(1-\rho)\sigma^2.$			

Figure 10.2 Structure of the anticipated variance, $Var(C)$, for a contrast with 3 weights: -1, 0.5 and 0.5 and assuming compound symmetry for ρ.

Weights	$W_0=-1$	$W_2=0.5$	$W_5=0.5$
$W_0=-1$	$W_0^2\sigma^2=\sigma^2$	$W_0W_2\rho^2\sigma^2=-0.5\rho^2\sigma^2$	$W_0W_5\rho^5\sigma^2=-0.5\rho^5\sigma^2$
$W_2=0.5$	$W_2W_0\rho^2\sigma^2=-0.5\rho^2\sigma^2$	$W_2^2\sigma^2=0.25\sigma^2$	$W_2W_5\rho^3\sigma^2=0.25\rho^3\sigma^2$
$W_5=0.5$	$W_5W_0\rho^5\sigma^2=-0.5\rho^5\sigma^2$	$W_5W_2\rho\sigma^2=0.25\rho^3\sigma^2$	$W_5^2\sigma^2=0.25\sigma^2$
$Var(C)=(1.5-\rho^2+0.5\rho^3-\rho^5)\,\sigma^2.$			

Figure 10.3 Structure of the anticipated variance, $Var(C)$, for a contrast with 3 weights: -1, 0.5 and 0.5 at 0, 2 and 5 years assuming $AR(1)$ with ρ being the per year intraclass correlation.

In the case of compound symmetry, θ_{lk} equals σ^2 when $l=k$ and equals $\rho\sigma^2$ when $l\neq k$. This then leads the corresponding multiplier for use in equation (10.7) as

$$R_{Weight}=Var(C)/\sigma^2. \tag{10.14}$$

An example of the structure of $Var(C)$ is given in **Figure 10.2**.

If, in the case when w post-randomisation observations are made and the weights are defined by $W_k=\dfrac{(t_k-\bar{t})}{\sum_k(t_k-\bar{t})^2}$, then this is essentially the situation when the slope is to be estimated. This therefore leads to the equivalent of the use of equation (10.11) for sample size purposes. Further in this situation with the weights $W_k=1/w$, then we have the situation of equation (10.9).

An alternative is to assume that the ICC, ρ, gets weaker the further apart in time the measurements are made. Commonly, it is assumed that this may decay geometrically so that observations between two successive observations taken T units of time apart have a correlation equal to ρ^T. This is known as the autoregressive order one, $AR(1)$, correlation. An example of how this affects $Var(C)$ is given in **Figure 10.3**.

10.3 Practicalities

When considering the special case $v=w=1$ in which there is only a single post-intervention assessment, the design effect of equation (10.8) reduces to $R=1-\rho^2$, which with $\rho=0.5$ gives $R=0.75$. Thus, the addition of a baseline to a single post-randomisation assessment design reduces the sample size required.

In general, by taking repeated measurements at regular time points, the required total sample size is considerably reduced. Nevertheless, there is a practical limit to increasing the number of post-randomisation assessments. Thus, with $v = 1$ but with w increasing to infinity, R approaches $\rho(1 - \rho)$. The maximum value of this occurs when $\rho = 0.5$ and $R_{Max} = 0.25$. Thus, the best we can do by increasing w is to reduce the sample size to a quarter of that of a design with the outcome measure assessed once with no (pre-randomisation) covariates involved.

Frison and Pocock (1992) have suggested that values of the intraclass correlation coefficient, ρ, between 0.60 and 0.75 are common in repeated measure designs.

Fitzmaurice, Laird and Ware (2011, p596) indicate that the assumption of a fixed slope is likely to give an underestimate of the sample size and should be regarded as a minimum requirement. They also discuss how missing assessments can be accounted for in the analysis by suggesting that if the proportion likely to drop out is W, then they advise increasing the initial estimate of the sample size by dividing it by $(1 - W)$.

10.4 Bibliography

Matthews, Altman, Campbell and Royston (1990) described the use of summary measures to analyse longitudinal data. Frison and Pocock (1992), see also Frison and Pocock (1997), describe equation (10.7) and they also discuss the relative merits of the use of analysis of covariance compared to change-from-baseline methods of analysis. Diggle, Heagerty, Liang and Zeger (2002) discuss the different types of models to analyse longitudinal data and give equation (10.11) when post-intervention slopes are to be compared. Fitzmaurice, Laird and Ware (2011. Equation (20.6)) describe equation (10.13).

10.5 Examples

Table 2.2
For two-sided test size, $\alpha = 0.05$, $z_{0.975} = 1.96$ For one-sided $1 - \beta = 0.8$ and 0.9, $z_{0.8} = 0.8416$ and $z_{0.9} = 1.2816$

Table 10.1 and Equations 10.7 and 10.8

Example 10.1   Repeated pre- and post-intervention observations - Phenylketonuria
Suppose a similar trial to that conducted by Levy, Milanowski, Chakrapani, *et al* (2007) in patients with phenylketonuria is planned. The new investigators anticipate a similar response profile (see **Figure 10.2**) but with mean lowering in blood phenylalanine with Sepropterin (*S*) as compared to Placebo (*P*) of about $\delta_{Plan} = 250$ rather than the earlier study's estimated difference of 300 µmol/L. They further assume $\sigma_{Plan} = 400$ µmol/L. However, although they plan to repeat the earlier design (omitting the initial screening) with $v = 3$ pre- and $w = 4$ post-randomisation assessments, they are uncertain as to the value of ρ (assuming compound symmetry) to adopt. Consequently, they use equation (10.8) to investigate a range of options for R and the impact of these on the subsequent trial size assuming 2-sided $\alpha = 0.05$, $\beta = 0.1$ and using equation (10.7). Their results are summarized in **Figure 10.4**.

Repeated measures design		$v=3$, $w=4$					
Planning assumptions		$\delta_{Plan}=250$, $\sigma_{Plan}=400$					
Statistical requirements		2-sided $\alpha=0.05$, Power $1-\beta=0.9$					
Planning values	ρ	0.001	0.05	0.1	**0.2**	0.3	0.4
Design effect	R	0.251	0.281	0.300	**0.314**	0.306	0.283
Sample size	N	28	32	34	**36**	34	32
Assessments	$A=N\times(v+w)$	196	224	238	**252**	238	224

Figure 10.4 Planning values assumed for a repeated measures design and consequential changes in the proposed sample size with compound symmetry for differing autocorrelation values.

Figure 10.4 suggests that as ρ increases the value of R increases to a maximum of 0.314 and thereafter falls in value. At this maximum, the corresponding sample size is $N=36$, implying 18 patients will be randomised to receive S and 18 P. Thus, the investigators judge it wise to be conservative in their choice and use this number for their trial, taking due account that this will imply that $A=252$ assessments will be necessary. Note that for a relatively wide range of values the specific correlation size chosen has little influence on the sample size.

If they were unable to make repeated measures, or the outcome was simply the last measurement, then the sample size increases. For example, for a single baseline, one further measure and keeping all the other parameters the same, then if $\rho=0.3$, $R=0.910$, $N=100$ subjects and $A=2\times100=200$ assessments are necessary. For $\rho=0.05$. $R=0.998$, $N=110$ subjects with $A=220$ assessments.

Table 10.1 and Equations 10.7 and 10.8

Example 10.2 Single pre- and repeated post-intervention observations - Lifestyle intervention for diabetes

In a randomised trial of a lifestyle intervention for type 2 diabetes, Davies, Heller, Skinner, *et al* (2008) measured HbA1c at times 0, 4, 8 and 12 months. This was a cluster randomised trial, but for the purpose of this example we will treat it as individually randomised. The authors included a baseline covariate in the analysis, but this was not allowed for in the sample size calculation.

Suppose 0.5% is regarded as a meaningful change in HbA1c, previous experience suggests a SD of 2.0%, and the same correlation between the measurements at any time point (compound symmetry) is assumed. Then with $\varphi=1$, 2-sided $\alpha=0.05$, $1-\beta=0.9$, $v=1$ and $w=3$, equation (10.8) or **Table 10.1** gives for $\rho=0.5$, $R=0.417$. From equation (10.7) we obtain the total number subjects required as $N=282$. For $\rho=0.2$, $R=0.427$ and $N=288$. Had the baseline observation been omitted, the values of R would increase to 0.667 and 0.467 and consequently the number of subjects required would increase to 450 and 316 respectively. In general, adding a baseline observation reduces sample size.

If only the 12-month outcome was of interest, implying $w = 1$, then with $v = 1$, $\rho = 0.5$, $R = 0.750$ and $N = 506$ while with $\rho = 0.2$, $R = 0.960$ and $N = 648$. The magnitude of the correlation now has a much greater influence on R and consequently the final sample size.

Equations 10.7 and 10.9

Example 10.3   Repeated assessments of the same radiographs - Hip osteoarthritis

Ornetti, Gossec, Laroche, *et al* (2015) looked at 50 radiographs obtained from patients with hip osteoarthritis. One experienced radiographer then measured, in a blinded and random fashion, the hip-joint space width, r_i ($i = 1, ..., 12$), from each radiograph on 12 successive occasions.

The difference between the first two readings, $d_1 = r_1 - r_2$, from each radiograph was calculated, from these the corresponding mean difference, $\bar{d}_1$, was obtained and the corresponding standard deviation of the differences was $SD_1 = 0.37$. Subsequently, $d_2 = (r_1 + r_2)/2 - (r_3 + r_4)/2$ was calculated and $\bar{d}_2$ and $SD_2 = 0.30$ obtained. The next calculations compared the first three and second three readings, and so on.

If the radiograph readings had been completely independent of each other, we would have expected that SD_2 would be reduced to $SD_1/\sqrt{2} = 0.2616$ rather than the calculated 0.30. In fact, from equation (10.9) with w increased from 1 to 2, the reduction in SD would be anticipated to be $\sqrt{R} = \sqrt{\dfrac{1+\rho}{2}}$. Equating this to the actual reduction, $\sqrt{[(1+\rho)/2]} = 0.30/0.37 = 0.8108$, and this implies $\rho = 0.3148$.

Using a clinically important difference of $\delta_{Plan} = 0.27$ mm and $\sigma_{Plan} = 0.37$ mm in radiographs from patients receiving S and T interventions, equation (10.7), with only one reading per radiograph so that $R = 1$, and setting $\varphi = 1$, 2-sided $\alpha = 0.05$, $1 - \beta = 0.8$ suggests that $N = 62$ radiographs would be required to be read for a potential independent groups comparative trial. However, increasing from a single reading to $w = 2$, 3 and 4 readings (by the same radiographer) with $\rho = 0.3148$ reduces R of equation (10.9) to 0.6574, 0.5432 and 0.4861 and therefore patient numbers to 42, 34 and 32 respectively.

If the radiographer measured exactly the same value each time, then $\rho = 1$ and consequently $R = 1$ whatever w, and there would be no reduction in sample size by increasing the number of readings. In fact Ornetti, Gossec, Laroche, *et al* (2015) recommended that at least three joint space width measurements were made for each radiograph

This example demonstrates that in situations where a measurement has considerable (observer) error, it is worth repeating the measurement and using the average to reduce the variability of the measure and thus the required sample size in any associated study. Clearly, these measurements should be made in a blinded fashion otherwise the person making the measurements could bias the results toward some common value, which would increase ρ and thus require the relevant study size also to be increased.

Equations 10.7, 10.10 and 10.11

Example 10.4   Linear decline - Blood pressure

Diggle, Heagerty, Liang and Zeger (2002) considered a hypothetical trial concerning a treatment to reduce blood pressure. It was thought that the blood pressure would go down steadily, and so the rate of decline was the key outcome variable. A negative slope of 0.5 mmHg per year was deemed clinically important. The measurements were to be made at baseline, 2 and 5 years. Thus, from equation (10.10), $D_t^2 = [0^2 + 2^2 + 5^2] - [0 + 2 + 5]^2 / 3 = 12.67$.

For ρ equal to 0.2, equation (10.11) gives $R_{Slope} = (1 - 0.2)/12.67 = 0.063$. For a 2-sided $\alpha = 0.05$, $1 - \beta = 0.8$, SD of the intercept of 10 mmHg equation (10.7) gives

$$N = 0.063 \times \left[\frac{(1+1)^2}{1} \frac{(1.96 + 0.8416)^2}{(0.5/10)^2} + \frac{1.96^2}{2} \right] = 0.063 \times 12,560.13 = 794 \text{ or } 800 \text{ subjects implying}$$

2,400 assessments. For $\rho = 0.5$ and $R_{Slope} = 0.039$, the corresponding sample size $N = 496$ or 500 subjects implying 1,500 assessments. In this example, the sample size reduces as the correlation ρ increases.

Equation 10.7, 10.12, 10.13, and 10.14

Example 10.5   Attaining a plateau - Blood pressure
Suppose the investigators of Example 10.4 thought that the benefit could be achieved in two years and thereafter plateau. This implies the weights of equation (10.12) to be those of **Figure 10.2**, that is $W_0 = -1$, $W_1 = W_2 = 0.5$ and, if compound symmetry is assumed, $Var(C) = 1.5 \times (1 - \rho) \sigma^2$. Thus, with $\rho = 0.2$, equations (10.13) and (10.14) lead to $R_{Weight} = 1.2$.

Keeping the other parameters the same (2-sided $\alpha = 0.05$, $1 - \beta = 0.8$, $SD = 10$ mmHg), then equation (10.7) becomes $N = 1.2 \times \left[\frac{(1+1)^2}{1} \frac{(1.96 + 0.8416)^2}{(2.5/10)^2} + \frac{1.96^2}{2} \right] = 1.2 \times 504.25 = 605.10$ or 606. In contrast, for $\rho = 0.5$, $R_{Weight} = 0.75$ and $N = 380$ subjects. Fewer subjects than those of Example 10.4 are needed because the benefit is assumed larger, being achieved at 2 rather than 5 years.

If the authors preferred to assume first order autocorrelation, $AR(1)$ of **Figure 10.3**, rather than compound symmetry, then for $\rho = 0.2$, $R_{Weight} = (1.5 - 0.2^2 + 0.5 \times 0.2^3 - 0.2^5) = 1.4637$ while for $\rho = 0.5$, $R_{weight} = 1.2813$. These values result in trials of planned 740 and 646 subjects respectively.

References

Technical
Diggle PJ, Heagerty P, Liang KY and Zeger AL (2002). *Analysis of Longitudinal Data* (2nd ed). Oxford University Press.
Fitzmaurice GM, Laird NM and Ware JH (2011). *Applied Longitudinal Analysis*. (2nd ed). Wiley, Hoboken.
Frison L and Pocock SJ (1992). Repeated measures in clinical trials: analysis using mean summary statistics and its implications for design. *Statistics in Medicine*, **11**, 1685–1704.
Frison L and Pocock SJ (1997). Linearly divergent treatment effects in clinical trials with repeated measures: efficient analysis using summary statistics. *Statistics in Medicine* **16**, 2855–2872.
Matthews JNS, Altman DG, Campbell MJ and Royston JP (1990). Analysis of serial measurements in medical research. *British Medical Journal*, **300**, 230–235.

Examples

Davies MJ, Heller S, Skinner TC, Campbell MJ, Carey ME, Cradock S, Dallosso HM, Daly H, Doherty Y, Eaton S, Fox C, Oliver L, Rantell K, Rayman G and Khunti K (2008). Effectiveness of the diabetes education and self management for ongoing and newly diagnosed (DESMOND) programme for people with newly diagnosed type 2 diabetes: cluster randomised controlled trial. *British Medical Journal*, **336**, 491–495.

Levy HL, Milanowski A, Chakrapani A, Cleary M, Lee P, Trefz FK, Whitley CB, Feillet F, Feigenbaum AS, Bebchuk JD, Christ-Schmidt H and Dorenbaum A (2007). Efficacy of sepropterin dihydrochloride (tetrahydrobiopterin, 6R-BH4) for reduction of phenylalanine concentration in patients with phenylketonuria: a phase III randomised placebo-controlled study. *Lancet*, **370**, 504–510.

Ornetti P, Gossec L, Laroche D, Combescure C, Dougados M and Maillfert J-F (2015). Impact of repeated measures of joint space width on the sample size calculation: An application of hip osteoarthritis. *Joint Bone Spine*, **82**, 172–176.

Table 10.1 Multiplying factor for repeated measures designs summarised by comparing post-intervention means from each of two groups [Equation 10.8]. *v*: number of pre-intervention assessments including baseline; *w*: number of post-intervention assessments.

v	*w*	ρ								
		0.1	0.2	0.3	0.4	0.5	0.6	0.7	0.8	0.9
0	1	1.000	1.000	1.000	1.000	1.000	1.000	1.000	1.000	1.000
	2	0.550	0.600	0.650	0.700	0.750	0.800	0.850	0.900	0.950
	3	0.400	0.467	0.533	0.600	0.667	0.733	0.800	0.867	0.933
	4	0.325	0.400	0.475	0.550	0.625	0.700	0.775	0.850	0.925
	5	0.280	0.360	0.440	0.520	0.600	0.680	0.760	0.840	0.920
1	1	0.990	0.960	0.910	0.840	0.750	0.640	0.510	0.360	0.190
	2	0.540	0.560	0.560	0.540	0.500	0.440	0.360	0.260	0.140
	3	0.390	0.427	0.443	0.440	0.417	0.373	0.310	0.227	0.123
	4	0.315	0.360	0.385	0.390	0.375	0.340	0.285	0.210	0.115
	5	0.270	0.320	0.350	0.360	0.350	0.320	0.270	0.200	0.110
2	1	0.982	0.933	0.862	0.771	0.667	0.550	0.424	0.289	0.147
	2	0.532	0.533	0.512	0.471	0.417	0.350	0.274	0.189	0.097
	3	0.382	0.400	0.395	0.371	0.333	0.283	0.224	0.156	0.081
	4	0.307	0.333	0.337	0.321	0.292	0.250	0.199	0.139	0.072
	5	0.262	0.293	0.302	0.291	0.267	0.230	0.184	0.129	0.067
3	1	0.975	0.914	0.831	0.733	0.625	0.509	0.388	0.262	0.132
	2	0.525	0.514	0.481	0.433	0.375	0.309	0.238	0.162	0.082
	3	0.375	0.381	0.365	0.333	0.292	0.242	0.188	0.128	0.065
	4	0.300	0.314	0.306	0.283	0.250	0.209	0.163	0.112	0.057
	5	0.255	0.274	0.271	0.253	0.225	0.189	0.148	0.102	0.052
4	1	0.969	0.900	0.811	0.709	0.600	0.486	0.368	0.247	0.124
	2	0.519	0.500	0.461	0.409	0.350	0.286	0.218	0.147	0.074
	3	0.369	0.367	0.344	0.309	0.267	0.219	0.168	0.114	0.058
	4	0.294	0.300	0.286	0.259	0.225	0.186	0.143	0.097	0.049
	5	0.249	0.260	0.251	0.229	0.200	0.166	0.128	0.087	0.044
5	1	0.964	0.889	0.795	0.692	0.583	0.471	0.355	0.238	0.120
	2	0.514	0.489	0.445	0.392	0.333	0.271	0.205	0.138	0.070
	3	0.364	0.356	0.329	0.292	0.250	0.204	0.155	0.105	0.053
	4	0.289	0.289	0.270	0.242	0.208	0.171	0.130	0.088	0.045
	5	0.244	0.249	0.235	0.212	0.183	0.151	0.115	0.078	0.040

11

Non-Inferiority and Equivalence

SUMMARY

If the null hypothesis is rejected in a comparative two-group clinical trial, then *superiority* is claimed for one of the groups. In contrast, the concern in this chapter is with situations in which the aim is to claim either therapeutic *non-inferiority* for the *Test* as compared to the *Standard* or, in appropriate circumstances, therapeutic *equivalence* – neither less nor more than the *Standard* as defined by a pre-specified margin. In these cases, if the confidence interval of the difference between the comparators is, for example, totally within the acceptable effectiveness margin, it may be inferred that the *Test* can essentially replace the *Standard*. Of particular relevance in the development of therapeutic agents is the concept of *bioequivalence*, which looks at whether two drugs have similar pharmacokinetic properties.

11.1   Introduction

Implicit when making a comparison between two groups is the presumption that if the null hypothesis is rejected then a difference between the groups is claimed. Then, if this comparison involves two interventions for a particular condition, the conclusion drawn is that one intervention is *superior* to the other irrespective of the magnitude or clinical importance of the difference observed. For this reason, they are termed 'Superiority' trials and the studies considered in earlier chapters are of this kind.

However, in some situations, a *Test* (T) intervention may bring certain advantages over the current *Standard* (S), possibly in a reduced side-effects profile, easier administration or lower cost, but it may not be anticipated to be better with respect to the primary endpoint of concern. One can never prove that T and S are the same, but one may be able to choose a margin within which T and S can be considered interchangeable. If T were better the S, then we would have no qualms about using it in place of S, so it is only the case of how much worse than S can T be before its collateral advantages are outweighed. Under such conditions, T may be required to be 'non-inferior' in efficacy to S if it is to replace it in future clinical use. For example, if the two interventions are for an acute, but not serious, condition, then the cheaper but potentially not so effective alternative may be an acceptable replacement for the current standard. What is needed is convincing evidence that T is 'not much worse' than S. This implies that 'non-inferiority' (or worse) is a pre-specified maximum reduction of T below S which, if observed to be less than this value after the clinical trial is conducted, would render T as

Sample Sizes for Clinical, Laboratory and Epidemiology Studies, Fourth Edition. David Machin, Michael J. Campbell, Say Beng Tan and Sze Huey Tan.
© 2018 John Wiley & Sons Ltd. Published 2018 by John Wiley & Sons Ltd.

non-inferior. The implication being that T could then replace S for routine clinical use. However when, for example, comparing alternative formulations of an oral contraceptive, we might require that T should be neither inferior (which might imply loss of effectiveness) nor superior (which might imply unacceptably high levels of the compound circulating in ovulating women) to S. In such trials one is seeking to verify whether or not the two formulations are essentially *bioequivalent* in terms of their pharmacodynamic (what the drugs do to the body) properties.

11.2 Hypotheses

When comparing T with S using, for example, the corresponding means from each in the context of a *superiority* trial, the null hypothesis is specified by H_0: $\delta = \mu_S - \mu_T = 0$ and the 2-sided alternative hypothesis is H_{Alt}: $\delta \neq 0$ as in **Figure 11.1(a)**. For a continuous endpoint and once the trial is concluded, the observed difference between interventions, $d = \bar{x}_S - \bar{x}_T$, is the estimate of δ and the corresponding 2-sided $(1-\alpha)\%$ CI is

$$d - z_{1-\alpha/2}SE(d) \text{ to } d + z_{1-\alpha/2} SE(d), \tag{11.1}$$

where $SE(.)$ is the standard error. In loose terms the CI covers a plausible range of values for δ and if this does not include '0' then, depending on the sign of d, *superiority* of one of S or T is claimed. It is important to emphasise, should '0' difference fall within the CI, that this does not imply that the two interventions are necessarily equally effective but rather that there may be insufficient evidence from the trial to distinguish between them.

	Type of trial	Hypotheses		Error probability		Confidence Interval
		Null	Alternative	Type I α	Type II β	$(1-\gamma)\%$
(a)	Superiority: The aim is to estimate the size of δ with a view to claiming a difference between groups. Requires δ_{Plan} to be pre-specified					
	Usual	$\delta = 0$	$\delta \neq 0$ Different	2-sided 0.05	1-sided 0.1 or 0.2	2-sided 95%
(b)	Non-inferiority: The aim is not to estimate δ but to judge if it is within the margin defined by η. Requires η to be pre-specified					
	Usual	$\delta > \eta$ Inferiority	$\delta \leq \eta$ Non-inferiority	1-sided 0.05	1-sided 0.1 or 0.2	1-sided 90 or 95%
(c)	Equivalence: The aim is not to estimate δ but to judge if it is within the margins defined by η. Requires η to be pre-specified					
	Usual	$\delta \leq -\eta$ or $\delta \geq \eta$ Not equivalent	$-\eta < \delta < \eta$ Equivalent	2-sided 0.05	Usually 2-sided* 0.1 or 0.2	2-sided 95%

*See end of Section 11.4

Figure 11.1 Hypotheses tested in parallel group trials for (a) superiority, (b) non-inferiority and (c) equivalence when comparing a test (*T*) with a standard (*S*), where $\delta = \mu_S - \mu_T$.

In the case of an *equivalence* trial, the null hypothesis has two components of *non-equivalence*, which are H_0: $\delta < -\eta$ and $\delta > +\eta$. The alternative hypothesis of equivalence is H_1: $-\eta < \delta < \eta$ as in **Figure 11.1(c)**. Again, once the trial is completed, d is obtained and the corresponding 2-sided CI is calculated. In this case, to demonstrate *equivalence* of S and T, the whole of the CI must be within the interval $-\eta$ to $+\eta$. In contrast, should the CI overlap either or both of these margins, then equivalence is not demonstrated.

In the more usual situation when only *non-inferiority* (as opposed to equivalence) is required, the null hypothesis has only one component of *inferiority* which is H_0: $\delta > \eta$. The alternative hypothesis of *non-inferiority* is H_1: $\delta \leq \eta$ as in **Figure 11.1(b)**. In this situation, a one-sided CI is required.

11.3 Non-Inferiority

A key concern at the planning stage of a non-inferiority trial is to define an appropriate value for η. In practice, η is usually small and represents a reduction in effectiveness that is considered clinically unimportant. For example, if the response rate of the standard but toxic drug S is $\pi_S = 0.50$ (50%) then this might be replaced by the less toxic T provided the associated response rate is not less than (say) $\pi_T = 0.45$ (45%). In this case the limit of non-inferiority $\eta = 0.50 - 0.45 = 0.05$. Non-inferiority implies that T is required to be, at most, only less effective than S by η. If it is better than S then it is clearly not inferior. However, should T be less effective than S by more than η then this would imply that it is *noticeably worse* and so cannot be recommended to replace S.

The way to interpret the results from a non-inferiority trial is by using CIs rather than significance tests and p-values. As we have indicated, a one-sided $100(1 - \alpha)$% CI for δ is appropriate. This takes the form of

$$\left[d - z_{1-\alpha} SE(d) \right] \text{ to } UL, \tag{11.2}$$

where $z_{1-\alpha}$ replaces $z_{1-\alpha/2}$ of a 2-sided CI. The upper confidence limit, UL, depends on the type of endpoint of concern and *not* on the data obtained from the trial. For a comparison of two proportions in a non-inferiority setting, $UL = +1$, while when comparing means, $UL = +\infty$. These correspond to the largest possible difference that can occur when comparing outcomes between two groups with binary and continuous endpoints respectively. The requirement for *non-inferiority* is that the lower limit, $LL = [d - z_{1-\alpha} SE(d)]$, of equation (11.2) lies above $-\eta$. It should be pointed out that the context determines whether, for example, $\mu_S - \mu_T < \eta$ or $\mu_T - \mu_S < \eta$ implies *non-inferiority*. In the latter case, $LL = -\infty$ and $UL = [d + z_{1-\alpha} SE(d)]$.

Illustration

In the trial conducted by Zongo, Dorsey, Rouamba, *et al* (2007) in patients with uncomplicated falciparum malaria, an increased risk of recurrent parasitaemia of no greater than 3% with artemether-lumefantrine (T) as compared to amodiaquine plus sulfadoxine-pyrimethamine (S) was set. Here the concern is to accept non-inferiority if $\pi_T - \pi_S < 0.03$.

In the event, the observed recurrence rate with T was 37/245 (15.10%) and with S 11/233 (4.72%). An adverse difference of $d = 0.1510 - 0.0472 = 0.1038$ with $SE(Difference)$

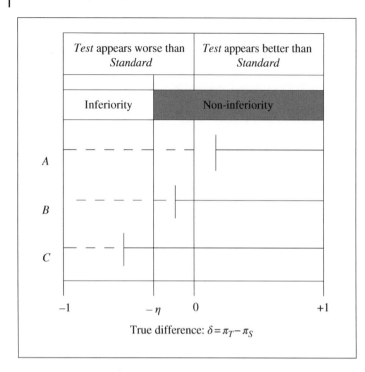

Figure 11.2 Schematic diagram to illustrate the concept of non-inferiority by using possible comparative trial outcomes as summarised by their 1-sided confidence intervals: Non-inferiority status: Trial A – Confirmed; Trial B – Confirmed; Trial C – Not accepted.

$$= \sqrt{\frac{0.1510(1-0.1510)}{245} + \frac{0.0472(1-0.0472)}{233}} = 0.0268.$$ For a 1-sided 90% CI, **Table 1.2** gives $z_{1-0.10} = z_{0.90} = 1.2816$ so that the upper limit corresponding to equation (11.2) becomes $0.1038 + (1.2816 \times 0.0268) = 0.1381$, while the lower limit is -1.

This CI suggests that the actual inferiority, as indicated by an increased rate of recurrent parasitaemia, with T over S may be as large as 13.81%. Thus the requirement for *non-inferiority*, that this should not exceed $\eta = 3\%$, is clearly violated. Consequently, T would not be suitable to replace S for clinical use.

The concept of *non-inferiority* is illustrated in **Figure 11.2** by considering the range of options possible for the one-sided CI for a comparison of two proportions that might result at the end of a trial comparing T with S. The 'non-inferior' limit, η, is set below no true difference between interventions or $\delta = 0$. In this illustration, both situations A and B represent *non-inferiority* so that the T could replace the S, while situation C represents *inferiority* in which case it would not.

Difference of Means

Independent groups

As previously indicated, when two means are compared, the *CI* of equation (11.2) has $UL = +\infty$. Thus if a comparison of two means is to be made, then the *UL* of all the corresponding *CI*s of **Figure 11.2** take this value. This is due to the fact that, in repeated sampling, we wish the interval to fail to cover δ only when this is less than the lower limit of the *CI*. Thus, to ensure *UL* is never less than δ, it is taken as $+\infty$.

If the two means are μ_S and μ_T, each with corresponding *SD* σ, and the non-inferiority limit is set as η, then the standardised effect size is $\Delta = (\mu_S - \mu_T)/\sigma$ and the standardised non-inferiority limit is $\varepsilon = \eta/\sigma$. The total sample size required, with patients randomised in the ratio 1:φ to S and T, for 1-sided Type I error, α, and 1-sided Type II error, β, is given by

$$N = \frac{(1+\varphi)^2}{\varphi} \frac{(z_{1-\alpha} + z_{1-\beta})^2}{(\Delta - \varepsilon)^2}.$$

(11.3)

The corresponding number randomised in each group is $n_S = N/(1+\varphi)$ and $n_T = \varphi N/(1+\varphi)$.

Sample sizes calculated from equation (11.3) for the situation $\varphi = 1$ are given in **Table 11.1** where the standardised effect size is expressed as a proportion of the non-inferiority limit, that is, $\Delta = \lambda \varepsilon$. It is important to note the asymmetric effect on the sample size for positive and negative values of λ. The sample size is inflated when the true mean difference moves towards the non-inferiority margin ($\lambda > 0$) and is reduced as the difference moves away ($\lambda < 0$).

Matched paired groups

For paired designs the unit of analysis is the difference in outcome experienced by the pair. Thus, if one member of the pair is termed A with endpoint measure x_A and the other is B with x_B, then their unit for analysis is $d = x_B - x_A$ and there will be N_{Pairs} of these differences. Similarly, if an individual is included in a cross-over trial and receives the sequence S followed by T (ST), then for that individual $d = x_S - x_T$, where measure x_S now represents that individual's observation after receiving S, and x_T that following intervention T.

As for the independent groups situation, the standardised effect size is $\Delta = (\mu_S - \mu_T)/\sigma$ and the standardised non-inferiority limit is $\varepsilon = \eta/\sigma$. The total sample size required, with patients randomised in the ratio 1:1 to ST and TS, for 1-sided α and 1-sided β, is given by:

$$N_{Pairs} = \frac{2(z_{1-\alpha} + z_{1-\beta})^2}{(\Delta - \varepsilon)^2}$$

(11.4)

This is similar in form to equation (11.3) but with $\varphi = 1$ and $N/2$ replaced by N_{Pairs}. Further, as the member(s) of each pair, either from a cross-over trial or from a matched design, are directly compared, this eliminates the between-subject variability present in an independent two group design. Consequently the standard deviation of the paired difference, d, will be correspondingly smaller than those of a parallel group design. Hence, sample sizes required for paired designs are also likely to be smaller.

In this context, N_{Pairs}, corresponds either to the number of matched-pairs required, N_{Match}, or for a two-period, two-group, cross-over trial it is $N_{Cross-over}$. In the latter case, subjects are usually randomised equally to ST and TS so that $n_{ST} = n_{TS} = N_{Cross-over}/2$.

Difference of Proportions

Independent groups

When the endpoint of the trial is assessed with a binary outcome, for example, 'cured' or 'not-cured', the respective true probabilities of success under S and T are denoted π_S and π_T. The total sample size

$$\bar{\pi}_{SD} = 2u\cos(w) - (b/3a), \quad \bar{\pi}_{TD} = \bar{\pi}_{SD} - \eta,$$

where $w = [\pi + \arccos(v/u^3)]/3$, and π is the irrational number 3.14159... and not a Binomial proportion.

Further, $v = b^3/(3a)^3 - bc/(6a^2) + d/(2a)$, $u = \text{sign}(v)\sqrt{[b^2/(3a)^2 - c/(3a)]}$, $a = 1 + \varphi$, $b = -[1 + \varphi + \pi_S + \varphi\pi_T + \eta(\varphi + 2)]$, $c = \eta^2 + \eta(2\pi_S + \varphi + 1) + \pi_S + \varphi\pi_T$ and $d = -\pi_S\eta(1 + \eta)$.

Figure 11.3 Maximum likelihood estimates of $\bar{\pi}_{SD}$ and $\bar{\pi}_{TD}$ of equation (11.5) (from Farrington and Manning, 1990).

required with patients randomised to the interventions in the ratio 1:φ, with anticipated proportions π_S and π_T, non-inferiority margin η, 1-sided α and 1-sided β, is:

$$N = \frac{(1+\varphi)}{\varphi} \frac{\left\{ z_{1-\alpha}\sqrt{\left[\phi\bar{\pi}_{SD}\left(1-\bar{\pi}_{SD}\right) + \bar{\pi}_{TD}\left(1-\bar{\pi}_{TD}\right) \right]} + z_{1-\beta}\sqrt{\left[\varphi\pi_S\left(1-\pi_S\right) + \pi_T\left(1-\pi_T\right) \right]} \right\}^2}{\left[\pi_S - \pi_T - \eta \right]^2},$$

(11.5)

giving for each group $n_S = N/(1+\varphi)$ and $n_T = \varphi N/(1+\varphi)$ subjects. Here $\bar{\pi}_{SD}$ and $\bar{\pi}_{TD}$ (see **Figure 11.3**) are the maximum likelihood estimates of the true values of π_S and π_T under the hypothesis that they differ by η. Sample sizes calculated from equation (11.5) for the situation $\varphi = 1$ are given in **Table 11.2**.

An approximate approach, which can be used to provide an easier check on the calculations, is to replace $\bar{\pi}_{SD}$ and $\bar{\pi}_{TD}$ in the numerator of (11.5) by π_S and π_T respectively, and this leads to

$$N = \frac{(1+\varphi)\left(z_{1-\alpha} + z_{1-\beta}\right)^2 \left[\varphi\pi_S\left(1-\pi_S\right) + \pi_T\left(1-\pi_T\right) \right]}{\varphi \left[\pi_S - \pi_T - \eta \right]^2}.$$

(11.6)

Matched paired groups

The results from a matched-pairs study or a two-period, two-intervention, cross-over clinical trial comparing S and T with a binary endpoint such as a Yes/No response can be summarised in the format of **Figure 11.4**. Here π_{00} corresponds to the proportion of subjects who would fail to respond with both S and T while π_{10} is the proportion who respond to S but fail with T, and π_{11} and π_{01} are similarly defined. The overall proportion responding to S is π_S and that for T is π_T.

The corresponding hypotheses for non-inferiority are H_0: $\pi_S - \pi_T \leq \delta$ versus H_1: $\pi_S - \pi_T > \delta + \eta$. Then, with subjects randomised to S and T in the ratio of 1: φ, 1-sided α and 1-sided β, the required sample size is:

$$N_{Pairs} = \frac{\left\{ z_{1-\alpha}\left[2\left(\pi_S - \pi_{11}\right) - \delta - \eta \right]\sqrt{\left(\pi_S - \pi_{11} - \delta\right)} + z_{1-\beta}\left[2\left(\pi_S - \pi_{11}\right) - \delta \right]\sqrt{\left(\pi_S - \pi_{11} - \delta - \eta\right)} \right\}^2}{\left(\pi_S - \pi_{11}\right)\left[2\left(\pi_S - \pi_{11}\right) - \delta - \eta \right]\eta^2}.$$

(11.7)

Standard Intervention	Test Intervention		Total	Anticipated proportion
	No ($j=0$)	Yes ($j=1$)		
No ($i=0$)	r (π_{00})	s (π_{10})	($r+s$)	$[1-\pi_S]$
Yes ($i=1$)	t (π_{01})	u (π_{11})	($t+u$)	$[\pi_S]$
Total	($r+t$)	($s+u$)	N_{Pairs}	
Anticipated proportion	$[1-\pi_T]$	$[\pi_T]$		$[1]$

Figure 11.4 The potential format of the results from a matched-pair or cross-over design.

To complete the calculation, the probability π_{11} has to be specified by the design team. It has been suggested that this can be defined by

$$\pi_{11} = \max\left\{\left[\pi_S - \delta - \eta - (1-\pi_S)/2\right], \left[(\pi_S - \delta - \eta)/2\right]\right\}. \tag{11.8}$$

However, if there is information on π_{11} from other related studies, then that may form a firmer basis for planning the current trial size.

In this context, N_{Pairs} corresponds to the number of matched-pairs required while, if a two-period, two group, cross-over trial is planned, $N_{Pairs} = n_{ST} + n_{TS}$, where n_{ST} is the number of patients receiving sequence ST with n_{TS} receiving TS. It is usual that subjects are randomised equally to ST and TS. Sample sizes calculated from equation (11.7) for the situation $\phi = 1$ are given in **Table 11.3**.

Hazard Ratio

Independent groups
Although the null and alternative hypotheses for a trial with a survival time endpoint, such as death, can be expressed by the difference between two instantaneous death rates (hazards) λ_S and λ_T, it is more usual to express the hypotheses in terms of the hazard ratio (HR), Θ, where

$$\Theta = \frac{\lambda_T}{\lambda_S}. \tag{11.9}$$

In this format, the hypotheses for a non-inferiority trial become H_0: $\Theta > \Theta_0$ and H_1: $\Theta \leq \Theta_1 = \eta\, \Theta_0$. Then, with subjects randomised to S and T in the ratio 1: φ, 1-sided α and 1-sided β, the required sample size is:

$$N = \left(\frac{1+\varphi}{\varphi}\right)\frac{\left(z_{1-\alpha} + z_{1-\beta}\right)^2}{\left(log\Theta_0 - log\Theta_1\right)^2}\left[\frac{\varphi g\left(\lambda_S, \xi\right)}{\lambda_S^2} + \frac{\varphi g\left(\Theta_1 \lambda_S, \xi\right)}{\Theta \lambda_S^2}\right], \tag{11.10}$$

from which $n_S = N/(1+\varphi)$ and $n_T = \varphi N/(1+\varphi)$ can be obtained.

Here $g(\lambda, \xi)$ depends on the anticipated duration of patient entry to the trial, a, the follow-up period beyond recruitment closure, f, and the anticipated loss to follow-up or censoring rate, ξ. If there is a constant recruitment rate over a and the censoring follows an Exponential distribution, then

$$g\left(\lambda,\xi\right)=\lambda^2\left\{\frac{\lambda}{\xi+\lambda}\left[1-\frac{exp\left[-f\left(\xi+\lambda\right)\right]-exp\left[-\left(a+f\right)\left(\xi+\lambda\right)\right]}{a\left(\xi+\lambda\right)}\right]\right\}^{-1}. \tag{11.11}$$

To evaluate this, it is necessary for the design team to specify a, f and ξ, then calculate equation (11.11) for each intervention separately by first setting $\lambda=\lambda_S$ and then $\lambda=\lambda_S\Theta_1=\lambda_S\eta\Theta_0=\eta\lambda_T$ respectively.

Note

In the situation where the survival can be assumed to follow an Exponential distribution (see **Figure 1.7**), the relationships between the hazard rate, λ, the proportion alive, π_τ, at a fixed point of time, τ, and the median survival time, M, can be summarised by

$$\lambda=\frac{-log\pi_\tau}{\tau}=\frac{-log0.5}{M}. \tag{11.12}$$

Thus if M_S and M_T can be assumed, then this equation can provide planning values for λ_S and λ_T in equations (11.10) and (11.11).

Regulatory Recommendations

Gupta (2011) provides a useful review of practical and regulatory aspects in relation to non-inferiority trials. Appropriate regulatory guidance is provided for the industry by the FDA (2010). The CPMP (2000) describes issues in switching between superiority and non-inferiority designs. The CPMP (2005) gives guidance on the choice of the non-inferiority margin.

11.4 Equivalence

For equivalence, one may want T to be *neither* less than S *nor* more than S within certain margins so the *equivalence* limit, η, is now set above and below the difference, δ. The concept of equivalence is illustrated, assuming $\delta=0$, in **Figure 11.5** by the range of possible options for the CIs that might result at the end of a trial comparing T with S.

In **Figure 11.5**, A clearly demonstrates an important difference between groups since even the lower limit of this CI is beyond $+\eta$. If a CI crosses a boundary (B and F), then one would be uncertain as to whether or not the interventions were equivalent, whereas if it were totally between the limits $-\eta$ to $+\eta$ (C, D, E), then equivalence would be claimed. The uncertain outcome of H would correspond to a trial of inadequate sample size, as the CI is so wide.

Neither C nor E of **Figure 11.5** cut the vertical lines at 0, $-\eta$ or $+\eta$ and so are indicative of a statistically significant difference between S and T. Thus it is quite possible to show a statistically *significant*

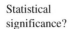

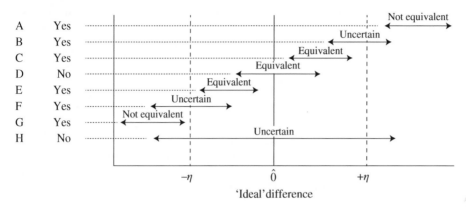

Figure 11.5 Schematic diagram to illustrate the concept of equivalence by using a series of possible comparative trial outcomes of a *Test* against a *Standard* intervention as summarised by their reported (2-sided) confidence intervals (after Jones, Jarvis, Lewis and Ebbutt, 1996).

difference between two treatments yet also demonstrate therapeutic *equivalence*. These are not contradictory statements but simply a realisation that there is evidence that one works better than the other. However, the magnitude of the *superiority* is less than η. As this margin will be small when testing for equivalence, the difference is unlikely to have clinical impact.

Sample Size

For *equivalence* trials the sample size formulae of **Section 11.3** derived for *non-inferiority* are still appropriate. However, in circumstances where, for example, the two means, μ_S and μ_T, or proportions, π_S and π_T, are assumed equal, the 1-sided α and 1-sided β for the *non-inferiority* designs are replaced by 2-sided values. Thus, α is replaced by $\alpha/2$ and (usually) β by $\beta/2$ in all the respective formulae as indicated in **Figure 11.1** and by, for example, Ganju, Izu and Anemona (2008, Equation 2) when describing sample size for equivalence in a vaccine lot consistency trial. Consequently in these situations, and with all other conditions held the same, the corresponding sample sizes for an equivalence design would all be larger than those based on a non-inferiority margin. On the other hand, if equality of the means is not assumed, then a 1-sided β is retained.

11.5 Bioequivalence

When, for example, a particular pharmaceutical compound or a vaccine is being developed for routine clinical use, small adjustments may be necessary to their formulation. Perhaps such a change may be needed when restricted supplies, initially packaged for successful early stage trials, are to be made available for routine clinical use and hence wider distribution. Alternatively, a rival manufacturer may wish to produce a generic copy of the drug in question. Thus, although these situations may involve only minor changes to the product, appropriate investigation to assess whether the new formulation is indeed *equivalent* to the reference product may be required. This assessment may be done by, for example, examination of the pharmacokinetics of the *Reference (R)* and *Test (T)* formulation. In this section, we use *R* rather than *S*, as the term *Reference* is widely used in the bioequivalence context. If the formulations have equal properties, then this implies equal clinical effectiveness in terms of both safety and efficacy and hence they are termed *bioequivalent*.

Cross-Over Design

Pharmacokinetic measures used to assess *bioequivalence* of drugs may concern their rate and extent of absorption as assessed by the area under a concentration/time curve, *AUC*, the maximum concentration, C_{max}, and the time of its occurrence, t_{max}. For many pharmaceutical compounds, a large between-subject variation exists and so cross-over designs are recommended for use in their evaluation. In such a trial, if formulation *T* is to be compared with *R*, then the subjects would be randomised between the two sequences *TR* and *RT* with an equal number of subjects per sequence.

Ratio of Means

In practice, the distributions of the continuous measures *AUC*, C_{max} and t_{max} are usually assumed to have a log-Normal form. Thus, comparisons between *T* and *R* are calculated using the logarithms of the relevant measure which implies the use of the ratio. Thus, when specifying the criteria for *bioequivalence*, the focus will be on $log\mu_T - log\mu_R$ or essentially the ratio $\Lambda = \mu_T/\mu_R$, where μ_T and μ_R are the anticipated mean values of the respective formulations. In this case the null hypothesis is $\Lambda_0 = 1$ and so *bioequivalence* is then concluded if the subsequently observed value, Λ_{Obs}, is contained wholly within a pre-specified 2-sided $100(1 - \gamma)\%$ CI surrounding the null value $\Lambda_0 = 1$. That is, Λ_{Obs} must lie between the predefined limits θ_L and θ_U, where $\theta_L < 1 < \theta_U$. Recommended limits are $\theta_L = 0.8$ and $\theta_U = 1.25$ as in **Figure 11.6**, which implies bioequivalence defined as $\Omega = 20\%$. Since $log1.25 = -log(0.8) = 0.2231$ and $log(1) = 0$, these limits are equidistant from unity on the logarithmic scale. Commonly a 2-sided 90% CI is chosen, so $\gamma = 0.1$.

μ_T and μ_R assumed equal	Hypothesis		Error Probability		Confidence Interval
	Null Not bioequivalent	Alternative Bioequivalent	Type I α	Type II β	$(1 - \gamma)\%$
$\Lambda = \mu_T/\mu_R = 1$	$\Lambda \leq -\theta_L$ or $\Lambda \geq \theta_U$	$-\theta_L < \Lambda < \theta_U$			
Example	Bioequivalence: $\Omega = 20\%$ $\theta_L = 0.8$, $\theta_U = 1.25$ with $log(1.25) = -log(0.8) = 0.22$		1-sided 0.05	2-sided 0.2	90%

Note: Here, in the symmetrical situation, when it is assumed in the planning that $\mu_T = \mu_R$, the Type II error, β, is taken as 2-sided. In contrast, for the asymmetric situations of $\mu_T > \mu_R$ or $\mu_T < \mu_R$, β is considered as 1-sided

Figure 11.6 Hypotheses tested in trials for bioequivalence when comparing a test (*T*) with a reference (*R*) in situations where μ_T and μ_R are assumed equal.

Although the statistical calculations for bioequivalence studies are conducted on the logarithmic scale, the resulting estimate of the ratio and corresponding upper and lower confidence limits are transformed back to the original scale for interpretation.

The number of subjects required, half to receive the sequence TR and half RT, in a *bioequivalence* cross-over design is, provided $\mu_T = \mu_R$, given by

$$N_{Pairs} = \frac{2(t_{df,1-\alpha} + z_{1-\beta})^2}{\{log\theta / \sigma_{Plan}\}^2},$$ (11.13)

and when $\mu_T \neq \mu_R$, this is replaced by

$$N_{Pairs} = \frac{2(t_{df,1-\alpha} + z_{1-\beta/2})^2}{\{[log(\mu_T/\mu_S) - log\theta]/\sigma_{Plan}\}^2},$$ (11.14)

where $\theta = \theta_L$ if $\mu_T/\mu_R < 1$ and $\theta = \theta_U$ if $\mu_T/\mu_R \geq 1$. Here $t_{df,1-\beta}$ and $t_{df,1-\beta/2}$ are obtained from **Table 1.3** of student's t-distribution with degrees of freedom, df.

The coefficient of variation ($CV = SD/$Mean) on the linear scale is related to the estimate of σ on the ratio scale by

$$CV_{Plan} = \sqrt{exp(\sigma_{Plan}^2) - 1}.$$ (11.15)

Further if σ_{Plan} is small, then $exp(\sigma_{Plan}^2) \approx 1 + \sigma_{Plan}^2$ and therefore $CV_{Plan} \approx \sigma_{Plan}$. Sample sizes for bioequivalence studies are given in **Table 11.4** but with σ_{Plan} replaced by CV_{Plan} in equations (11.13) and (11.14).

Degrees of freedom (df)

Besides depending on α, the term $t_{df,1-\alpha}$ in equation (11.13) depends on the number of degrees of freedom, df, utilised to estimate them within subject SD in the final analysis. For a two-period cross-over design, with $N_{Pairs} = n_{TR} + n_{RT}$ sequences with $n_{TR} = n_{RT}$, using a paired t-test for analysis of the mean of the differences, there are $df = N_{Pairs} - 2$ degrees of freedom.

Iteration

However, at the design stage we do not know the actual value of N_{Pairs} (and hence df) as we are using the sample size equation to determine this. As a consequence, to obtain the sample size from equations (11.13) and (11.14) an iterative procedure is required. This starts by first assuming that the degrees of freedom is very large, that is, $df_0 = \infty$, so that $z_{1-\alpha}$ can replace $t_{df,1-\alpha}$. With this in place the calculation, when rounded up to the next integer, gives an initial estimate of the sample size, N_{Pairs}^0. This is then used to obtain a revised value for the degrees of freedom as $df_1 = N_{Pairs}^0 - 2$. The value of $t_{df1,1-\alpha}$ can now be determined by reference to **Table 1.3**. Substituting this in either equation (11.13) or (11.14) as appropriate provides a second estimate of the sample size, N_{Pairs}^1, from which the revised $df_2 = N_{Pairs}^1 - 2$ can be obtained. The iteration is then repeated again to obtain N_{Pairs}^2. This process continues until convergence, that is, when two successive integer values of N_{Pairs} are obtained which do not differ from each other.

Regulatory Recommendations

In the context of *bioequivalence*, β, which is the probability of erroneously concluding bio-inequivalence, is often called the 'producer risk', while α, which is the probability of erroneously accepting bioequivalence, is termed the 'consumer risk'. Balancing these risks has led regulatory bodies to detail rules for the conduct of bioequivalence studies (FDA, 2003; CPMP, 2010;). Thus, the 80/20 rule specifies that a test of *bioequivalence* must have at least 80% power of detecting a 20% ($\Omega = 0.2$) difference between the endpoint of interest, and use of a 90% CI is also suggested (**Figure 11.6**).

We caution, however, that regulatory guidelines are continuously updated, so investigators are advised to check on their current status during the course of the design of a study.

11.6   Practical Issues

Intention-to-Treat or Per Protocol

Intention to treat (ITT)

In a randomised controlled trial (RCT), despite every effort to commence treatment as soon after randomisation as possible, there will be circumstances when the patient nevertheless refuses the treatment allocated or may even request the alternative option. In double-blind trials requesting the other option, at an early stage post-randomisation, would be very unlikely, but in an open trial where the patient is fully aware (and can recognise the option), this will be more of a problem. However, even if a patient commences the intervention in question, they may subsequently refuse to continue with it and even wish to withdraw from the trial entirely.

The intention-to-treat (ITT) principle is that once randomised the patient is retained in the allocated group for analysis regardless of whatever occurs. The application of the ITT principle to a *superiority* trial is a conservative procedure. Thus ITT will tend to dilute the difference between the randomised interventions (since the two groups become more similar whenever a participant, for example, refuses the randomised option and then receives the alternative) and thereby reduces the chance of demonstrating efficacy should it exist. In general, careless or inaccurate measurement, poor follow-up of patients, poor compliance with study procedures and medication all tend to bias results towards no difference between treatment groups.

However, Piaggio and Pinol (2001) point out that for *non-inferiority* and *equivalence* trials, the dilution caused by ITT will not act conservatively as in these cases any dilution will tend to favour, as appropriate, the non-inferiority or equivalence hypothesis. Hence, the conduct of such trials demands especially high compliance of the patients with respect to the treatment protocol. Consequently, although analysis and interpretation can be quite straightforward, the design and management of non-inferiority and equivalence trials is often especially demanding.

Per-protocol (PP)

Jones, Jarvis, Lewis and Ebbutt (1996) suggest that a per-protocol (PP) analysis may be relevant when reporting the results of non-inferiority or equivalence randomised trials. In a PP summary of the results, the comparison is made only in those patients who comply with the treatment allocated. If a PP analysis is considered appropriate, then the trial protocol should state that such an analysis is intended from the onset.

11.7 Bibliography

Walker and Nowcki (2010) give a non-technical discussion of issues relating to non-inferiority and equivalence testing and cite an earlier version of Piaggio, Elbourne, Pocock, *et al* (2012), who set standards for the reporting of non-inferiority and equivalence trials.

When comparing proportions, Roebruck and Kuhn (1995) recommend the Farrington and Manning (1990) approach of equation (11.5) in determining the sample size for a parallel group non-inferiority or equivalence design. The corresponding methodology for a paired design, whether matched or cross-over, of equation (11.7) is taken from Lu and Bean (2004, p1834), who utilise equation (11.8) first suggested by Lachenbruch (1992). Julious and Campbell (2012) review aspects of non-inferiority and equivalence trials.

Sample size calculations for time-to-event data for a parallel group design are described by Crisp and Curtis (2008), who give equations (11.10) and (11.11). They also discuss the situation when the recruitment is assumed to follow a truncated Exponential distribution rather than occurring at a uniform rate and give an illustrative example of this situation. This requires a further parameter to be provided at the design stage.

Although not discussed explicitly in this text, Piaggio, Carolli, Villar, *et al* (2001) describe methodological considerations with respect to equivalence trials using cluster, as opposed to individual subject, randomised designs.

Julious (2004) and Julious, Tan and Machin (2010) discuss aspects related to bioequivalence and point out that, in situations covered by equations (11.13) and (11.14), alternative methods may be needed when sample sizes turn out to be very small. These make use of the non-central t (NCT) distribution of **Chapter 1** and equations (5.2) and (5.3) while Cousineau and Laurencelle (2011, equations 8a, b, c) provide an approximation which is useful in calculating probabilities from such distributions. In practice, these refinements make little practical difference to, for example, the entries of **Table 11.4**. Julious (2004, page 1960) develops the approximation (11.15). Chow and Wang (2001, equation 4) also note that, in contrast to using a 1-sided β when $\mu_T \neq \mu_R$, a 2-sided value is required when $\mu_T = \mu_R$ is assumed.

11.8 Examples

Table 1.2
For one-sided $\alpha = 0.1$, 0.05 and 0.025; $z_{0.9} = 1.2816$, $z_{0.95} = 1.6449$ and $z_{0.975} = 1.96$. For two-sided $\alpha = 0.1$; $z_{0.95} = 1.6449$. For one-sided $1 - \beta = 0.8$, 0.9 and 0.99, $z_{0.8} = 0.8416$; $z_{0.9} = 1.2816$ and $z_{0.99} = 2.3263$. For two-sided $1 - \beta = 0.8$ and 0.9; $z_{0.9} = 1.2816$ and $z_{0.95} = 1.6449$.

Non-Inferiority

Table 11.1 and Equation 11.3
Example 11.1 Non-inferiority of means - Home or institutional care for the elderly
Eranti, Mogg, Pluck, *et al* (2007) observed that patients with severe depression following electroconvulsive therapy (*ECT*) had a mean Hamilton Rating Scale (HAM-D) of 10 units at the end of their

treatment. Their non-inferiority trial compared *ECT* with repetitive transcranial magnetic stimulation (*rTMS*) and concluded that this approach was inferior as the margin of increased score they specified was exceeded. From their results, one can deduce that HAM-D has a SD of approximately 9 units. Suppose that a similar trial is planned, perhaps with what is thought to be improved *rTMS*, and the clinical team regards this to be *non-inferior* provided HAM-D is not more than 5 points more (which implies $\eta = -5$) than those receiving *ECT*.

Assuming $\mu_{rTMS} = \mu_{ECT} = 10$, then $\delta = \mu_{ECT} - \mu_{rTMS} = 0$ and $\Delta = 0$. Further, as $\sigma_{Plan} = 9$ and $\eta = -5$, $\varepsilon = -5/9 = -0.556$. Then with $\varphi = 1$, 1-sided $\alpha = 1$, 1-sided $\beta = 0.2$, equation (11.3) gives

$$N = \frac{(1+1)^2}{1} \frac{(1.2816 + 0.8416)^2}{(0 + 0.556)^2} = 58.33.$$ Thus a total of 60 patients with severe depression would

then be randomised half to receive *ECT* and half *rTMS*. Use of **Table 11.1** with 1-sided $\alpha = 0.1$, 1-sided $\beta = 0.2$, $\lambda = 0$ (since $\Delta = 0$), but $\varepsilon = 0.5$ (rather than 0.556) gives $N = 74$ and for $\varepsilon = 0.6$, $N = 52$ with a mid-value close to 64.

If the investigators thought that *rTMS* would be slightly better than *ECT*, with $\mu_{rTMS} = 9.75$, so that $\Delta = (10 - 9.75)/9 = +0.028$, then, with the same standardised margin $\varepsilon = -0.556$,

$$N = \frac{(1+1)^2}{1} \frac{(1.2816 + 0.8416)^2}{[0.028 + 0.556]^2} = 52.99$$ or 54. In this situation a smaller trial would be required.

To use **Table 11.1**, $\Delta = 0.028$ and $\varepsilon = -0.556$ imply $\lambda = 0.028/-0.556 = -0.05$. Entry into the -5% column of **Table 11.1** with 1-sided $\alpha = 0.1$, 1-sided $\beta = 0.2$, $\varepsilon = 0.5$ and 0.6 give *N* as 66 and 46 respectively with a mid-value of 56 patients.

On the other hand, if the investigators thought that *rTMS* would be slightly worse than *ECT*, with $\mu_{rTMS} = 10.5$, so that $\Delta = (10 - 10.25)/9 = -0.028$, then, with the same standardised margin $\varepsilon = -0.556$, the number of patients required increases to $N = 66$. Entry into the $+5\%$ column of **Table 11.1** with 1-sided $\alpha = 0.1$, 1-sided $\beta = 0.2$, $\varepsilon = 0.5$ and 0.6 gives *N* as between 80 and 56 respectively with a mid-value of 68 patients.

In the original trial, 46 patients were randomised. Such a trial size would result from setting $\Delta = 0$ with $\eta = -5.7$. This appears to be a very large margin for a non-inferiority trial.

Table 11.1 and Equation 11.4
Example 11.2 Cross-over trial - Non-inferiority of means - Type 2 diabetes
King (2009) compared, in a randomised double-blind cross-over design, once daily insulin detemir (*D*) with insulin glargine (*G*) for providing glycaemic control in patients with type 2 diabetes. The results of this trial indicate a mean of approximately 130 mg/dl for the 24-h glucose levels with a SD = 20 mg/dl.

Assume a non-inferiority trial of the same design, with patients randomised equally to the two sequences *DG* and *GD*, is planned with $\mu_G = \mu_D$ and $\eta = 5$. Hence $\Delta = 0$ and $\varepsilon = 5/20 = 0.25$. For 1-sided $\alpha = 0.05$ and 1-sided $\beta = 0.2$, equation (11.4) gives $N_{Pairs} = \dfrac{2(1.6449 + 0.8416)^2}{(0 - 0.25)^2} = 197.85$ or 200 sequences with 100 patients randomised to each sequence.

Alternatively, use may be made of **Table 11.1** with 1-sided $\alpha = 0.05$ and 1-sided $\beta = 0.2$, $\lambda = \Delta = 0$, $\varepsilon = 0.2$ and 0.3 to give sample sizes of 620 and 276 respectively with an average of 448. However, sample sizes given by equation (11.4) are half those of equation (11.3), hence $N_{Pairs} \approx 448/2$ or 224 sequences.

Table 11.2 and Equations 11.5 and 11.6

Example 11.3 Non-inferiority of proportions - HIV infections

Eron, Yeni, Gathe, *et al* (2006) describe a non-inferiority trial which compared fosamprenavir-ritonavir (*F*) to lopinavir-ritonavir (*L*) (which is regarded as the preferred protease inhibitor), each in combination with abacavir-lamivudine for the initial treatment of HIV infection. They assumed a 72% success rate with *L* and anticipated a reduced rate of 70% with *F*, a 1-sided $\alpha = 0.025$, 1-sided $\beta = 0.1$ and set the limit of non-inferiority as $\eta = 12\%$.

For both equations (11.5) and (11.6), $\pi_L - \pi_F - \eta = 0.72 - 0.70 - 0.12 = -0.10$. Further, as the calculation of $\bar{\pi}_{LD}$ and $\bar{\pi}_{FD}$ are complex, we use equation (11.6) to obtain, as the authors did,

$$N = \frac{(1+1)}{1} \times \frac{(1.96 + 1.2816)^2 \left[1 \times 0.72 \times (1 - 0.72) + 0.70(1 - 0.70) \right]}{-0.012} = 864.98 \text{ or } 866 \text{ to allow a 1:1 ran-}$$

domisation. In the event, 887 individuals were randomised by the investigators. The more precise calculations provided by equation (11.5) in $\boxed{^SS_S}$ give $N = 864$.

Had the success rates been assumed as 70% for both *F* and *L*, and the investigators had set a larger non-inferiority limit as 15% together with a less stringent 1-sided $\alpha = 0.05$, 1-sided $\beta = 0.2$, then with $\pi_S = \pi_T = 0.7$, $\eta = 0.15$, equation (11.6) gives $N = 232$ whereas **Table 11.2**, which uses equation (11.5), gives $N = 230$.

Equations 11.5 and 11.6

Example 11.4 Non-inferiority of proportions - Breast cancer

In planning a non-inferiority trial of targeted intraoperative radiotherapy (*IRT*) versus whole breast radiotherapy (*WBRT*) for breast cancer, Vaidya, Joseph, Tobias, *et al* (2010) for the TARGIT group of investigators anticipated a 5-year local recurrence rate of 6% with *WBRT* and an acceptable non-inferiority recurrence rate increase of $\eta = 0.025$ (2.5%). They further set $\varphi = 1$, $\pi_{WBRT} = \pi_{IRT} = 0.06$, 1-sided $\alpha = 0.05$ and 1-sided $\beta = 0.2$.

Use of equation (11.6) gives $N = \left(\frac{1+1}{1} \right) \dfrac{(1.6449 + 0.8416)^2 \left[1 \times 0.06 \times (1 - 0.06) + 0.06 \times (1 - 0.06) \right]}{[0 - 0.025]^2} =$

2,231.66 or 2,232 which they obtained. In the event, the trial recruited exactly this number over a 9 year period but with $n_{WBRT} = 1,119$ and $n_{IRT} = 1,223$ respectively. The more precise calculations provided by equation (11.5) in $\boxed{^SS_S}$ require a slightly larger trial size of $N = 2,282$.

An interesting aspect of this trial was that, at the planning stage, a 5-year local recurrence rate of 6% was assumed when making the sample size calculations. However, on successfully completing the trial some 10 years later, TARGIT compared this with the 1.5% that they actually found from their results. Then, assuming again $\alpha = 0.05$, $\beta = 0.2$ and $\eta = 0.025\%$ as before, they found in their Table 6 that if a trial were to be conducted currently then only 585 patients would be required. This can be confirmed by the use of equation (11.6). However, the more accurate equation (11.5) in $\boxed{^SS_S}$ suggests a considerably larger trial of 752 patients. This indicates that the approximation provided by equation (11.5) is unreliable when the proportions to be compared are very small.

Table 11.3 and Equations 11.7 and 11.8

Example 11.5 Non-inferiority of matched paired proportions

In describing their method, Lu and Bean (1995) tabulate sample sizes for different combinations of α, β, δ, η and π_S. For example, when 1-sided $\alpha = 0.025$, 1-sided $\beta = 0.1$, $\delta = \pi_S - \pi_T = 0$, $\eta = 0.1$ and

$\pi_S = 0.9$, equation (11.8) gives $\pi_{11} = \max\{[0.9-0-0.1-(1-0.9)/2],\ [(0.9-0-0.1)/2]\} = \max\{0.75, 0.40\} = 0.75$.

Then with $\pi_S - \pi_{11} = 0.9 - 0.75 = 0.15$, equation (11.7) gives $N_{Pairs} =$

$$\frac{\left\{1.96 \times \left[(2 \times 0.15)-0.1\right]\sqrt{0.15} + 1.2816 \times \left[2 \times 0.15\right]\sqrt{(0.15-0.1)}\right\}^2}{0.15 \times \left[(2 \times 0.15)-0.1\right] \times 0.1^2} = 188.49 \text{ or } 189,$$ which agrees with Lu

and Bean (1995, Table III). This is then rounded to give 190 pairs.

However, with the same assumptions $\delta = 0$, $\eta = 0.1$, $\pi_S = 0.9$ and 1-sided $\beta = 0.1$, but with the less stringent 1-sided $\alpha = 0.05$, **Table 11.3** gives $N_{Pairs} = 152$.

Changing π_S to 0.8 and 0.7 reduces π_{11} to 0.6 and 0.45 respectively with the corresponding N_{Pairs} from $^S S_S$ equal to 302 and 410 respectively.

Equations 11.9, 11.10, 11.11 and 11.12

Example 11.6 Non-inferiority – Recurrence free survival times – Breast cancer

The TARGIT-A trial of Vaidya, Joseph, Tobias, *et al* (2010) anticipated a 5-year local recurrence rate of breast tumours under whole breast radiotherapy (*WBRT*) as 6% and an acceptable non-inferiority recurrence rate increase of $\eta = 2.5\%$ with targeted intraoperative radiotherapy (*IRT*).

Although (see Example 11.4) the investigators used the anticipated local recurrence rate of the breast tumours under *WBRT* of 6% as a (binomial) proportion when determining the sample size, the trial analysis used 'time-to-local recurrence' as the endpoint measure and reported the Kaplan-Meier estimates of the local recurrence rates for *WBRT* and *IRT* in their publication.

In strict terms for sample size determination purposes, it would seem more appropriate to use the approach of equations (11.10) and (11.11), but this requires the design team to make assumptions about recruitment patterns which are often problematic. In fact, their recruitment extended over $a = 9$ years, with extended follow up of $f = 0.5$ years beyond.

The investigators set $\pi_{WBRT} = \pi_{IRT} = 0.06$ with the corresponding instantaneous recurrence rate $\lambda_{WBRT} = -[log0.06]/5 = 0.5627$ determined from equation (11.12) and the acceptable non-inferior rate $\lambda_{IRT} = -[log(0.06+0.025)]/5 = 0.4930$. Hence, using equation (11.9) H_0: $\Theta_0 = 0.4930/0.5627 = 0.8761$ and H_1: $\Theta_1 = 1$.

They further set $\varphi = 1$ and $\pi_{WBRT} - \pi_{IRT} = 0$. With these values, and $a = 9$, $f = 0.5$, an assumed low censoring rate of $\xi = 0.001$, so that $a + f = 9.5$ and $\lambda_{WBRT} + \xi = 0.5637$. With $\varphi = 1$, 1-sided $\alpha = 0.05$ and 1-sided $\beta = 0.2$, equation (11.11) gives g_{WBRT} (0.5627,0.001) $=$

$$0.5627^2 \left\{ \frac{0.5627}{0.5637} \left[1 - \frac{exp\left[-0.5 \times 0.5637\right] - exp\left[-9.5 \times 0.5637\right]}{9 \times 0.5637} \right] \right\}^{-1} = 0.3688 \text{ and, as } \Theta_1 = 1, \text{ exactly the}$$

same for g_{IRT}.

Equation (11.10) then gives $N = \left(\frac{1+1}{1}\right) \frac{(1.6449+0.8416)^2}{(log0.8761 - log1)^2} \left[\frac{1 \times 0.3688}{(1 \times 0.5627)^2} + \frac{0.3688}{(0.5627)^2} \right] = 1649.21$

and therefore approximately $N = 1{,}650$ women are required.

Example 11.7 Non-inferiority – Cardiovascular morbidity and mortality – Type 2 diabetes

In the RECORD trial of Home, Pocock, Beck-Nielson, *et al* (2009), cardiovascular outcomes in patients with type 2 diabetes were randomly assigned (if already on sulfonylurea) to the addition of rosiglitazone or metformin or (if already on metformin) to rosiglitazone or sulfonylurea. The arms including rosiglitazone are denoted T and the others S. The objective was to demonstrate non-inferiority of T with respect to the compound primary outcome which was time to cardiovascular hospitalisation or cardiovascular death.

The limit of non-inferiority for T was set as a $HR = 1.2$ with an 11% event rate per year for S, and duration of recruitment was set at 2 years with follow-up continuing for 6 years and allowing a 2% annual loss to follow-up. Further, the design team set $\varphi = 1$, 1-sided $\alpha = 0.01$ and a small 1-sided $\beta = 0.01$.

Thus, $\Theta_0 = 1.2$ and they set $\Theta_1 = 1$, $\lambda_S = 0.11$, $a = 2$, $f = 6$, and $\xi = 0.02$ so that $a + f = 8$ and $\lambda_S + \xi = 0.11 + 0.02$

$$= 0.13, \text{ and equation (11.11) gives } g_s(0.11, 0.02) = 0.11^2 \left\{ \frac{0.11}{0.13} \left[1 - \frac{exp[-6 \times 0.13] - exp[-8 \times 0.13]}{8 \times 0.13} \right] \right\}^{-1}$$

$= 0.0159$ for S and exactly the same for T as $\Theta_1 = 1$. Then equation (11.10) gives

$$N = \left(\frac{1+1}{1} \right) \frac{(2.3263 + 2.3263)^2}{(log 1.2 - log 1)^2} \left[\frac{1 \times 0.0159}{(1 \times 0.11)^2} + \frac{0.0159}{(0.11)^2} \right] = 3,425.23 \text{ or approximately 3,500 patients.}$$

In the event, the trial recruited 4,447 patients and concluded that rosiglitazone does not increase the risk of overall cardiovascular morbidity or mortality compared to standard glucose-lowering drugs.

Equivalence

Equations 11.5 and 11.6

Example 11.8 Comparing proportions - Head louse infestation

Burgess, Brown and Lee (2005) conducted a clinical trial to test whether dimenticone lotion (T) was as effective as phenothrin (R) for young people and adults with head louse infestation. They state: 'The trial was designed to demonstrate therapeutic equivalence with an equivalence margin of 20%.'

Assuming $\varphi = 1$, a 2-sided $\alpha = 0.05$, 2-sided $\beta = 0.1$ and an overall response rate of 75%, which had been demonstrated in the Burgess, Brown and Lee (2005) trial, what would be a realistic sample size if the trial were to be repeated?

Here, $\pi_S = \pi_T = 0.75$ and $\eta = 0.2$, then use of equation (11.5) with $^S S_S$ gives $N = 246$. A check on this calculation is provided by utilising equation (11.6) to give $N =$

$$\left(\frac{1+1}{1} \right) \frac{(1.96 + 1.6449)^2 \left[1 \times 0.75 \times (1 - 0.75) + 0.75 \times (1 - 0.75) \right]}{0.2^2} = 243.66 \text{ and } N = 244. \text{ This is very close}$$

to the former value.

Had $\pi_S = \pi_T = 0.65$ been assumed, then the number of subjects required would be increased to 296 with equation (11.6) and 292 with (11.5) through $^S S_S$.

At the end of their trial, Burgess, Brown and Lee (2005) reported, following an intention-to-treat (ITT) analysis based on 252 subjects, a deficit in cure rate with dimenticone of -5% with a two sided 95% CI of -16% to $+6\%$ compared to phenothrin. A per-protocol (PP) analysis reported by Sedgwick (2013), excluding 18 of the subjects from the previous analysis, suggested a larger deficit of -8% with CI of -19% to $+3\%$.

Bioequivalence

Table 11.4 and Equations 11.13 and 11.15

Example 11.9 Cross-over trial - Ratio scale - Estimating C_{max}

Julious, Tan and Machin (2010, Page 150) give an example of data from bioequivalence trials in which for C_{max}, on the difference scale, the $CV = 0.27$. From this information, equation (11.15) implies

$$\sigma_{Plan} = \sqrt{\log(CV^2 + 1)} = \sqrt{\log(0.27^2 + 1)} = 0.265 \text{ or close to the } CV \text{ itself. Further if the upper limit of}$$

the ratio of means, $\Lambda = \mu_T / \mu_S$, is set as $\theta_U = \log(1.25) = 0.2231$ as suggested in **Figure 11.6** and assumed $\Lambda = 1$. With 1-sided $\alpha = 0.05$, 2-sided $\beta = 0.1$ and $df_0 = \infty$, **Table 1.2** or the final row of **Table 1.3** gives

$t_{\infty, 1-\alpha} = 1.6449$ and $t_{\infty, 1-\beta/2} = 1.6449$. Hence, equation (11.13) gives $N_{Pairs}^0 = \dfrac{2(1.6449 + 1.6449)^2}{\left[\log(1.25)/0.265\right]^2} = 30.54$

or 31 as the initial estimate of sample size.

Now setting $df_1 = 31 - 2 = 29$, **Table 1.3** gives for 1-sided $\alpha = 0.05$, $t_{29, 0.9} = 1.6991$. Using this gives

$$N_{Pairs}^1 = \dfrac{2(1.6991 + 1.6449)^2}{\left[\log(1.25)/0.265\right]^2} = 31.55 \approx 32.$$ The next iteration will have $df_2 = 32 - 2 = 30$, which leads to

$t_{30, 0.9} = 1.6973$. This implies $N_{Pairs}^2 = 31.52$, and, as this results in only a decimal point change from the previous situation, the design is set with $N_{Pairs} = 32$.

Direct entry into **Table 11. 4** with $\Omega = 20\%$, $\Lambda = 1$, 1-sided $\alpha = 0.05$, 2-sided $\beta = 0.1$, and CV equal to 0.25 and 0.30 gives 29 and 41 pairs respectively. The mean of these values suggests $N_{Pairs} = 35$, which is quite close to the more precise earlier calculation.

If it is assumed that $\mu_R = 0.98$ while $\mu_T = 1.02$, then since $\Lambda = \mu_T / \mu_R = 1.02/0.98 = 1.04 > 1$, equation (11.13) with $\theta_U = 1.25$ is needed for sample size purposes. This gives

$$N_{Pairs}^0 = \dfrac{2(1.6449 + 1.6449)^2}{\left\{\left[\log(1.04) - \log(1.25)\right]/0.265\right\}^2} = 44.95 \text{ or } 45.$$ Now setting $df_1 = 45 - 2 = 43$, **Table 1.3** gives

$t_{43, 0.9} = 1.6811$. Using these gives $N_{Pairs}^1 = \dfrac{2(1.6811 + 1.6449)^2}{\left\{\left[\log(1.04) - \log(1.25)\right]/0.265\right\}^2} = 45.95.$ or 46. The next

iteration will have $df_2 = 46 - 2 = 44$, which leads to $t_{44, 0.9} = 1.6802$ and $N_{Pairs}^2 = 45.93$ indicating little change, and therefore the design is set with $N_{Pairs} = 46$.

Direct entry into the corresponding entries of **Table 11.4** with $\Lambda = 1.05$ for CV equal to 0.25 and 0.30 gives 37 and 52 pairs respectively. The mean of these values suggests $N_{Pairs} \approx 45$, which is very close to the more precise calculation above.

References

Technical

Cousineau D and Laurencelle L (2011). Non-central *t* distribution and the power of the *t* test: A rejoinder. *Tutorials in Quantitative Methods in Psychology*, **7**, 1–4.

Crisp A and Curtis P (2008). Sample size estimation for non-inferiority trials of time-to-event data. *Pharmaceutical Statistics*, **7**, 236–244.

Farrington CP and Manning G (1990). Test statistics and sample size formulae for comparative binomial trials with null hypothesis of non-zero risk difference or non-unity relative risk. *Statistics in Medicine*, **9**, 1447–1454.

Ganju J, Izu A and Anemona A (2008). Sample size for equivalence trials: A case study from a vaccine lot consistency trial. *Statistics in Medicine*, **27**, 3743–3754.

Chow S-C and Wang H (2001) On sample size calculation in bioequivalence trials. *Journal of Pharmacokinetics and Pharmacodynamics*, **28**, 155–169.

Gupta SK (2011). Non-inferiority clinical trials: Practical issues and current regulatory perspective. *Indian Journal of Pharmacology*, **43**, 371–374.

Jones B, Jarvis P, Lewis JA and Ebbutt AF (1996). Trials to assess equivalence: the importance of rigorous methods. *British Medical Journal*, **313**, 36–39.

Julious (2004). Sample sizes for clinical trials with Normal data. *Statistics in Medicine*, **23**, 1921–1986.

Julious SA and Campbell MJ (2012). Tutorial in biostatistics: sample sizes for parallel group clinical trials with binary data. *Statistics in Medicine*, **31**, 2904–2936.

Julious SA, Tan S-B and Machin D (2010). *An Introduction to Statistics in Early Phase Trials*. Wiley-Blackwell, Chichester.

Lachenbruch PA (1992). On the sample size for studies based upon McNemar's test. *Statistics in Medicine*, **11**, 1521–1525.

Lu Y and Bean JA (1995). On the sample size for one-sided equivalence of sensitivities based upon McNemar's test. *Statistics in Medicine*, **14**, 1831–1839.

Piaggio G, Carolli G, Villar J, Pinol A, Bakketeig L, Lumbiganon P, Bergsjø P, Al-Mazrou Y, Ba'aqeel H, Belizán JM, Farnot U and Berendes H (2001). Methodological considerations on the design and analysis of an equivalence stratified cluster randomization trial. *Statistics in Medicine*, **20**, 401–416.

Piaggio G, Elbourne DR, Pocock SJ, Evans SJW and Altman DG for the CONSORT Group (2012). Reporting of noninferiority and equivalence randomized trials: Extension of the CONSORT 2010 statement. *Journal of the American Medical Association*, **308**, 2594–2604. doi:10.001/jama.2012.87802

Piaggio G and Pinol APY (2001). Use of the equivalence approach in reproductive health trials. *Statistics in Medicine*, **20**, 3571–3587.

Roebruck P and Kühn A (1995). Comparison of tests and sample size formulae for proving therapeutic equivalence based on the difference of binomial probabilities. *Statistics in Medicine*, **14**, 1583–1594.

Walker E and Nowcki AS (2010). Understanding equivalence and noninferiority testing. *Journal of General Internal Medicine*, **26**, 192–196.

Guidelines

[Note that Regulatory Guidlines are continually updated, so for reference purposes the list below should be crosschecked with any later versions.]

CPMP (2000) *Points to Consider when Switching between Superiority and Non-Inferiority*. EMEA, London.

CPMP (2005). *Guideline on the Choice of the Non-inferiority Margin*. EMEA, London.

CPMP (2010). *Guideline on the Investigation of Bioequivalence*. EMEA, London.

FDA (2003). *Guidance for Industry. Bioavailability and Bioequivalence Studies for Orally Administered Drug Products – General Considerations*. Food and Drug Administration, Rockville, MD.

FDA (2010). *Guidance for Industry, Non-inferiority Clinical Trials*. Food and Drug Administration, Rockville, MD.

Examples

Burgess IF, Brown CM and Lee P (2005). Treatment of head louse infestation with 4% dimeticone lotion: randomised controlled equivalence trial. *British Medical Journal*, **330**, 1423–1425.

Eranti S, Mogg A, Pluck G, Landau S, Purvis R, Brown RG, Howard R, Knapp M, Philpot M, Rabe-Hesketh S, Romeo R, Rothwell J, Edwards D and McLoughlin DM (2007). A randomized, controlled trial with 6-month follow-up of repetitive transcranial magnetic stimulation and electroconvulsive therapy for severe depression. *American Journal of Psychiatry*, **164**, 73–81.

Eron J, Yeni P, Gathe J, Estrada V, DeJesus E, Staszewski S, Lackey P, Katlama C, Young B, Yau L, Sutherland-Phillips D, Wannamaker P, Vavro C, Patel L, Yeo J and Shaefer M, (2006). The KLEAN study of fosamprenavir-ritonavir versus lopinavir-ritonavir, each in combination with abacavir-lamivudine, for initial treatment of HIV infection over 48 weeks: a randomised non-inferiority trial. *Lancet*, **368**, 476–482.

Home PD, Pocock SJ, Beck-Nielson H, Curtis PS, Gomis R, Hanefeld M, Jones NP, Komajda M, McMurray JJV for the RECORD Study Team (2009). Rosiglitazone evaluated for cardiovascular outcomes in oral agent combination therapy for type 2 diabetes (RECORD): a multicentre, randomised, open-label trial. *Lancet*, **373**, 2125–2135.

King (2009). Once-daily insulin detemir is comparable to once-daily insulin glargine in providing glycaemic control over 24 h in patients with type 2 diabetes: a double-blind, randomized, crossover study. *Diabetes, Obesity and Metabolism*, **11**, 69–71.

Sedgwick P (2013). Equivalence trials. *British Medical Journal*, **346**:f184 doi:10.1136/bmj.f184.

Vaidya JS, Joseph DJ, Tobias JS, Bulsara M, Wenz F, Saunders C, Alvarado M, Flyger HL, Massarut S, Eiermann W, Keshtgar M, Dewar J, Kraus-Tiefenbacher U, Süttterlin M, Esserman L, Holtveg HMR, Roancadin M, Pigorsch S, Metaxas M, Falzon M, Matthews A, Corica T, Williams NR and Baum M (2010). Targeted intraoperative radiotherapy versus whole breast radiotherapy for breast cancer (TARGIT-A trial): an international, prospective, randomised, non-inferiority phase 3 trial. *Lancet*, **376**, 91–102.

Zongo I, Dorsey G, Rouamba N, Tinto H, Dokomajilar C, Guiguemde RT, Rosenthal P and Ouedraogo JB (2007). Artemether-lumefantrine versus amodiaquine plus sulfadoxine-pyrimethamine for uncomplicated falciparum malaria in Burkina Faso: a randomised no-inferiority trial. *Lancet*, **369**, 491–498.

Table 11.1 Sample Sizes for testing the non-inferiority of two means from two groups of equal size [Equation 11.3]. For pair matched designs each entry is divided by 2 [Equation 11.4]. Standardised Difference: $\Delta = \lambda\varepsilon\%$. Each cell gives the total number of subjects required, N.

Standardised Non-inferiority limit ε	$\lambda\%$								
	−10	−7.5	−5	−2.5	0	2.5	5	7.5	10
	1-sided $\alpha = 0.1$, 1-sided $\beta = 0.2$								
0.1	1492	1562	1636	1718	1804	1898	1998	2108	2228
0.2	374	392	410	430	452	476	500	528	558
0.3	166	174	182	192	202	212	222	236	248
0.4	94	98	104	108	114	120	126	132	140
0.5	60	64	66	70	74	76	80	86	90
0.6	42	44	46	48	52	54	56	60	62
0.7	32	32	34	36	38	40	42	44	46
0.8	24	26	26	28	30	30	32	34	36
0.9	20	20	22	22	24	24	26	28	28
1.0	16	16	18	18	20	20	20	22	24
	1-sided $\alpha = 0.1$, 1-sided $\beta = 0.1$								
0.1	2172	2274	2384	2502	2628	2766	2912	3072	3246
0.2	544	570	596	626	658	692	728	768	812
0.3	242	254	266	278	292	308	324	342	362
0.4	136	144	150	158	166	174	182	192	204
0.5	88	92	96	102	106	112	118	124	130
0.6	62	64	68	70	74	78	82	86	92
0.7	46	48	50	52	54	58	60	64	68
0.8	34	36	38	40	42	44	46	48	52
0.9	28	30	30	32	34	36	36	38	42
1.0	22	24	24	26	28	28	30	32	

(Continued)

Table 11.1 (Continued)

Standardised Non-inferiority limit ε	λ%								
	−10	**−7.5**	**−5**	**−2.5**	**0**	**2.5**	**5**	**7.5**	**10**
			1-sided $\alpha = 0.05$, 1-sided $\beta = 0.2$						
0.1	2044	2140	2244	2354	2474	2602	2742	2892	3054
0.2	512	5336	562	590	620	652	686	724	764
0.3	228	238	250	262	276	290	306	322	340
0.4	128	134	142	148	156	164	172	182	192
0.5	82	86	90	96	100	106	110	116	124
0.6	58	60	64	66	70	74	78	82	86
0.7	42	44	46	50	52	54	56	60	64
0.8	32	34	36	38	40	42	44	46	48
0.9	26	28	28	30	32	34	34	36	38
1.0	22	22	24	24	26	28	28	30	32
			1-sided $\alpha = 0.05$, 1-sided $\beta = 0.1$						
0.1	2832	2966	3108	3262	3426	3604	3796	4004	4230
0.2	708	742	778	816	858	902	950	1002	1058
0.3	316	330	346	364	382	402	422	446	470
0.4	178	186	196	204	216	226	238	252	266
0.5	114	120	126	132	138	146	152	162	170
0.6	80	84	88	92	96	102	106	112	118
0.7	58	62	64	68	70	74	78	82	88
0.8	46	48	50	52	54	58	60	64	68
0.9	36	38	40	42	44	46	48	50	54
1.0	30	30	32	34	36	38	38	42	44

Table 11.2 Total sample sizes for testing the non-inferiority of two proportions from two groups of equal size – reference group π_S, anticipated difference $\pi_S - \pi_T$, non-inferiority limit η: 1-sided $\alpha = 0.05$, 1-sided $\beta = 0.2$ [Equation 11.5].

π_S	η	$\pi_S - \pi_T$										
		−0.05	−0.04	−0.03	−0.02	−0.01	0	0.01	0.02	0.03	0.04	0.05
0.1	0.05	280	334	406	510	664	914	1360	2292	4868	18260	–
	0.10	130	144	162	184	210	244	286	346	428	548	740
	0.15	78	84	90	98	106	116	128	142	158	180	206
	0.20	52	54	58	62	664	706	74	80	86	92	100
0.2	0.05	434	528	656	842	1124	1588	2432	4234	9320	36424	–
	0.10	194	220	2528	290	338	402	486	602	768	1020	14342
	0.15	110	120	132	146	162	180	204	232	266	3082	364
	0.20	72	764	82	88	96	104	112	122	134	148	166
0.3	0.05	544	666	834	1080	1456	2078	3214	5652	12578	49740	–
	0.10	242	274	316	368	434	520	634	794	1026	1380	1962
	0.15	136	150	164	184	204	230	262	300	348	410	490
	0.20	86	94	100	110	118	130	142	156	174	194	218
0.4	0.05	604	744	938	1220	1654	2372	3690	6528	14612	58134	–
	0.10	268	306	354	414	490	592	726	914	1188	1608	2304
	0.15	150	166	184	206	230	262	298	344	402	476	572
	0.20	96	104	112	122	132	146	160	178	198	224	252
0.5	0.05	616	762	964	1260	1716	2470	3858	6856	15414	61592	–
	0.10	274	314	364	428	508	616	760	960	1252	1704	2450
	0.15	152	170	188	212	238	272	312	362	424	504	608
	0.20	96	106	114	126	138	152	168	186	210	236	268
0.6	0.05	580	720	914	1200	1640	2372	3720	6636	14982	60110	–
	0.10	258	296	346	408	486	592	732	930	1218	1662	2400
	0.15	144	160	180	202	228	262	300	350	412	492	596
	0.20	92	100	110	120	132	146	162	182	204	230	262
0.7	0.05	494	616	788	1040	1430	2078	3274	5870	13318	53690	–
	0.10	220	256	300	354	426	520	646	824	1084	1488	2158
	0.15	124	140	156	176	202	230	266	312	368	442	538
	0.20	80	88	96	106	116	130	144	162	182	208	238
0.8	0.05	362	456	588	782	1084	1588	2524	4562	10424	42340	–
	0.10	164	192	226	270	326	402	502	646	854	1180	1722
	0.15	96	106	120	138	156	180	210	246	294	354	432
	0.20	62	68	76	84	92	104	116	130	148	168	194
0.9	0.05	188	242	320	434	612	914	1480	2720	6322	26092	–
	0.10	94	110	132	160	196	244	308	400	536	748	1104
	0.15	58	66	76	86	100	116	136	160	192	234	288
	0.20	40	44	50	56	62	70	78	88	102	116	134

(*Continued*)

Table 11.2 (Continued)

π_S	η	$\pi_S - \pi_T$										
		−0.05	−0.04	−0.03	−0.02	−0.01	0	0.01	0.02	0.03	0.04	0.05
0.1	0.05	384	458	560	702	916	1262	1878	3166	6726	25260	–
	0.10	178	198	222	250	286	332	392	472	584	750	1012
	0.15	104	112	122	132	144	156	172	192	214	242	276
	0.20	70	74	78	82	88	92	100	106	114	124	134
0.2	0.05	600	730	908	1164	1556	2200	3368	5864	12906	50448	–
	0.10	270	304	346	400	468	554	670	832	1062	1412	1984
	0.15	152	166	182	202	224	250	280	318	366	426	502
	0.20	98	106	112	122	132	142	154	168	186	204	228
0.3	0.05	752	920	1156	1496	2018	2878	4450	7830	17424	68902	–
	0.10	334	380	438	508	600	720	878	1100	1422	1912	2720
	0.15	188	206	228	254	284	320	362	416	484	568	680
	0.20	120	130	140	150	164	180	196	216	240	268	302
0.4	0.05	854	1054	1336	1746	2376	3422	5346	9498	21352	85322	–
	0.10	378	434	504	592	704	852	1052	1330	1736	2362	3396
	0.15	212	234	262	294	332	376	432	502	588	698	844
	0.20	134	146	160	174	190	210	232	260	290	328	372
0.5	0.05	854	810	1026	1340	1826	2628	4106	7294	16396	65486	–
	0.10	292	336	390	456	544	658	812	1026	1340	1820	2616
	0.15	164	182	204	228	258	292	336	390	456	542	654
	0.20	72	80	86	94	104	114	126	140	156	176	200
0.6	0.05	802	996	1266	1662	2272	3286	5154	9194	20754	83270	–
	0.10	356	410	478	564	674	820	1014	1288	1688	2304	3328
	0.15	200	222	248	280	318	362	418	486	572	682	826
	0.20	128	138	152	166	184	202	224	252	282	320	364
0.7	0.05	684	854	1092	1440	1980	2878	4536	8132	18448	74376	–
	0.10	306	354	414	490	590	720	896	1142	1504	2062	2990
	0.15	172	192	216	244	278	320	370	432	510	612	744
	0.20	110	120	132	146	162	180	200	224	254	288	330
08	0.05	500	630	814	1082	1500	2200	3496	6316	14440	58648	–
	0.10	226	264	312	372	452	554	696	892	1184	1634	2384
	0.15	130	146	166	188	216	250	290	340	406	488	598
	0.20	84	94	104	114	128	142	160	180	204	232	268
0.9	0.05	258	332	438	596	844	1262	2044	3760	8748	36126	–
	0.10	126	150	180	218	266	332	422	550	738	1030	1522
	0.15	76	88	100	116	134	156	184	218	262	320	394
	0.20	52	58	66	74	82	92	106	120	136	158	182

Table 11.3 Number of pairs, N_{Pairs}, required for testing the non-inferiority of two proportions in a matched pair design [Equation 11.7].

		1-sided $\alpha=0.1$					
		1-sided $\beta=0.2$			1-sided $\beta=0.1$		
		π_S					
$\delta=\pi_S-\pi_T$	η	0.7	0.8	0.9	0.7	0.8	0.9
0.0	0.1	176	130	82	256	186	116
	0.2	54	42	28	76	58	38
	0.3	28	22	16	40	30	22
	0.4	18	14	10	24	20	14
0.1	0.1	154	110	68	220	156	94
	0.2	48	38	26	68	52	34
	0.3	26	20	14	36	28	20
	0.4	14	14	10	18	18	14
0.2	0.1	140	100	62	200	142	84
	0.2	46	34	24	64	48	32
	0.3	20	20	14	26	26	18
	0.4	10	14	10	12	18	12
		One-sided $\alpha=0.05$					
0.0	0.1	244	180	114	334	246	152
	0.2	74	58	40	100	76	52
	0.3	38	30	22	52	40	28
	0.4	24	20	16	32	26	20
0.1	0.1	212	154	96	288	206	126
	0.2	68	52	36	90	68	46
	0.3	36	28	22	48	38	26
	0.4	20	20	14	24	24	18
0.2	0.1	194	140	88	262	188	114
	0.2	62	48	34	84	64	42
	0.3	28	28	20	34	34	24
	0.4	14	18	14	18	24	18

Table 11.4 Sample sizes for cross-over bioequivalence studies – ratio of two paired means, Λ: 1-sided $\alpha = 0.05$, $\beta = 0.1$. When the ratio $\mu_T/\mu_R = 1$, it is assumed the power is 2-sided, otherwise it is 1-sided [Equation 11.13].

			Bioequivalence acceptance criterion, Ω		
			15%	20%	25%
			90% CI		
CV	β	Λ	0.85 to 1.18	0.80 to 1.25	0.75 to 1.33
10		0.90	54	14	7
		0.95	16	8	5
	2-sided	1	10	6	5
		1.05	15	8	5
		1.10	40	12	6
15		0.90	120	29	13
		0.95	33	15	9
	2-sided	1	20	11	8
		1.05	31	14	9
		1.10	87	25	12
20		0.90	211	51	22
		0.95	57	25	14
	2-sided	1	34	19	12
		1.05	55	24	14
		1.10	153	44	20
25		0.90	329	79	34
		0.95	88	38	21
	2-sided	1	53	29	18
		1.05	84	37	20
		1.10	239	67	31
30		0.90	474	113	48
		0.95	126	54	29
	2-sided	1	75	41	25
		1.05	121	52	29
		1.10	343	96	43
35		0.90	644	153	65
		0.95	171	73	39
	2-sided	1	102	55	34
		1.05	164	71	38
		1.10	466	130	58
40		0.90	841	199	84
		0.95	223	94	51
	2-sided	1	133	71	43
		1.05	214	92	50
		1.10	609	169	76

12

Cluster Designs

SUMMARY

Cluster randomised trial designs are growing in popularity in many clinical areas, and parallel statistical developments are numerous. Nevertheless, reviews suggest that design issues associated with cluster randomised trials are often poorly appreciated, and there remain inadequacies in how the associated results are presented. In addition, there is an apparent lack of understanding of how to plan for an appropriate trial size. We focus on parallel two-group designs, although cross-over and matched pairs designs are also considered, with the primary purpose of comparing two interventions with respect to binary, ordered categorical, continuous, incidence and time-to-event outcome variables. Issues of aggregate and non-aggregate cluster trials, adjustment for variation in cluster size and subject and/or cluster losses are detailed. The problem of establishing the anticipated magnitude of between- and within-cluster variation to enable planning values of the intra-cluster correlation coefficient and the coefficient of variation are also described.

12.1   Introduction

In contrast to clinical trials in which individual subjects are each randomised to receive one of the therapeutic options or interventions under test, the distinctive characteristic of a cluster trial is that specific groups or blocks of subjects (the clusters) are first identified and these units are assigned at random to the interventions. The term 'cluster' in this context may be a household, school, clinic, care home or any other relevant grouping of individuals. When comparing the interventions in such *cluster randomised trials*, account must always be made of the particular cluster from which the data item is obtained.

We assume that the objective of the trial design is to compare two interventions and that several clusters have been identified. Each cluster is then assigned at random to one of the interventions. Sample sizes are required for both the number of clusters per intervention and the number of subjects to be recruited from each cluster.

Sample Sizes for Clinical, Laboratory and Epidemiology Studies, Fourth Edition. David Machin, Michael J. Campbell, Say Beng Tan and Sze Huey Tan.
© 2018 John Wiley & Sons Ltd. Published 2018 by John Wiley & Sons Ltd.

12.2 Design Features

In, for example, the context of an individually randomised trial comparing two interventions, *Standard* (*S*) and *Test* (*T*), using a continuous outcome measure, we have shown in **Chapter 5** that the number of patients required is given by equation (5.4), that is

$$N = \left[\frac{(1+\varphi)^2}{\varphi} \right] \left[\frac{(z_{1-\alpha/2} + z_{1-\beta})^2}{(\delta_{Plan}/\sigma_{Plan})^2} + \frac{z_{1-\alpha/2}^2}{2} \right], \tag{12.1}$$

from which $n_S = \dfrac{N}{1+\varphi}$ and $n_T = \dfrac{\varphi N}{1+\varphi}$. Here α is the 2-sided test size, $1 - \beta$ the power, δ_{Plan} the anticipated effect size, σ_{Plan} the corresponding planning standard deviation (SD) and $1:\varphi$ the required randomisation ratio.

When the randomised allocation applies to the clusters, the basic principles for sample size calculation still apply, although modifications are required. To illustrate these we describe the *t*-test, for comparing means from samples of two populations with means μ_S and μ_T, using linear regression terminology with intercept μ_S and slope δ, that is,

$$y_i = \mu_S + \delta x + \varepsilon_i, \tag{12.2}$$

where the subjects are $i = 1, 2, ..., N$; $x = 0$ for S and $x = 1$ for T. Further, ε_i is a random variable with mean zero and, within each intervention group, assumed to have the same variance, σ^2. If this regression model is fitted to the data, then $d = \bar{y}_T - \bar{y}_S$ estimates $\delta = \mu_T - \mu_S$ and the null hypothesis remains $\delta = 0$. However, the analysis must now take account of the cluster to which an individual subject belongs. When we compare two interventions, $N (= n_S + n_T)$, patients will be recruited who will come from clusters of equal size m with therefore $k_S = n_S/m$, $k_T = n_T/m$ and $K = k_S + k_T$ clusters in total.

To allow for the clusters, model (12.2) is extended to

$$y_{ik} = \mu_S + \delta x + \gamma_k + \varepsilon_{ik}. \tag{12.3}$$

Here, the clusters are $k = 1, 2, ..., K$ and the subjects $i = 1, 2, ..., m$ in each cluster. The cluster effects, γ_k, are assumed to vary at random within each intervention about a mean of zero, with a variance $\sigma_{Between-Cluster}^2$. Further, the ε_{ik} are also assumed to have mean zero but with variance $\sigma_{Within-Cluster}^2$ and both random variables, γ_k and ε_{ik}, are assumed to be Normally distributed.

Although the format of the (random-effects) model (12.3) will change depending on the outcome measure of concern, all will contain random terms accounting for the cluster design.

The sample size formula (12.1) is essentially determined as a consequence of model (12.2), while the formulae which follow for cluster trials are based on (12.3).

Intra-Cluster Correlation – (ICC) Continuous Outcome

A feature of all cluster trials is that subjects recruited from within the same cluster cannot be regarded as acting independently of each other in terms of their response to the intervention received. For a continuous outcome, the magnitude of this within-cluster dependence is quantified by the intra-cluster correlation coefficient (ICC), ρ, which is interpreted in a similar way to Pearson correlation.

With each subject in every cluster providing an outcome measure, the ICC is the proportion of the combined sum of the within- and between-cluster variances, σ^2_{Total}, accounted for by the between-cluster variation, that is

$$\rho = \frac{\sigma^2_{Between-Cluster}}{\sigma^2_{Total}} = \frac{\sigma^2_{Between-Cluster}}{\sigma^2_{Between-Cluster} + \sigma^2_{Within-Cluster}}. \tag{12.4}$$

Thus, since variances cannot be negative, the ICC cannot be negative. A major challenge in planning the sample size is identifying an appropriate value for ρ.

The Design Effect (*DE*)

The impact of the ICC on the planned trial size will depend on its magnitude and on the number of subjects recruited per cluster, m, through the so-called design effect (*DE*),

$$DE = 1 + (m-1)\rho. \tag{12.5}$$

Table 12.1 gives *DE* for a range of values of m and ρ. In all situations, *DE* will be ≥ 1 since $m > 1$ and $\rho \geq 0$. The *DE* is then multiplied by the total sample size, $N_{Non-Cluster}$, obtained from (say) equation (12.1) to give that required for a cluster design, N, and the total number of clusters required, $K = N/m$. However, as the value of *DE* depends on ρ, whose value may not be firmly established, it is advisable to try different values of the ICC and investigate how sensitive the sample size estimates are to these changes.

In practice there may be substantial variation from cluster to cluster in size. To allow for any such variation, the *DE* can be modified to

$$DE = 1 + \left\{ \left[CV(m)^2 \left(\frac{K-1}{K} \right) + 1 \right] \bar{m} - 1 \right\} \rho, \tag{12.6}$$

where $\bar{m}$ is the anticipated mean cluster size and, $CV(m) = \dfrac{SD(m)}{\bar{m}}$ is the coefficient of variation. At the initial stages of determining the sample size, the values of K may be uncertain, and equation (12.6) can be replaced by

$$DE = 1 + \left\{ \left[CV(m)^2 + 1 \right] \bar{m} - 1 \right\} \rho. \tag{12.7}$$

Another option may be to increase the total number of clusters initially planned to

$$K_{Adjusted} = \frac{K}{\left\{ 1 - \left[CV(m) \right]^2 \xi (1-\xi) \right\}}, \tag{12.8}$$

where $\xi = \dfrac{\bar{m}\rho}{\bar{m}\rho + (1-\rho)}$.

However, the maximum possible value of $\xi(1-\xi) = \dfrac{1}{4}$ and so the largest adjustment to K corresponds to $1/\{1 - [CV(m)]^2/4\}$ in equation (12.7). This implies that the maximum adjustment occurs if $\rho = 1/(\bar{m}+1)$. Further, since the $CV(m)$ is usually less than 0.7, the inflation of K necessary to allow for varying m is at most about 14%. If $CV(m) = 0.35$ then the inflation is at most 3%.

Potential attrition

For many different reasons, the eventual numbers of clusters and/or subjects recruited may be less than those planned.

Clearly, the loss of all information from a cluster has greater impact than the loss of (a few) subjects within a cluster. Thus, as a precaution, the initial number of clusters, K, indicated by the preliminary sample size calculations may need to be increased. Relevant experience of the design group, or reference to published trials reporting such losses, may provide guidance on the extent of potential loss.

Suppose we anticipated that of a possible N subjects we may only achieve $N\theta$, the remaining $N(1 - \theta)$ being lost to follow-up and thereby failing to have the outcome measured. In that case, it would be a sensible precaution to recruit N/θ initially. However, this tends to *overestimate* the sample size required since the DE is based on the number of subjects per cluster before attrition.

An alternative is first to modify the DE using $m\theta$ in place of m, obtain the total sample size by the appropriate means, and then divide this figure by θ to obtain the revised sample size. This process tends to *underestimate* the sample size required since it is unlikely that the drop-out rate is equal in each cluster. The consequential variation in cluster size will result in loss of statistical power, which will need to be compensated for by increasing the trial size perhaps through the use of equation (12.7).

Consequently, a compromise sample size mid-way between the two approaches may be sought. Any change in N may lead the design team to reconsider m, K or both.

12.3   Sample Size for Cluster Trials

Non-aggregate and Aggregate Designs

A *non-aggregate* design uses the individual observations as the unit of analysis. The objective of the sample size calculation is then to determine the appropriate number of *subjects* required per intervention, n_S and n_T, and the number of *clusters*, k_S and k_T, is determined by how many subjects, m, are anticipated per cluster.

An *aggregate* design is one in which a summary measure from each cluster is obtained. For example, with continuous data and $n = mk$ subjects in each intervention, the trial will provide k cluster means $\bar{y}_{01}, \bar{y}_{02}, ..., \bar{y}_{0k}$ (each based on m observations) with a mean of means $\bar{\bar{y}}_0$ for intervention $x = 0$ and $\bar{\bar{y}}_1$ for the k clusters of intervention $x = 1$. The randomised interventions are then compared using $d = \bar{\bar{y}}_1 - \bar{\bar{y}}_0$. In this situation, m is fixed by the design team and the sample size calculation provides the required number of *clusters*, $K = k_S + k_T$.

Continuous Outcome

Non-aggregated design
The variance for individuals in each cluster within each intervention group is assumed the same, and of the form

$$Var(y_{ij}) = \sigma^2_{Between-Cluster} + \sigma^2_{Within-Cluster} = \sigma^2_{Total}. \tag{12.9}$$

If planning values for $\sigma_{Between\text{-}Cluster}$ and $\sigma_{Within\text{-}Cluster}$ can be provided, then the planned values for σ_{Total} (denoted σ_{Plan}) and the ICC can be obtained from equation (12.4). Alternatively, values for the ICC may be gained from previous experience. In either case, although m needs to be pre-specified, DE can be determined from (12.5), and the sample size is

$$N = DE \times \left\{ \left[\frac{(1+\varphi)^2}{\varphi} \right] \frac{\left(z_{1-\alpha/2} + z_{1-\beta} \right)^2}{\left(\delta_{Plan}/\sigma_{Plan} \right)^2} + \frac{z_{1-\alpha/2}^2}{2} \right\}, \tag{12.10}$$

and $n_S = \dfrac{N}{1+\varphi}$ and $n_T = \dfrac{\varphi N}{1+\varphi}$. Hence, the total number of clusters required is $K = N/m$ with $k_S = \dfrac{K}{1+\varphi}$ and $k_T = \dfrac{\varphi K}{1+\varphi}$.

Aggregated design
If an aggregated design is considered, then the summary mean, $\bar{y}_i$, calculated from the m subjects within the cluster i, is the endpoint of concern. In this case

$$Var\left(\bar{y}_i \right) = \sigma_{Between-Cluster}^2 + \frac{\sigma_{Within-Cluster}^2}{m} = \frac{DE\sigma_{Total}^2}{m}. \tag{12.11}$$

A value for this provides the required σ_{Plan}, and the corresponding calculation now refers to the number of clusters required. Thus, since the ICC is taken account of through the DE in equation (12.11), equation (12.1) is used for the sample size estimation but with k_S, k_T and K replacing n_S, n_T and N.

Binary Outcome

Non-aggregated design
For a binary outcome, the dependent variable y_{ij} only takes the values 0 or 1 with the probability π_i that $y_{ij} = 1$, and this probability is assumed to be the same for each subject within a cluster.

In order to calculate a sample size, the anticipated proportions responding in each intervention group, π_S and π_T, need to be anticipated, from which $\delta_{Plan} = \pi_T - \pi_S$, and it is usual to assume that

$$\sigma_{Plan} = \sigma_{Total} = \sqrt{\frac{\left[\pi_T \left(1 - \pi_T \right) + \pi_S \left(1 - \pi_S \right) \right]}{2}} \approx \sqrt{\bar{\pi}\left(1 - \bar{\pi} \right)}, \tag{12.12}$$

where $\bar{\pi} = \dfrac{\pi_T + \pi_S}{2}$.

Also required is the ICC, ρ_{Binary}, for use in the expression for DE of equations (12.6) or (12.7). If the eventual comparison between the observed proportions p_S and p_T is to be made using the z-test (or equivalently the χ^2 test), then the null hypothesis is expressed as H_0: $\delta = \pi_T - \pi_S = 0$, in which case the expression for the ICC is

$$\rho_{Binary} = \frac{\sigma_{Between-Cluster}^2}{\sigma_{Total}^2} = \frac{\sigma_{Between-Cluster}^2}{\bar{\pi}\left(1 - \bar{\pi} \right)}. \tag{12.13}$$

On the other hand, if a logistic regression model is to be used for analysis, which would often be necessary if covariates are also to be considered, then H_0: $\log(OR) = \log\left[\dfrac{\pi_T / (1 - \pi_T)}{\pi_S / (1 - \pi_S)}\right] = 0$. In this case the ICC becomes

$$\rho^*_{Binary} = \bar{\pi}(1 - \bar{\pi})\sigma^{*2}_{Between-Cluster}. \tag{12.14}$$

Note, since the data are analysed in different ways, that $\sigma^{*2}_{Between-Cluster}$ will not take the same value as $\sigma^2_{Between-Cluster}$. Finally, the sample size for both situations is calculated from equation (12.10) using the effect size, $\delta_{Plan} = \pi_T - \pi_S$, and σ_{Plan}, as specified in equation (12.12). The estimate of the sample size may have to be revised to account for possible variation in cluster size, non-participation of some of the clusters, and/or reduced numbers of individuals completing the assessments.

Aggregated design

In an aggregated design, each cluster within each intervention provides a single proportion, p_i, calculated from the m patients within that cluster. These proportions correspond to the $\bar{y}_i$ of the continuous measure situation albeit now taken over a restricted range of values from 0 to 1.

The corresponding variance of each cluster proportion, p_i, is

$$Var(p_i) = \sigma^2_{Between-Cluster} + \frac{\bar{\pi}(1 - \bar{\pi})}{m} = \frac{DE\sigma^2_{Total}}{m}. \tag{12.15}$$

The sample size for this situation is calculated from equation (12.1), or (12.10) with $DE = 1$, but with k_S, k_T and K replacing n_S, n_T and N. The influence of the ICC, in the form of $\rho Binary$, is taken account of by the DE component of equation (12.15).

Ordinal Outcome

In some situations, a binary outcome may be extended to comprise an ordered categorical variable of κ (>2) groups. In principle, if the underlying measure is categorical, then any comparisons between groups will be more sensitive than if a binary outcome is chosen. Consequently, for given Type I and Type II errors, the numbers of patients required will usually be smaller. Further, only *non-aggregate* designs are likely as individual cluster summaries (needed for an *aggregate* design) take the form of a κ-group tabulation rather than a single measure. In practice, there is little statistical benefit to be gained by having more than $\kappa = 5$ ordered categories.

Combining the DE from equations (12.5), (12.6) or (12.7), as appropriate, with equations (4.3) and (4.4) of **Chapter 4**, the expression for calculating sample sizes for comparing two interventions using clusters with individual subject responses from κ possible ordered categories is

$$N = DE \times \left\{ \Gamma \times \left[\frac{(1 + \varphi)^2}{\varphi} \right] \frac{(z_{1-a/2} + z_{1-\beta})^2}{(\log OR_{Plan})^2} \right\}, \tag{12.16}$$

where

$$\Gamma = 3 / \left[1 - \sum_{i=1}^{\kappa} \bar{\pi}_i^3 \right] \tag{12.17}$$

and $\bar{\pi}_i = \left(\pi_{Si} + \pi_{Ti} \right) / 2$. Finally, $n_S = \dfrac{N}{1 + \varphi}$ and $n_T = \dfrac{\varphi N}{1 + \varphi}$.

Rate Outcome

In some situations, all the m individuals within each cluster are followed-up for a fixed period (say F years) and the number of occurrences of a specific event is recorded among the individuals. If r_j individuals in cluster i experience the event, then the event rate per-person-years is estimated by $\lambda_j = r_j / (m \times F)$. In other situations, each of the m subjects within cluster j may have individual follow-up times, say, f_{ij}, in which case the incidence rate for cluster j is $\lambda_j = r_j / Y_j$, where $Y_j = \sum_i f_{ij}$ is the anticipated total follow-up time recorded in the cluster. In practice, the incidence rate may be expressed as per-person, per-100-person or per-1000-person days, years or other time frames depending on the context.

An *aggregate* design is the usual option as it is the rate provided from each cluster which will be the unit for analysis. In this case an alternative to the ICC, as a measure of how close individual responses are within a cluster, is the coefficient of variation for the aggregated outcome of concern:

$$cv(\lambda) = \frac{SD \Big(Cluster\ Rates\ within\ an\ Intervention \Big)}{Mean \Big(Rate\ for\ that\ Intervention \Big)}. \tag{12.18}$$

This should not be confused with $CV(m)$ of the individual cluster sizes defined previously and used in equation (12.7).

In designing a cluster trial, the investigators would need to specify planning values λ_S and λ_T for the mean incidence rates of the interventions, the corresponding cv_S and cv_T (often assumed equal), as well as the maximum duration of follow-up, F, of the individuals in the clusters. The number of clusters required is

$$K = (1 + \varphi) \left\{ \left(\frac{\lambda_S + \varphi \lambda_T}{mF\varphi} \right) + \left(cv_S^2 \right) \lambda_S^2 + \left(cv_T^2 \right) \lambda_T^2 \right\} \frac{\left(z_{1-\alpha/2} + z_{1-\beta} \right)^2}{\left(\lambda_S - \lambda_T \right)^2} + \left[\frac{z_{1-\alpha/2}^2}{2} \right], \tag{12.19}$$

and $k_S = \dfrac{K}{1 + \varphi}$ and $k_T = \dfrac{\varphi K}{1 + \varphi}$. If subjects are only followed up to when the event of interest occurs, then mF in equation (12.19) may be replaced by Y, the stipulated total follow-up time to be recorded in every cluster.

Time-to-Event Outcome

Non-aggregated design
Rather than merely counting the number of events (as for the incidence rate), if the individual times to the event (often termed survival times) are recorded and used in the analysis, the usual summary

for each intervention is the Kaplan-Meier survival curve. The comparison between interventions is then made using a Cox proportional hazards regression model including a random effects term to account for the cluster design. This analysis provides an estimate of the corresponding hazard ratio (HR) which summarises the relative survival difference between the groups. A $HR = 1$ corresponds to the null hypothesis of no difference.

For planning purposes, it is usual to specify γ_S and γ_T, which are the anticipated proportions of subjects alive at a fixed time-point beyond the date their cluster was randomised. Once the design team has specified these, then the planning HR can be calculated from

$$HR_{Plan} = \frac{\log \gamma_T}{\log \gamma_S}. \tag{12.20}$$

The number of subjects required, using the DE of (12.5), is

$$N = DE \times \left(\frac{1+\varphi}{\varphi} \right)\left(\frac{1+\varphi HR}{1-HR} \right)^2 \frac{\left(z_{1-\alpha/2} + z_{1-\beta} \right)^2}{\left[\left(1-\gamma_S \right) + \varphi \left(1-\gamma_T \right) \right]}, \tag{12.21}$$

with $n_S = \dfrac{N}{1+\varphi}$ and $n_T = \dfrac{\varphi N}{1+\varphi}$.

Aggregated design

For an aggregated design, it may be appropriate to consider the survival rate at a fixed time following randomisation, say at the 1-year follow-up. The planning values of these, γ_S and γ_T, may then be taken as π_S and π_T and used in much the same way as for sample size calculations for a cluster trial with either a binary or rate endpoint as discussed previously.

Matched Designs

In the preceding sections each cluster participating in the trial has been identified and then randomised (say) in equal numbers to receive the S or T intervention. However, there is a limit to how well randomisation can balance potentially prognostic factors especially since the number of clusters in a cluster trial is often limited. An alternative design is the matched pairs design, whereby clusters are first matched in pairs. If the clusters themselves are of variable size, then an efficient method of matching is to create cluster pairs of a similar size. Options other than size may be used to create the matched pairs, the choice being perhaps related to features of the clusters concerned, such as their location in rural or urban areas. Once these *matched pairs* are identified, the allocation of T is made at random to one of the pair and the other is then automatically assigned to S.

Once the trial is complete, a simple method of analysis is to compare the difference in summary measure from each matched pair of clusters. This *matched* design implies an *aggregate* analysis. Thus, for example, if the endpoint is continuous, this measure will be the difference, $d_k = \bar{y}_{Tk} - \bar{y}_{Sk}$, for each of the cluster pairs, $k = 1, 2, ..., K_{Pairs}$. From these values the mean difference $\bar{d}$ is obtained, and this estimates the true difference between the interventions, δ. The paired t-test then tests the null hypothesis $\delta = 0$.

In this situation, the number of cluster pairs required is

$$K_{Pairs} = DE \times \left\{ \frac{2\left(z_{1-\alpha/2} + z_{1-\beta}\right)^2}{\left(\delta_{Plan}/\sigma_{Plan}\right)^2} + \frac{z_{1-\alpha/2}^2}{2} \right\}. \tag{12.22}$$

Here σ_{Plan} is the anticipated SD of the differences, d_i, obtained from the cluster pairs.

Cross-over Designs

In a cluster-based cross-over trial, the interventions are allocated in the sequence ST or TS with (usually) half the clusters randomised to ST, while for the remaining clusters the opposite sequence TS would be used. Thus, all subjects in a cluster allocated ST will receive S in Period I and then T in Period II. Similarly, all subjects in a cluster allocated TS will receive T in Period I and then S in Period II. The usual situation is to introduce a no-intervention interval, termed the washout, between the two periods in which the interventions are activated.

A full analysis of such trials estimates the intervention effect and examines the influence of the period in which the intervention was given and whether the influence of the first intervention given carries over into the second.

The implication of allocating the sequences by cluster is that the design team needs to be aware of the presence of both intra-class and inter-period correlations. Thus, the m subjects receiving the intervention of Period I share a common correlation, here η, and this same correlation will also be present in their Period II. Further, there will be a correlation, ω, between the two responses (one from Period I, the other from Period II) of a patient, consequently the DE of equation (12.5) is modified, assuming a fixed m, to become

$$DE_{Cross} = 1 + (m - 1)\eta - m\omega. \tag{12.23}$$

Table 12.2 gives DE_{Cross} for $\omega = 0.005$ and 0.01 for a range of values of m and η. Further since a 1:1 randomisation is preferred for a cross-over trial, $\varphi = 1$. For values of η greater than ω the $DE > 1$. Combining these changes, equation (12.9) is modified, for a continuous outcome, to give the number of subjects required as:

$$N_{Cross} = DE_{Cross} \times \left\{ \frac{2\left(z_{1-\alpha/2} + z_{1-\beta}\right)^2}{\left(\delta_{Plan}/\sigma_{Plan}\right)^2} + \frac{z_{1-\alpha/2}^2}{2} \right\} \tag{12.24}$$

This implies that $n_{ST} = n_{TS} = N_{Cross}/2$ subjects receive each sequence. In expression (12.23) the component $m\omega$, with $\omega > 0$, will reduce the size of the DE as compared to that given by equation (12.5). Thus, the inflation in sample size caused by using a cluster design for a cross-over trial may be less than in the situations discussed previously.

12.4 Baseline Observations

In the situation when the endpoint variable is continuous and a baseline observation is feasible, the DE for a given design can be modified by multiplying the design effect by $(1 - r^2)$, where r is the correlation of the cluster means between baseline and the follow-up assessment. In general, this will lead to a reduction in the corresponding sample size.

12.5   Number of Clusters Fixed

The methods above are predicated on a fixed cluster size and the investigator is free to increase the number of clusters to obtain the requisite power. If the number of clusters is fixed, and we wish to increase the cluster size to increase the sample size to achieve a given significance level and power, then to find the required cluster size we use.

$$m = \frac{m'(1-\rho)}{1-m'\rho},$$

(12.25)

where $m' = N_{Ind}/K$ is the number of subjects per cluster required for an individually randomised trial. The fact that m'ρ must be less than unity leads to the fact that the minimum number of clusters, for a cluster trial with ICC, ρ, is

$$K_{Min} = N_{Ind}\rho$$

(12.26)

If the number of clusters the investigators have available is less than K_{Min}, then they will never achieve the required power at the given significance level and effect size, since they would require infinitely large cluster sizes. Even when the actual number of clusters available is only slightly larger than K_{Min} leads to infeasibly large cluster sizes and the investigators options are to recruit yet more clusters, accept a larger effect size or to accept a reduced power.

12.6   Practicalities

Cluster trials consume considerable logistical and other resources, so a critical factor is to determine the appropriate size for the trial in question. In some instances, the number of clusters available may be fixed, in others the number of subjects per cluster is fixed or possibly both may be open to choice. Although 1:1 allocation of interventions is usual, there is nevertheless a decision to be made with respect to this ratio.

Also, in the cluster trial situation, an ICC (or some other measure of the lack of independence of the subjects within a cluster) will need to be specified. In some situations, cluster trials may have been done in similar circumstances to the one in planning so that the magnitude of such measures may be well documented. For example, the ICC from 1039 variables obtained by Adams, Gulliford, Ukoumunne, et al (2004) ranges from 0 to 0.840 with a median value of 0.010, while Hade, Murray, Pennell, et al (2010) detail 51 values from screening studies for breast, cervical, colon and prostate cancers with a median value of 0.0355 with a range from essentially zero to 0.292. However, in most situations some (often considerable) judgment is required as to what is an appropriate value. Carter (2009) stresses the importance of considering the potential variation in cluster size. Whatever the situation, the design team will need to consider the impact on sample size of a range of options for these (and other design features) before deciding the final trial size.

A review by Ivers, Taljaard, Dixon, et al (2011) concluded that the methodological quality of cluster trials often remains suboptimal. Investigators should verify what will be required by CONSORT (Campbell, Piaggio, Elbourne and Altman, 2012) for reporting their cluster trial to ensure all that is needed with respect to design and sample size issues are in place *before* the trial commences.

12.7 Bibliography

This chapter is an expansion of the material contained in Gao, Earnest, Matchar, *et al* (2015). The books by Hayes and Moulton (2009), Eldridge and Kerry (2012) and Campbell and Walters (2014) include detailed discussion of the design, analysis and reporting of cluster trials.

Eldridge, Ashby and Kerry (2006) suggested the modified *DE* of equations (12.6) and (12.7) to allow for variation in cluster size while van Breukelen and Candel (2012) derive equation (12.8), which adjusts the number of clusters required after first assuming a fixed cluster size in the calculations.

Equation (12.19) for calculating sample sizes when comparing rates, taking into account variation of cluster rates within an intervention through equation (12.18), is given by Hayes and Moulton (2009), who also provide equation (12.22), which defines the necessary *DE* for a cluster pair-matched design.

Equation (12.21) for survival time studies is given by Xie and Waksman (2003), while Giraudeau, Ravaud and Donner (2008, 2009) show how the *DE* is modified in equation (12.23) when considering a cross-over trial design. For a continuous endpoint variable, Teerenstra, Eldridge, Graff, *et al* (2012) show how the *DE* can be reduced, and hence also the sample size, by including a baseline assessment into the study design.

Hemming and Taljaard (2016) describe a unified approach to sample size calculations for cluster trials and the stepped wedge designs (SWD) of Chapter 13. Campbell (2014) and Moberg and Kramer (2015) provide brief histories of the cluster randomised trial and Hemming, Eldridge, Forbes et al (2017) provide useful advice on the efficient design of cluster trials. Some aspects related to computational methods are included in the computing section of the references (Chapter 12.7).

12.8 Examples

Numerical Accuracy

When calculating sample sizes, it is usual to obtain a non-integer from the appropriate algebraic expression and then *automatically* round this upwards to give a convenient integer value. However, as we indicated in **Chapter 1.8**, when considering the number of clusters some care is needed as the rounding up may result in an unacceptable study size as each additional cluster adds a further m (which may be quite large) subjects to the study.

Table 1.2
For two-sided test size, $\alpha = 0.05$, $z_{0.975} = 1.96$.   For one-sided $1 - \beta = 0.80$ and 0.90, $z_{0.80} = 0.8416$ and $z_{0.90} = 1.2816$ respectively.

Equations 12.5 and 12.9

Example 12.1   Non-aggregate design - Comparing two means - Outdoor time for children
Suppose a design team is planning a confirmatory *non-aggregate* cluster randomised trial, based on the trial of Ngo, Pan, Finkelstein, *et al* (2014, Table 3), to see if a revised incentive-based strategy (T)

in addition to information on the health benefits of physical activity (S) would increase outdoor time in children age 6-12 years. Families of varying numbers of children within the age group concerned were randomised on a 1:1 basis. One outcome of concern was the number of outdoor hours spent per week measured 6 months post-randomisation. Previous experience suggests that in the control children have a mean outdoor time of 12.40 hours with SD = 6.94 and that the effect of T would be considered important if this increased by 3.5 hours per week.

These lead to planning values $\delta_{Plan} = 3.5$ and $\sigma_{Plan} = 6.94$. Previous experience suggests selecting only those families with 2 or more children within the age group concerned so that an achievable cluster size is $m = 2$ and ICC = 0.025 so that equation (12.5) gives $DE = 1 + [(2-1) \times 0.025] = 1.025$. Further, the investigators set a 2-sided $\alpha = 0.05$, $\beta = 0.1$ and $\varphi = 1$, and so the sample size required from equation (12.9) is $N = 1.025 \times \left\{ \left[\frac{(1+1)^2}{1} \right] \times \frac{(1.96+1.2816)^2}{(3.5/6.94)^2} + \frac{1.96^2}{2} \right\} = 1.025 \times 167.17 = 171.35$. The planned total sample size is therefore $N = 172$ children, and with $m = 2$, this implies $K = 172/2 = 86$, which allows a 1:1 randomisation to assign to each intervention 43 families (each of two children).

If the ICC assumed was set as $\rho = 0.1$ or 0.2, then these would increase N to 184 and 204 respectively.

Table 12.1 and Equations 12.5, 12.6, 12.7, 12.8 and 12.9

Example 12.2   Non-aggregate design - Comparing two means - Daily exercise

Suppose a design team is planning a confirmatory *non-aggregate* cluster randomised trial, based on the trial of Munro, Nicholl, Brazier, *et al* (2001), to see if a daily exercise regime delivered by personal trainers at the suggestion of their general practitioner for a year (*PT*) would lead to improved quality of life compared to no intervention (*NI*) in older men. The primary outcome was the Physical Function (PF) dimension of the SF-36 measure at 1-year. Previous experience suggests that such men have a mean score of 66.4 units, with $\sigma_{PF} = 29.5$ units, and the effect of the daily exercise regime would be considered important if it increased the PF score by at least 10 units.

These lead to planning values $\delta_{Plan} = 10$ and $\sigma_{Plan} = 29.5$. However, due to the high cost of providing personal trainers, the new design team decides on a 3:2 randomisation in favour of *NI*, that is $\varphi = 2/3 = 0.6667$. This implies that K will have to be a multiple of 5 if the clusters are to be randomised in this ratio. Previous experience suggests that an achievable cluster size is $m = 25$ and $\rho = 0.01$ so that **Table 12.1** and equation (12.5) give $DE = 1 + [(25-1) \times 0.01] = 1.240$. **Table 12.1** indicates that, for $m = 25$, the DE is quite sensitive to the choice of ρ and attains a value of 3.400 when $\rho = 0.1$. The value of DE steadily increases as m increases.

The investigators set a 2-sided $\alpha = 0.05$, $\beta = 0.1$, and so the sample size required from equation (12.9) is $N = 1.240 \times \left\{ \left[\frac{(1+0.6667)^2}{0.6667} \right] \times \frac{(1.96+1.2816)^2}{(10/29.5)^2} + \frac{1.96^2}{2} \right\} = 1.240 \times 382.92 = 474.82 \, \text{or} \, 475$.

If there was a concern that the cluster size may vary about a mean of $\bar{m} = 25$, with $SD(m) = 2.5$, then $CV(m) = \frac{2.5}{25} = 0.1$ and use of equation (12.7) gives $DE = 1 + \{[(0.1^2 + 1) \times 25] - 1\} \times 0.01 = 1.2425$. This increases the initial value of N to 475.78 or 480 and the number of clusters to $K = 480/25 = 19.2$ or 20. Since K is now established, this allows the use of equation (12.6) to give a modified $DE = 1 + \left\{ \left[0.1^2 \left(\frac{20-1}{20} \right) + 1 \right] \times 25 - 1 \right\} \times 0.01 = 1.2424$. This is very close to the former value for the DE and hence has no additional impact on the sample size for the design chosen.

Further, if the adjustment of (12.8) is examined, then with $m=25$, $SD(m)=2.5$, $\xi = \dfrac{25\times0.01}{(25\times0.01)+(1-0.01)} = 0.2016$, and $K_{Adjusted} = \dfrac{20}{\left\{1-[0.01]^2\times0.2016\times(1-0.2016)\right\}} = 20.03$. This too has little influence on the overall design as the investigators are unlikely to round this upwards to 21. Finally, if the investigators set $k_{NI}=12$ and $k_{PT}=8$, then the stipulated randomisation ratio of 3:2 is achieved and this requires 500 men to be recruited.

There are clearly many options for the design team to consider.

Equations 12.1, 12.4, 12.9 and 12.10

Example 12.3 Aggregate design - Comparing two means - Daily exercise

Had *Example 12.2* been designed as an *aggregated* cluster trial, then with the information provided as $\sigma_{Total}=29.5$ and $\rho=0.01$, equation (12.4) can be used to obtain $\sigma^2_{Between-Cluster} = \rho\times\sigma^2_{Total} = 0.01\times(29.5)^2 = 8.70$ and $\sigma^2_{Within-Cluster} = \sigma^2_{Total} - \sigma^2_{Between-Cluster} = (29.5)^2 - 8.70 = 861.6$. Hence, if we now assume $m=30$, using equation (12.15) implies $\sigma_{Plan} = \sqrt{8.70+\dfrac{861.6}{30}} = 6.12$ and, from equation (12.1) (or equation (12.9) with $DE=1$) with $\varphi=2/3$, 2-sided $\alpha=0.05$, $\beta=0.1$, $K = \left\{\left[\dfrac{(1+2/3)^2}{2/3}\right]\times\dfrac{(1.96+1.2816)^2}{(10/6.12)^2}+\dfrac{1.96^2}{2}\right\} = 18.32$ or 19 clusters. Consequently, $k_S = K/[1+(2/3)] = 19\times(3/5) = 11.4$ or 12 while $k_T = [(2/3)K]/[1+(2/3)] = 19\times(2/5) = 7.6$ or 8 clusters, giving a revised total of $K=20$ clusters.

Some judgement is required as to whether 11.4 and 7.6 are rounded down to 11 and 7 or up to 12 and 8 as every extra cluster requires a further $m=30$ patients to be recruited.

Equations 12.5, 12.8, 12.10 and 12.12

Example 12.4 Non-aggregate - Comparing two proportions - Hypertension and hypercholesterolemia

The STITCH2 randomised cluster design trial of Dresser, Nelson, Mahon, *et al* (2013) involving 35 primary care practices (PCP) compared Guidelines (*G*) for intervention with the same guidelines with an initial use of single-pill combination (*SPG*) to improve management of participants with both hypertension and dyslipidemia.

Assuming a repeat trial is planned with $m=50$ subjects from each PCP, with the planning value for *G*, the proportion achieving target, as 0.40 while that for *SPG* is 0.52. From these, $\delta_{Plan}=0.52-0.40=0.12$, and from (12.12) $\bar{\pi} = \dfrac{0.52+0.40}{2} = 0.46$ and $\sigma_{Plan} = \sqrt{0.46(1-0.46)} = 0.4984$. Further assuming $\rho_{Binary}=0.071$ (see *Example 12.5* below) and using equations (12.5) and (12.10) with 2-sided $\alpha=0.05$, $\beta=0.2$ and $\varphi=1$,

$$N_{Clus} = DE\times N_{Ind} = \left[1+(50-1)\times0.071\right]\times\left\{\left[\dfrac{(1+1)^2}{1}\right]\dfrac{(1.96+0.8416)^2}{(0.12/0.4984)^2}+\dfrac{1.96^2}{2}\right\} = 4.4790\times543.50 =$$

2,434.33, implying $N_{Clus}=2{,}436$ subjects in total as compared to an individually randomised design with $N_{Ind}=544$. The corresponding number of clusters $K=2{,}436/50\approx49$.

If the number recruited per PCP was likely to vary, as was indeed the case in STITCH2, then a conservative application of equation (12.8) would lead to increasing this number by 14%. Hence, the number of clusters becomes $K = 49 \times 1.14 = 55.9$ or 56. Thus the total number of patients required is thereby increased to $N = 56 \times 50 = 2,800$.

Only 44 (85%) of the 52 PCPs identified for the STITCH2 trial eventually participated in the trial. Thus, in planning a future trial, the initial K might be increased by 15%, suggesting here that $56 \times 1.15 \approx 64$ PCPs might need to be approached.

Further, as a precautionary measure to account for potential patient (not cluster) loss (see equation (7.18), **Chapter** 7), an approximate 15% increase in this number may be adopted, in which case $N = 2,800/(1 - 0.15) \approx 3,300$ need to be targeted.

Should all three possibilities arise, the planned trial size may be designed to recruit up to (say) 4,000 individuals with consequent increases in either, m, K or both.

Equations 12.10, 12.13 and 12.15

Example 12.5   Aggregate design - Comparing two proportions - Hypertension and hypercholesterolemia

The report of the STITCH2 trial of Dresser, Nelson, Mahon, *et al* (2013) states 'The primary analysis compared the proportion of participants achieving targets [for example, specified blood pressure levels] between the two treatment groups using a two-sample t-test at the level of the cluster ... '. This clearly indicates an aggregated design was planned.

In addition to the planning values indicated in *Example 12.4*, they also specify $\sigma_{Total} = 0.15$, which is taken as σ_{Plan}, and this provides, using equation (12.15) with $\bar{\pi} = 0.46$, $\sigma^2_{Between-Cluster} = 0.15^2 - \dfrac{0.46(1 - 0.46)}{50} = 0.017$. Further from equation (12.13), $\rho_{Binary} = 0.017/(0.46 \times 0.54) = 0.071$ as we had noted earlier.

Then from equation (12.10) with $DE = 1$, the number of clusters required assuming $\varphi = 1$, 2-sided $\alpha = 0.05$, $\beta = 0.2$ is $K = \dfrac{(1+1)^2}{1} \dfrac{(1.96 + 0.8416)^2}{(0.12/0.15)^2} + \dfrac{1.96^2}{2} = 50.98$ or 52, implying 26 per intervention.

Equations 4.3, 12.5, 12.16 and 12.17

Example 12.6   Aggregate design - Ordinal outcome - Intimate partner violence

Assume investigators plan a cluster trial with women who have experienced intimate partner violence on the basis of the information of **Figure 4.3** obtained from the S group of the WEAVE trial of Hegarty, O'Doherty, Taft, *et al* (2013) and with anticipated effect size $OR_{Plan} = 1.5$ in favour of a new intervention strategy, T. In which case, log $OR_{Plan} = 0.4055$, equation (12.17) gives $\Gamma = 3.5129$. Then, with $\varphi = 1$, 2-sided $\alpha = 0.05$ and $\beta = 0.2$, equation (4.3) in *Example 4.3* gives $N_4 = 670.74$.

Further assuming the cluster size is $m = 30$ and $\rho = 0.001$, then from equation (12.5), $DE = 1 + (29 \times 0.001) = 1.029$. The results from equations (4.3) with (12.1) and (12.17) combined lead to the required number of subjects as $N = 1.029 \times 670.74 = 690.19$. To be divisible by $m = 30$, this is rounded down to give $K = 690/30 = 23$ clusters, which would need to be increased to 24 to allow a 1:1 allocation.

Equation 12.19

Example 12.7   Aggregate design – Rate outcome - Left ventricular systolic dysfunction

The results from a trial conducted by Lowrie, Mair, Greenlaw, *et al* (2012) concerned with attempts to improve the outcome for patients with left ventricular systolic dysfunction suggested that *Usual* care (*U*) was associated with a rate of 7.2 deaths per 100 years ($\lambda_U = 0.072$). It is hoped that *Enhanced* care (*E*) might reduce this by 20% ($\lambda_E = 0.0576$). A 1:1 cluster trial is planned with 2-sided $\alpha = 0.05$, $\beta = 0.2$, $m = 12$, $F = 5$ years, and $cv_U = cv_E = 0.1$. Use of equation (12.19) results in $K = (1+1)$

$$\left\{ \left(\frac{0.072 + (1 \times 0.0576)}{12 \times 5 \times 1} \right) + (0.1 \times 0.072)^2 + (0.1 \times 0.0576)^2 \right\} \frac{(1.96 + 0.8416)^2}{(0.072 - 0.0576)^2} + \left[\frac{1.96^2}{2} \right] = 171.88 \text{ or } 172.$$

Hence, $k_U = k_E = K/2 = 86$ clusters. Had more variation been anticipated, perhaps $cv_U = cv_E = 0.2$, then $K = 192$.

Equations 12.5, 12.20 and 12.21

Example 12.8 Non-aggregate design - Survival times - Heart dysfunction

In the Trial of Education And Compliance in Heart (TEACH) dysfunction trial of Gwadry-Sridhar, Guyatt, O'Brien, *et al* (2008), the investigators anticipated that the 1-year rate of re-hospitalisation following earlier hospital admission for heart problems (*Standard care, S*) would be about 75%. It was further anticipated that this could be reduced to 60% using enhanced education on their condition from their home pharmacist (*HP*). Thus, with $\gamma_S = 0.75$ and $\gamma_{HP} = 0.60$ representing the anticipated proportions re-admitted at 1-year, equation (12.20) gives $HR = \dfrac{\log 0.60}{\log 0.75} = 1.7757$. Further, if we take $m = 2$, $\varphi = 1$, 2-sided $\alpha = 0.05$ and $\beta = 0.2$, then, for this non-aggregate design using (12.5), equation

(12.21) becomes $N = \left[1 + (2-1)\rho \right] \times \left(\dfrac{1+1}{1} \right) \left(\dfrac{1+1.7757}{1-1.7757} \right)^2 \dfrac{(1.96 + 0.8416)^2}{\left[(1-0.60) + (1-0.75) \right]} = 309.23 \times (1 + \rho).$

Setting ρ equal to 0.05 and 0.10, as the investigators did, gives the respective values of $N = 326$ and 342 with the corresponding total number of pharmacies (clusters) required as $K = 326/2 = 163$ and 171 respectively. To allow a 1:1 randomisation, these are then increased to 164 and 172 to give either 82 or 86 pharmacies per intervention.

Equations 12.5 and 12.22

Example 12.9 Aggregate design - Matched clusters - Daily exercise

Suppose a second trial of a similar design to that of Munro, Nicholl, Brazier, *et al* (2001) described in *Example 12.2* was to involve communities with very diverse socio-economic characteristics, then the design team might wish to create cluster pairs with similar features. The anticipated improvement in physical function (PF) anticipated with *PT* over *NI* is assumed the same with $\delta_{Plan} = 10$ units. However, the previous trial provided a $\sigma_{Plan} = 6.12$ units, whereas for a matched design this might be anticipated to be smaller than this to an extent depending on the numbers to be recruited per cluster, *m*. Thus, a range of values for σ_{Plan}, as well as the intra-class correlation, ρ, are investigated.

As a first step, the investigators take $\rho = 0.01$ and $\sigma_{Plan} = 6.12$ and, from equations (12.23) and (12.24), with $m = 30$, 2-sided $\alpha = 0.05$ and $\beta = 0.1$, obtain $DE_{Pairs} = \left[1 + (30 - 1) \times 0.01 \right] = 1.29$,

$$K_{Pairs} = 1.29 \times \left\{ \frac{2(1.96 + 1.2816)^2}{(10/6.12)^2} + \frac{1.96^2}{2} \right\} = 1.29 \times 9.79 = 12.63 \text{ or } 13. \text{ This implies 26 clusters are}$$

required, which are then matched into 13 pairs. If $\eta = 0.05$ then the number of cluster pairs increases to $K_{Pairs} = 24$. A reduced $\sigma_{Plan} = 3.06$ results in $K_{Pairs} = 6$ and 10 for $\rho = 0.01$ and 0.05 respectively.

Table 12.2 and Equations 12.23 and 12.24

Example 12.10 Non-aggregate design - Cross-over trial - Surgical hand preparation

Nthumba, Stepita-Poenaru, Poenaru, *et al* (2010) describe the results from a randomised cluster cross-over trial designed to compare the efficacy of plain soap and water (*W*) versus alcohol-based (*A*) rub for surgical hand preparation. Their trial involved 10 surgical teams (the clusters), 5 of which were randomised to the sequence *WA* and 5 to *AW*. Their planning value for the rate of surgical-site infection (SSI) in their patients using *W* was anticipated to be 0.15.

Different investigators planning a repeat trial in similar circumstances set $m = 200$ patients per clinical team but are unclear of reasonable planning values for δ_{Plan}, σ_{Plan}, ρ and ω. Consequently, they investigate a range of options beginning with 2-sided $\alpha = 0.05$, $\beta = 0.2$, a reduction in SSI rate of $\Delta = \delta_{Plan}/\sigma_{Plan} = -0.25$, $\eta = 0.05$ and $\omega = 0.01$.

Use of equation (12.23) or **Table 12.2** gives $DE_{Cross} = 1 + [(200 - 1) \times 0.05] - [200 \times 0.01] = 12.95$, and

hence equation (12.24) results in $N_{Cross} = 8.95 \times \left\{ \dfrac{2(1.96 + 0.8416)^2}{(-0.25)^2} + \dfrac{1.96^2}{2} \right\} = 8.95 \times 253.09 = 2{,}265.16$.

Thus, $K_{Cross} = 2{,}265.16/\ 200 = 11.33$ or a total of 12 clusters.

Further investigation, by setting $\omega = 0.02$, reduces the required sample size quite dramatically to $N_{Cross} = 1{,}759$, requiring $K_{Cross} = 9$, which might be increased to give 5 clusters for each sequence *WA* and *AW*.

Equations 12.25 and 12.26

Example 12.11 Restricted number of clusters

The STITCH2 trial of Example 12.4 required 544 patients if the trial were not clustered. Given $\rho = 0.071$, the minimum number of Primary Care Practices (PCPs) for a cluster trial that can achieve the same power as an individually randomised one from (12.26) is $N_{Ind}\rho = 544'0.071 = 38.6$. Thus STITCH2 cannot achieve the desired power with fewer than 39 clusters.

If the investigators chose $K = 40$ PCPs then $m' = 544/40 = 13.6$ or 14 and from equation (12.25) the revised $m = 14(1 - 0.071)/[1 - (14'0.071)] = 2{,}167$ subjects per cluster or 86,680 subjects in total. This is not a feasible number since it is bigger than most clinical trials ever conducted!

However, if the investigators could persuade 44 PCPs to join, as in the original trial of Dresser, Nelson, Mahon, *et al* (2013), then about $m = 94$ subjects per cluster or 4,136 subjects in total are needed. This contrasts with the much fewer 2,436 subjects, comprising $K = 49$ PCPs with $m = 50$ subjects in each cluster suggested by Example 12.4. The investigators would have to weigh up the costs of nearly doubling the numbers of subjects per PCP versus increasing the number of PCPs by only 5. This effect is bigger when ρ is relatively large, as in Example 12.4 and one would normally expect the number of available clusters to be much bigger than K_{Min}.

Thus equation (12.25) is only really useful if the normal procedure (where the cluster size drives the number of clusters), suggests that the number of clusters required is greater than the number available. Given that the number available is greater than *KMin*, the investigators may wish to see how much bigger the cluster sizes have to be to achieve the required sample size for the power stipulated with the design.

References

Technical

Adams G, Gulliford MC, Ukoumunne OC, Eldridge S, Chinn S and Campbell MJ (2004). Patterns of intra-cluster correlation from primary care research to inform study design and analysis. *Journal of Clinical Epidemiology*, **57**, 785–794.

Campbell MJ and Walters SJ (2014). *How to Design, Analyse and Report Cluster Randomised Trials in Medicine and Health Related Research*. Chichester, Wiley.

Campbell MK, Piaggio G, Elbourne DR and Altman DG (2012). Consort 2010 statement: extension to cluster randomized trials. *British Medical Journal*, **345**, e5661. doi:10.1136/bmj.e5661.

Carter B (2010). Cluster size variability and imbalance in cluster randomized controlled trials. *Statistics in Medicine*, **29**, 2984–2993.

Eldridge SM, Ashby D and Kerry S (2006). Sample size for cluster randomized trials: effect of coefficient of variation of cluster size and analysis method. *International Journal of Epidemiology*, **35**, 1202–1300.

Eldridge SM and Kerry S (2012). *A Practical Guide to Cluster Randomised Trials in Health Services Research*. Chichester, Wiley-Blackwell.

Gao F, Earnest A, Matchar DB, Campbell MJ and Machin D (2015). Sample size calculations for the design of cluster randomized trials: a review. *Contemporary Clinical Trials*, **42**, 41–50.

Giraudeau B, Ravaud P and Donner A (2008, 2009). Sample size calculation for cluster randomized cross-over trials. *Statistics in Medicine*, **27**, 5578–5585 (Correction, **28**, 720).

Hemming K, Eldridge S, Forbes G, Weijer C, Taljaard M (2017) How to design efficient cluster randomised trials. *BMJ*. 358:j3064.

Hemming K and Taljaard M (2017). Sample size calculations for stepped wedge and cluster randomised trials: a unified approach. *Journal of Clinical Epidemiology*, **69**, 137–146.

Hade EM, Murray DM, Pennell ML, Rhoda D, Paskett ED, Champion VL, Crabtree BF, Dietrich A, Dignan MB, Farmer M, Fenton JJ, Flocke S, Hiatt RA, Hudson SV, Mitchell M, Monahan P, Shariff-Marco S, Slone SL, Stange K, Stewart SL and Strickland PAO (2010). Intraclass correlation estimates for cancer screening outcomes: estimates and applications in the design of group-randomized cancer screening studies. *Journal of the National Cancer Institute Monographs*, **40**, 90–107.

Hayes RJ and Moulton L (2009). *Cluster Randomised Trials*. Boca Raton, Chapman and Hall/CRC.

Hemming K, Eldridge S, Forbes G, Weijer C and Taljaard M (2017) How to design efficient cluster randomised trials. *British Medical Journal*, **358**:j3064.

Ivers NM, Taljaard M, Dixon S, Bennett C, McRae A, Taleban J, Skea Z, Brehaut JC, Boruch RF, Eccles MP, Grimshaw JM, Weijer C, Zwarenstein M and Donner A (2011). Impact of CONSORT extension for cluster randomized trials on quality of reporting and study methodology: review of random sample of 300 trials, 2000-8. *British Medical Journal*, **343**, d5886.

Teerenstra S, Eldridge S, Graff M, de Hoop E and Born GF (2012). A simple sample size formula for analysis of covariance in cluster randomized. *Statistics in Medicine*, **31**, 2169–2178.

Van Breukelen GJP and Candel MJJM (2012). Comments on 'Efficiency loss because of varying cluster size in cluster randomized trials is smaller than literature suggests'. *Statistics in Medicine*, **31**, 397–400.

Xie T and Waksman J (2003). Design and sample size estimation in clinical trials with clustered survival times as the primary endpoint. *Statistics in Medicine*, **22**, 2835–2846.

Computing

Batistatou E, Roberts C and Roberts S (2014). Sample size and power calculations for trials and quasi-experimental studies with clustering. *The Stata Journal*, **14**, 159–175.

Campbell MJ and Walters SJ (2014). *How to Design, Analyse and Report Cluster Randomised Trials in Medicine and Health Related Research*. Chichester, Wiley.

Hemming K and Marsh J (2013). A menu-driven facility for sample-size calculations in cluster randomized controlled trials. *The Stata Journal*, **13**, 114–135.

IBM Corp (2013). IBM SPSS Statistics for Windows, Version 22. Armonk, NY, IBM Corp.

Rotondi M and Donner A (2012). Sample size estimation in cluster randomized trials: An evidence-based perspective. *Computation Statistics and Data Analysis*, **56**, 1174–1187.

Examples

Dresser GK, Nelson SA, Mahon JL, Zou G, Vandervoort MK, Wong CJ, Feagan BG and Feldman RD (2013). Simplified therapeutic intervention to control hypertension and hypercholesterolemia: a cluster randomized controlled trial (STITCH2). *Journal of Hypertension*, **31**, 1702–1713.

Gwadry-Sridhar F, Guyatt G, O'Brien B, Arnold JM, Walter S, Vingilis E and MacKeigan L (2008). TEACH: Trial of Education And Compliance in Heart dysfunction chronic disease and heart failure (HF) as an increasing problem. *Contemporary Clinical Trials*, **29**, 905–918.

Hegarty K, O'Doherty L, Taft A, Chondros P, Brown S, Valpied J, Astbury J, Taket A, Gold L, Feder G and Gunn J (2013). Screening and counselling in the primary care setting for women who have experienced intimate partner violence (WEAVE): a cluster randomised controlled trial. *Lancet*, **382**, 249–258.

Lowrie R, Mair FS, Greenlaw N, Forsyth P, Jhund PS, McConnachie A, Rae B, and McMurray JJV (2012). Pharmacist intervention in primary care to improve outcomes in patients with left ventricular systolic dysfunction. *European Heart Journal*, **33**, 314–324.

Munro JF, Nicholl JP, Brazier JE, Davey R and Cochrane T (2004). Cost effectiveness of a community based exercise programme in over 65 year olds: cluster randomised trial. *Journal of Epidemiology and Community Health*, **58**, 1004–1010.

Ngo CS, Pan C-W, Finkelstein EA, Lee C-F, Wong IB, Ong J, Ang M, Wong T-Y and Saw S-M (2014). A cluster randomized controlled trial evaluating an incentive-based outdoor physical activity programme to increase outdoor time and prevent myopia in children. *Opthalmic & Physiological Optics*, **34**, 362–368.

Nthumba PM, Stepita-Poenaru E, Poenaru D, Bird P, Allegranzi B, Pittet D and Harbarth S (2010). Cluster-randomized, crossover trial of the efficacy of plain soap and water *versus* alcohol-based rub for surgical hand preparation in a rural hospital in Kenya. *British Journal of Surgery*, **97**, 1621–1628.

History

Campbell MJ (2014). Challenges of cluster randomised trials. *Journal of Comparative Effectiveness*, **3**, 271–278.

Moberg J and Kramer M (2015). A brief history of the cluster randomised trial design. *Journal of the Royal Society of Medicine*, **108**, 192–198.

Table 12.1 The Design Effect [Equation 12.5].

ICC	Number of subjects per cluster, m					
ρ	10	25	50	75	100	200
0.005	1.045	1.120	1.245	1.370	1.495	1.995
0.010	1.090	1.240	1.490	1.740	1.990	2.990
0.015	1.135	1.360	1.735	2.110	2.485	3.985
0.020	1.180	1.480	1.980	2.480	2.980	4.980
0.025	1.225	1.600	2.225	2.850	3.475	5.975
0.030	1.270	1.720	2.470	3.220	3.970	6.970
0.035	1.315	1.840	2.715	3.590	4.465	7.965
0.040	1.360	1.960	2.960	3.960	4.960	8.960
0.045	1.405	2.080	3.205	4.330	5.455	9.955
0.050	1.450	2.200	3.450	4.700	5.950	10.950
0.075	1.675	2.800	4.675	6.550	8.425	15.925
0.100	1.900	3.400	5.900	8.400	10.900	20.900

Table 12.2 The Design Effect for Cluster Crossover Trials [Equation 12.23].

Response correlation ω	Period correlation η	Number of subjects per cluster, m					
		10	25	50	75	100	200
0.005	0.005	0.995	0.995	0.995	0.995	0.995	0.995
	0.010	1.040	1.115	1.240	1.365	1.490	1.990
	0.015	1.085	1.235	1.485	1.735	1.985	2.985
	0.020	1.130	1.355	1.730	2.105	2.480	3.980
	0.025	1.175	1.475	1.975	2.475	2.975	4.975
	0.030	1.220	1.595	2.220	2.845	3.470	5.970
	0.035	1.265	1.715	2.465	3.215	3.965	6.965
	0.040	1.310	1.835	2.710	3.585	4.460	7.960
	0.045	1.355	1.955	2.955	3.955	4.955	8.955
	0.050	1.400	2.075	3.200	4.325	5.450	9.950
	0.075	1.625	2.675	4.425	6.175	7.925	14.925
	0.100	1.850	3.275	5.650	8.025	10.400	19.900
0.010	0.005	0.945	0.870	0.745	0.620	0.495	–

(Continued)

Table 12.2 (Continued)

Response correlation ω	Period correlation η	Number of subjects per cluster, m					
		10	25	50	75	100	200
	0.010	0.990	0.990	0.990	0.990	0.990	0.990
	0.015	1.035	1.110	1.235	1.360	1.485	1.985
	0.020	1.080	1.230	1.480	1.730	1.980	2.980
	0.025	1.125	1.350	1.725	2.100	2.475	3.975
	0.030	1.170	1.470	1.970	2.470	2.970	4.970
	0.035	1.215	1.590	2.215	2.840	3.465	5.965
	0.040	1.260	1.710	2.460	3.210	3.960	6.960
	0.045	1.305	1.830	2.705	3.580	4.455	7.955
	0.050	1.350	1.950	2.950	3.950	4.950	8.950
	0.075	1.575	2.550	4.175	5.800	7.425	13.925
	0.100	1.800	3.150	5.400	7.650	9.900	18.900

13

Stepped Wedge Designs

SUMMARY

One type of cluster trial is that in which the clusters are maintained over successive periods of time during which, for example, all will commence on the standard intervention for the condition concerned and, as periods go by, more of the clusters will receive the test intervention. Typically, in the final period all clusters will be utilising the test intervention. Such trials have what is termed a stepped wedge design (SWD). The determination of an appropriate study size involves multiplying the sample size calculation for an independent, parallel, two-group trial by a design effect (DE). The DE has a component to take account of the cluster design, the specific structure of the SWD, and whether this is a cross-sectional or a closed-cohort design.

13.1 Introduction

The cluster designs of **Chapter 12** can be extended to the situation when all potential clusters are identified and then each of these will be monitored sequentially over blocks of time. Initially, the randomisation to (say) the *Intervention* (*I-Yes*) will be confined to a small proportion of the clusters with the remainder allocated to the control or *No-Intervention* (*I-No*). Those allocated to *I-Yes* will continue with this intervention in the next period of time, and further randomisation to *I-Yes* will again be confined to a proportion of the other clusters with the remainder continuing with *I-No*. Thus the key feature of a stepped wedge design (SWD) is that the *I-Yes* intervention is rolled-out to the clusters in a stepwise manner. Thus SWD trials are 'Phased implementation designs'.

The idea behind such designs is that there is some imperative that all subjects should receive *I-Yes* at some stage. In this a parallel group trial, where some clusters will never receive the intervention within the trial implementation period, is not a design option. In an SWD the clusters are sequentially allocated to *I-Yes*, until eventually all clusters are usually receiving this option. The clusters receiving *I-No* act as controls until such time as they are randomised to receive *I-Yes*.

Two SWD types, generally termed *cross-sectional* and *closed-cohort*, are described.

13.2 Basic Structure

The basic design of an SWD is given in **Figure 13.1** and, in that example, $\lambda = 2$ interventions are randomised into $A = 3$ groups of $g = 2$ clusters at each time point beyond Time 0. It is commonly

Sample Sizes for Clinical, Laboratory and Epidemiology Studies, Fourth Edition. David Machin, Michael J. Campbell, Say Beng Tan and Sze Huey Tan.
© 2018 John Wiley & Sons Ltd. Published 2018 by John Wiley & Sons Ltd.

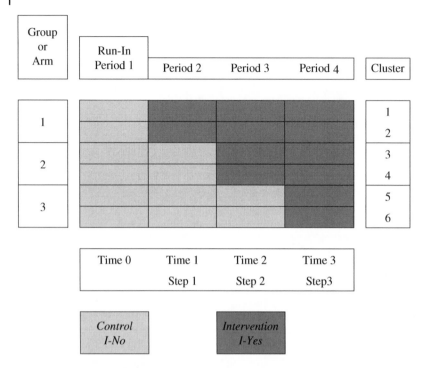

Figure 13.1 Schema of a full SWD trial with $\lambda = 2$ interventions, *I-No* and *I-Yes*, $K = 6$ clusters with $P = 4$ periods, $A = 3$ arms with $g = 2$ clusters randomised at each of $S = 3$ steps. (*See insert for color representation of the figure.*)

assumed that g is constant but this does not have to be the case. In this design all clusters received *I-No* in Period 1. Following that, Clusters 1 and 2 receive, in Periods 2, 3 and 4, *I-Yes*. Clusters 3 and 4 continue with *I-No* in Period 2 but thereafter receive *I-Yes*, while Clusters 5 and 6 continue with *I-No* during Period 3 and have *I-Yes* in Period 4. Thus, all clusters commence with *I-No* for a single run-in period (Time 0), hence $b = 1$, and all end up eventually with *I-Yes*. The number of subsequent steps following Time 0 is $S = 3$, and the number of periods is $P = b + S = 4$. There are $K = g \times A = 6$ clusters and a total of $C = g \times A \times P = 2 \times 4 \times 3 = 24$ cells.

In **Figure 13.1** all clusters receive the *I-No* during Period 1, and the randomised allocation only begins for Period 2 when some of the clusters are allocated *I-Yes* and the remainder continue on *I-No*. For this situation we term Period 1 as a 'run-in' period (as clusters in this period do receive one of the comparator interventions at this stage), although confusingly this is sometimes referred to as a 'baseline'. Note, Day (2007) defines baseline as 'the moment in time that subjects are randomized … to their study medication. It is also used to refer to periods of time after a study has started but before randomization has occurred'. In non-SWD situations, the second part of this definition usually corresponds to a period in which a (baseline) characteristic is recorded or the trial endpoint variable determined *before* any of the interventions are implemented. For an SWD trial the baseline endpoint variable is determined *following I-No* having been implemented in the run-in. The design of **Figure 13.1** includes the run-in of Period 1 (equivalently those groups at Time 0), and we term this a full design in which case the number of periods, P, equals the number of steps plus 1, that is, $S + 1$, and all clusters receive *I-Yes* in the final Period. A Reduced or Incomplete design has no 'run-in', in which case $b = 0$ and $P = S$. The notation for an SWD is reviewed in **Figure 13.2**.

	Notation	Figure 13.1	Poldervaart, *et al* (2013)	Mhurchu, *et al* (2013)
Design Type			*Cross-Sectional (CS)*	*Closed Cohort (CC)*
Number of different arms (randomisation sequences 1, for each step)	A	3	10	4
Total number of clusters allocated	$K (\geq A)$	6	10 clinics	16 schools
Number of interventions	λ	2	2	2
Number of run-in periods on *I-No*	b	1	1 of 1 month	0
Number of *post-randomisation* Steps or Times	S or T	3	10 of 1 month	4 school terms
Total number of periods (may be termed cross-sections, or blocks)	$P = b + S$	4	11	4
Number of clusters allocated *I-Yes* at each step	g	2	1	3 or 4 schools per term
Number of cells (including any run-in)	$C = K \times P$	24	$10 \times 11 = 110$	$16 \times 4 = 64$
Number of participants per cell	m	-	60	25
Anticipated total number of participants	N	-	6,600	400

Figure 13.2 Notation used for describing an SWD with examples from the literature.

There are many possible variations of the basic SWDs. One common variation is the Incomplete design just referred to where there is no run-in included, and another variation is when there are insufficient resources available to implement the *I-Yes* repeatedly in a cluster so that, for example, Period 4 for Clusters 1 and 2 in **Figure 13.1** is omitted.

13.3 Cross-Sectional Design

In a *cross-sectional* (CS) SWD a *different* group of m participants is recruited within each cell of every cluster so that by the end of the trial a total of mP participants is recruited per cluster and from whom the individual outcome variable is assessed.

Illustration

Figure 13.3 outlines the structure of a full SWD trial conducted by Poldervaart, Reitsma, Hoffijberg, *et al* (2013). The trial was designed to investigate the effect of introducing a policy promoting the use of a scoring system to guide clinical decisions for patients with acute chest pain on arrival at hospital emergency departments. Clinics are the clusters who start with a period of 'usual care' (*U*) and are then randomised in their timing of when to switch to 'intervention care' (*H*). The latter involves the calculation of the HEART score for each patient to guide the clinical decision: Reassurance and discharge of patients with low HEART scores and Intensive monitoring and early intervention in-patients with high scores. The primary outcome is occurrence of major adverse cardiac events (MACE), including acute myocardial infarction, revascularisation or death within 6 weeks after

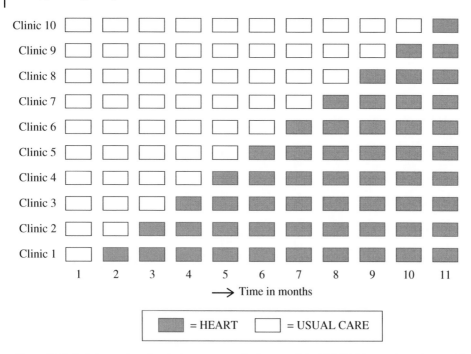

Figure 13.3 Full stepped wedge design to assess the impact of the HEART risk score in patients with acute chest pain (from Poldervaart, Reitsma, Hoffijberg, *et al*, 2013, Figure 1).

presentation. Ten clinics were included in the trial and each month one switched from U to continue on H.

Thus for the planned full SWD trial of Poldervaart, Reitsma, Hoffijberg, *et al* (2013) there are: $\lambda = 2$ interventions, $A = 10$ arms, $K = 10$ clusters, $b = 1$ run-in, $S = 10$ steps, $g = 1$ allocation of H per period, $P = 11$ periods, hence $C = K \times P = 110$ cells. This *CS* design anticipated $m = 60$ patients with acute chest pain per cell requiring $N = C \times m = 6,600$ individuals in total to provide individual (*non-aggregate*) data.

As we have indicated, there are many variations possible of the basic SWD. For example if $g = 2$ clinics rather than $g = 1$ clinic, they are allocated to H in **Figure 13.3** at each step and then, as the allocation progresses, the design would eventually require $A = 6$ arms, with $b = 1$ and only $S = 5$ further steps so $P = 6$, then with $K = 10$ there would be $C = 10 \times 6 = 60$ cells, and hence $N = 60 \times 60 = 3,600$ participants.

Design Features

The associated statistical model for a *CS* SWD extends that of equation (12.3) of **Chapter 12** for a cluster design. Thus with a continuous endpoint comparing *I-No* with *I-Yes*, the model now accounts for an estimation of the fixed-effect of time, θt, to become

$$y_{itkl} = \mu_{I-No} + \delta x_{lt} + \theta_t + \gamma_{kl} + \eta_{tkl} + \varepsilon_{itkl}. \tag{13.1}$$

Here $l = 1, 2, ..., A$ are the trial arms; $k = 1, 2, ..., K$ the clusters, the steps (assuming $b = 1$ at $t = 0$) are taken at times $t = 1, ..., T$ consisting of $i = 1, 2, ..., m$ individuals, $x_{lt} = 0$ if *I-No* is allocated at t, and $x_{lt} = 1$ if *I-Yes*.

Total variance:	$\sigma^2_{Total} = \sigma^2_{Error} + \sigma^2_{Time|Cluster} + \sigma^2_{Cluster}$
Intra Class Correlation (ICC):	$\rho = \left(\sigma^2_{Time|Cluster} + \sigma^2_{Cluster}\right) / \sigma^2_{Total}$
Cluster auto-correlation:	$\omega = \sigma^2_{Cluster} / \left(\sigma^2_{Time|Cluster} + \sigma^2_{Cluster}\right)$
If $\sigma^2_{Time|Cluster} = 0$, then $\rho = \sigma^2_{Cluster} / \sigma^2_{Total}$ and $\omega = 1$	

Figure 13.4 Extension of the definition of ICC, ρ, together with the cluster autocorrelation, ω, for a cross-sectional design.

The terms (two random effects and one error term), γ_{kl}, η_{tkl} and ε_{itkl} respectively, of equation (13.1) are assumed to have independent Normal distributions with mean 0, and corresponding variances, $\sigma^2_{Cluster}$, $\sigma^2_{Time|Cluster}$ and σ^2_{Error}. There are now two cluster components, $\sigma^2_{Cluster}$ and $\sigma^2_{Time|Cluster}$. Consequently, the quantities of **Figure 13.4** are obtained and these can be seen to involve an extension of the definition of the ICC of equation (12.4) of **Chapter 12**.

In general, the SWD can be described in the form of an $A \times P$ design matrix **D** with elements $\{x_{lt}\}$. Thus, for the full SWDs of **Figures 13.1 and 13.3**, the corresponding design matrices are given in **Figure 13.5**.

Sample Size

Design effect
The *design effect* (*DE*) for an SWD is

$$DE_{SWD}(r) = \frac{A^2(1-r)(1+Sr)}{4\left[AE - G + \left(E^2 + SAE - SG - AF\right)r\right]}, \tag{13.2}$$

where

$$E = \sum_{lt} x_{lt}, \quad F = \sum_l \left(\sum_t x_{lt}\right)^2, \quad G = \sum_t \left(\sum_l x_{lt}\right)^2. \tag{13.3}$$

For the full designs of the type of **Figure 13.1**, these take the values $gS(S+1)/2$, $gS(S+1)(2S+1)/6$ and $g^2 S(S+1)(2S+1)/6$ respectively.

In equation (13.2) r, for a CS design, is set equal to

$$r_{CS} = \frac{m\rho\omega}{1+(m-1)\rho}. \tag{13.4}$$

The corresponding DE is denoted DE^{CS}_{SWD}.

However, the fact that a cluster structure is included in the planned design also needs to be taken into account. This requires the use of equation (12.5), which we repeat here for convenience:

$$DE_{Cluster} = \left[1 + (m-1)\rho\right]. \tag{13.5}$$

(a)

$$D\ (6\times4) = \begin{bmatrix} 0 & 1 & 1 & 1 \\ 0 & 1 & 1 & 1 \\ 0 & 0 & 1 & 1 \\ 0 & 0 & 1 & 1 \\ 0 & 0 & 0 & 1 \\ 0 & 0 & 0 & 1 \end{bmatrix}$$

(b)

$$D\ (10\times11) = \begin{bmatrix} 0 & 0 & 0 & 0 & 0 & 0 & 0 & 0 & 0 & 0 & 1 \\ 0 & 0 & 0 & 0 & 0 & 0 & 0 & 0 & 0 & 1 & 1 \\ 0 & 0 & 0 & 0 & 0 & 0 & 0 & 0 & 1 & 1 & 1 \\ 0 & 0 & 0 & 0 & 0 & 0 & 0 & 1 & 1 & 1 & 1 \\ 0 & 0 & 0 & 0 & 0 & 0 & 1 & 1 & 1 & 1 & 1 \\ 0 & 0 & 0 & 0 & 0 & 1 & 1 & 1 & 1 & 1 & 1 \\ 0 & 0 & 0 & 0 & 1 & 1 & 1 & 1 & 1 & 1 & 1 \\ 0 & 0 & 0 & 1 & 1 & 1 & 1 & 1 & 1 & 1 & 1 \\ 0 & 0 & 1 & 1 & 1 & 1 & 1 & 1 & 1 & 1 & 1 \\ 0 & 1 & 1 & 1 & 1 & 1 & 1 & 1 & 1 & 1 & 1 \end{bmatrix}$$

Figure 13.5 Design matrices, D, corresponding to the full SWD of (a) Figure 13.1 and (b) Figure 13.3.
a) $A=3, \lambda=2, g=2, K=6, b=1, S=3, P=4$
b) $A=10, \lambda=2, g=1, K=10, b=1, S=10, P=11$

Finally, combining DE_{SWD}^{CS} with $DE_{Cluster}$ gives

$$DE_{Full}^{CS} = DE_{SWD}^{CS} \times DE_{Cluster} \tag{13.6}$$

as the required DE for sample size estimation purposes.

Sample size

If the outcome variable is continuous, the number of subjects required for a two-group individually randomised trial, N_0, is given by equation (5.4). However, as there will be $P=S+1$ periods in the SWD, this will be increased to $N_0 \times P$. Thus the planned total sample size is

$$N_{SWD}^{CS} = DE_{Full}^{CS} \times (S+1) \times N_0. \tag{13.7}$$

The corresponding number of clusters is estimated by

$$K_{SWD}^{CS} = DE_{Full}^{CS} \times \frac{N_0}{m}. \tag{13.8}$$

Table 13.1 illustrates, with the cluster-correlation $\omega = 1$, how DE_{Full}^{CS}, and the corresponding inflation in the sample size required change with differing values of, m, S, and the ICC ρ as compared to the independent two-group comparative trial.

Figure 13.6 Design matrix, *D*, for a full *A* by *P* SWD with *g* = 1 allocated to *I-Yes* in each post run-in period.

$$D\,(A\times P)=\begin{bmatrix} 0 & 1 & 1 & \dots & \dots & 1 & 1 \\ 0 & 0 & 1 & \dots & \dots & 1 & 1 \\ 0 & 0 & 0 & \dots & \dots & 1 & 1 \\ \dots & \dots & \dots & \dots & \dots & \dots & \dots \\ \dots & \dots & \dots & \dots & \dots & \dots & \dots \\ 0 & 0 & 0 & \dots & \dots & 0 & 1 \end{bmatrix}$$

Specific Examples

Single run-in (*b* = 1) and *S* further steps

For a single run-in with all receiving *I-No* and *S* further steps, the design matrix, $D\,(A\times P)=\{\,x_{lt}\,\}$, takes the form shown in **Figure 13.6**.

Crossover design

For a crossover design there is no baseline (run-in) before randomisation to the *A* = 2 sequences *I-NoI-Yes* or *I-YesI-No*; hence *b* = 0. Further, $T=S=2$, $D=\begin{bmatrix} 1 & 0 \\ 0 & 1 \end{bmatrix}$ and hence, from equation (13.3), $E=F=G=2$. Using equation (13.2), $DE_{SWD}(r)=\dfrac{1-r}{2}$. Then, using equation (13.4), and combining with (13.5),

$$DE_{cross}=\frac{1}{2}\left[1+(m-1)\rho-m\rho\omega\right].\tag{13.9}$$

Single run-in and one post-randomisation assessment

For a design with a baseline (run-in) receiving *I-No*, before randomisation to *I-No* or *I-Yes*, for a single period: $A=2$, $b=1$, $S=1$, $D=\begin{bmatrix} 0 & 0 \\ 0 & 1 \end{bmatrix}$. Hence, from equation (13.3), $E=F=G=1$ and using equation (13.2) the corresponding combined DE is

$$DE=\left(1-r_{CS}^2\right)\times\left[1+(m-1)\rho\right].\tag{13.10}$$

Design with each cluster within each period to be assessed on *τ* occasions and *b* run-in periods and *ω* = 1

This design implies that each column of the basic design matrix, **D**, is repeated *τ* times. In this situation, the combination of the *DE*s for the SWD and for the cluster are pooled to give

$$DE=\frac{1+\rho(mS\tau+bm-1)}{1+\rho\left(\dfrac{mS\tau}{2}+bm-1\right)}\cdot\frac{3(1-\rho)}{2\tau\left(S-\dfrac{1}{S}\right)}.\tag{13.11}$$

The sample size is given by

$$N=DE\times N_0\times(S+1).\tag{13.12}$$

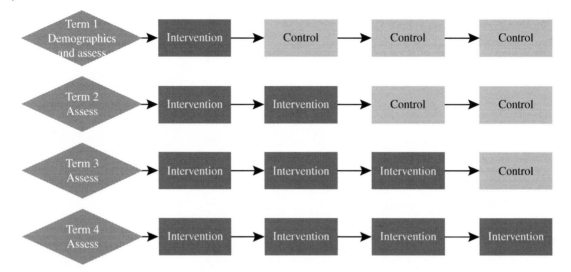

Figure 13.7 Stepped wedge cluster design for evaluating a free school breakfast programme involving 14 schools. Each sequence (denoted Term) was allocated to either 3 or 4 schools (from Mhurchu, Gorton, Turley, *et al*, 2013, Figure 1).

13.4 Closed-Cohort Design

In a closed-cohort (*CC*) design, the *same* group of *m* participants is retained within each cell of a cluster in every period. Thus, although a total of *m* $(b + S)$ endpoint variable assessments will be made, the same participants remain as *m* per cluster.

Illustration

In the SWD of **Figure 13.7** described by Mhurchu, Gorton, Turley, *et al*, (2013) for evaluating a *Free Breakfast (FB)* as the *Intervention*, against *No Free Breakfast (NoFB)* as the *Control*, schools formed the clusters and the periods were school terms.

As indicated in **Figure 13.2**, the trial design anticipated $K = 16$ clusters, $S = 4$ steps, $g = 3$ or 4 allocated at each step to *FB* (*Intervention*) while any remainder continued as *NoFB*, $P = 4$ periods and $C = K \times P = 64$ cells. The design anticipated *m* students per school and these same students would provide an *aggregate* unit of assessment for each of the four periods.

Design Features

In a closed-cohort (*CC*) design, the *same* group of *m* participants are retained within each cluster at every step thus, although a total of *m* $(b + S)$ assessments will be made, the number of participants remains at *m* per cluster. In which case, the model of equation (13.1) for a continuous endpoint SWD comparing *I-No* and *I-Yes*, is extended to account for the individual autocorrelation. Thus

$$y_{itkl} = \mu_{I-No} + \delta x_{lt} + \theta_t + \gamma_{kl} + \zeta_{ikl} + \eta_{tkl} + \varepsilon_{itkl}. \tag{13.13}$$

Total variance:	$\sigma^2_{Total} = \sigma^2_{Error} + \sigma^2_{Indiv|Cluster} + \sigma^2_{Time|Cluster} + \sigma^2_{Cluster}$
Intra Class Correlation (ICC):	$\rho = \left(\sigma^2_{Time|Cluster} + \sigma^2_{Cluster} \right) / \sigma^2_{Total}$
Cluster auto-correlation:	$\omega = \sigma^2_{Cluster} / \left(\sigma^2_{Time|Cluster} + \sigma^2_{Cluster} \right)$
Individual auto-correlation	$\pi = \sigma^2_{Indiv|Cluster} / \left(\sigma^2_{Error} + \sigma^2_{Indiv|Cluster} \right)$

Figure 13.8 Extension of the definitions of ICC, ρ, the cluster auto-correlation, ω, and individual auto-correlation, π, for a closed-cohort SWD.

The additional random effects term, ζ_{ikl}, is assumed to have Normal distribution with mean 0 and variance $\sigma^2_{Indiv|Cluster}$. The corresponding auto-correlation terms are defined in **Figure 13.8**.

Sample Size

Design effect

The design effect takes the same form as that for a *CS* design as described in equations (13.2) and (13.3). However r is now taken as

$$r_{CC} = \frac{m\rho\omega + (1-\rho)\pi}{1 + (m-1)\rho}. \tag{13.14}$$

and the corresponding DE is denoted DE^{CC}_{SWD}.

However, the fact that a cluster structure is planned requires the use of $DE_{Cluster}$ to be considered. Hence combining DE^{CC}_{SWD} with $DE_{Cluster}$ from equation (13.5) gives

$$DE^{CC}_{Full} = DE^{CC}_{SWD} \times DE_{Cluster} \tag{13.15}$$

as the required DE for the sample size estimation. **Table 13.2** gives the multiplier (DE^{CC}_{Full}) required for sample size adjustment for a full Closed-Cohort SWD for differing intra-class correlation (ρ) cluster and individual auto-correlations (w and π), S and m, as compared to the case of an independent two-group comparative trial.

Sample size

If the outcome variable is continuous, the number of subjects required for a two-group individually randomised trial, N_0, is given by equation (5.4). However, as there will be the same individuals concerned in each period of a *CC* design, the planned total sample size is given by

$$N^{CC}_{SWD} = DE^{CC}_{Full} \times N_0. \tag{13.16}$$

	v, Prior to Intervention all receiving *I-No*	*w*, Post-Intervention randomised equally to *I-No* and *I-Yes*
$\boldsymbol{D}=$	$\begin{matrix} 0 & 0 & \ldots & 0 \\ 0 & 0 & \ldots & 0 \end{matrix}$	$\begin{matrix} 0 & 0 & \ldots & 0 \\ 1 & 1 & \ldots & 1 \end{matrix}$

Figure 13.9 Design matrix, *D*, for a 2 by $(v+w)$ repeated measures design of Chapter 10 in which it is assumed that all subjects in the prior intervention period receive *I-No*.

13.5 Link with a Repeated Measures Design

Consider the design effect of equation (10.8) of **Chapter 10**, which describes independent two-group designs with repeated measures on the same individuals before and after allocation to the two interventions under study. In that situation the *DE* is given by

$$R=\left[-\frac{v\rho^2}{\left[1+(v-1)\rho\right]}+\frac{1+(w-1)\rho}{w}\right], \tag{13.17}$$

where v represents the number of baseline observations, w is the number of post-allocation to the intervention groups and ρ is the correlation between pairs of observations from one individual.

The corresponding 2 rows by $(v+w)$ columns design correlation matrix is given in **Figure 13.9**. Thus with $A=2$ and $S=1$, the elements of equation (13.3) are: $E=w, F=w^2, G=w$. These in turn imply

$$DE_{Repeat}=\frac{1-\rho^2}{w\left[1+(2-w)\rho\right]}. \tag{13.18}$$

13.6 Bibliography

A comprehensive review of sample size issues for SWDs is given by Hooper, Teerenstra, de Hoop, *et al* (2016). Woertman, de Hoop, Moerbeek, *et al* (2013) derive equation (13.11). Hemming and Taljaard (2016) describe a unified approach to sample size calculations for SWDs and the cluster trials of Chapter 12.

13.7 Examples

Numerical Accuracy

When calculating sample sizes it is usual to obtain a non-integer from the appropriate algebraic expression and then *automatically* round this upwards to give a convenient integer value. However, as we indicated in **section 1.8 of Chapter 1**, when considering the number of clusters, the rounding up may result in an unacceptable study size as each additional cluster adds a further m (which may be quite large) subjects to the study.

Table 1.2
For two-sided test size, $\alpha = 0.05$, $z_{0.975} = 1.96$. For one-sided $1 - \beta = 0.85$, $z_{0.85} = 1.0364$.

Equations 11.3, 12.2, 13.2 and 13.3

Example 13.1   Stepped wedge design - Cross-sectional - Acute chest pain

The trial of Poldervaart, Reitsma, Hoffijberg, *et al* (2013) is summarised in **Figures 13.2 and 13.3**. The aim of the trial was to demonstrate non-inferiority of H as compared to U. The authors state: 'Our sample size calculation is ... based on demonstrating that proportion of patients with MACE is not inferior to the proportion observed with usual care. The proportion MACE expected during usual care is 17%. The non-inferiority margin is based on clinical judgement and available literature as 3%, thus accepting an upper limit of the 95% confidence interval (CI) during the intervention period of 20%. With 10 hospitals, inclusion of 60 patients per hospital per month, a between-hospital variation in incidence of 16 to 18%, a one-sided alpha of 5% and a power of 80%, 6600 patients with chest pain should be included in total.'

It is not entirely clear how they arrived at the total sample size, but using equation (11.3) for a non-inferiority trial with $\varphi = 1$ and a continuous outcome (we assume the aggregate outcome per hospital, and a percentage, can be regarded as continuous) gives an initial estimate of the sample size, $N_0 = 4{,}568$ subjects. Assuming the postulated between-hospital variation in outcome of 16% to 18% represents approximately $4\sigma_{Cluster}$, then $\sigma_{Cluster} = 0.02 / 4 = 0.005$.

Further assuming $\sigma^2_{Time|Cluster} = 0$ and taking the proportion $\pi_U = 0.17$ for $\bar{\pi}$ in equation (12.12) gives the ICC of **Figure 13.5** as $\rho = \dfrac{\sigma^2_{Cluster}}{\bar{\pi}(1 - \bar{\pi})} = \dfrac{0.005^2}{0.17 \times 0.83} = 0.00018$.

If we assume the cluster auto-correlation $\omega = 1$, then with $m = 60$ equation (13.4) gives $r_{CS} = \dfrac{60 \times 0.00018 \times 1}{1 + (60 - 1) \times 0.00018} = 0.0107$. As the SWD has a full design, equation (13.3) with $S = 10$ gives, with $g = 1$, $E = \dfrac{S(S+1)}{2} = 55$ and $F = G = \dfrac{S(S+1)(2S+1)}{6} = 385$. Then the use of equations (13.2) and (13.4) lead to $DE^{CS}_{SWD} = 0.1575$ and $DE_{Cluster} = 1.0106$ from which equation (13.6) gives $DE^{CS}_{Full} = DE^{CS}_{SWD} \times DE_{Cluster} = 0.1592$. The final sample size from equation (13.7) is $N^{CS}_{SWD} = 0.1592 \times (10 + 1) \times 4{,}568 = 7{,}998.06$ or 8,000. With $C = 110$ cells in the design of **Figure 13.2**, this would imply a revised value of $m \approx 70$ might be considered.

Equations 3.2, 13.2, 13.5, 13.14, 13.15 and 13.16

Example 13.2   Stepped wedge design - Closed-cohort – Provision of school breakfast

The intention of the trial of Mhurchu, Gorton, Turley, *et al* (2013), summarised in **Figures 13.2 and 13.7**, was to evaluate the provision of a *Free Breakfast* (*FB*) in schools as compared to no breakfast provision (*NoFB*). The authors stated, with respect to their sample size calculation: 'The target sample size was 16 schools (four per sequence) and an average of 25 students per school, that is, 400 participants. Assuming an intra-cluster correlation coefficient of 0.05, this would provide at least

85% power, with a 2-sided significance level of 0.05, to detect a 10% absolute change in the proportion of students with a school attendance rate of 95% or higher.'

As, on the whole, the same ($m \approx 25$) children will be attending the school over the 4 terms, this is a *CC* design. The trial was planned to include children from 16 schools and the design did not include a baseline ($b = 0$) so that **Figure 13.2** indicates $A = 4$ arms, $P = 4$ periods, $S = 4$ steps and $K = 16$ schools. They further assumed $\rho = 0.05$ so that, from equation (13.5), $DE_{Cluster} = [1 + (25 - 1) \times 0.05] = 2.2$ and equation (13.14) suggests, with $\omega = 1$, that $r_{CC} = \dfrac{(25 \times 0.05) + (1 - 0.05)\pi}{1 + \left[(25 - 1) \times 0.05\right]} = 0.5682 + 0.4318\pi$.

Although the planning values for the two interventions for the proportions of children attending school are not given, the results of OR = 0.93 imply that about 52% ($p_{NoFB} = 0.52$) of children with *NoFB* would have satisfactory attendance. With an absolute change of 10%, this is anticipated to increase to $p_{FB} = 0.62$. Thus with 2-sided $\alpha = 0.05$ and $\beta = 0.15$, equation (3.2) with $\varphi = 1$ of **Chapter 3** or $^{|S}S_{S|}$ gives $N_0 = 868$. If $\pi = 0.4$ is assumed, $r_{CC} = 0.7409$ and using (13.2) with $r = r_{CC}$, $DE_{SWD}^{CC} = 0.1171$, which when combined with $DE_{Cluster}$ gives, from (13.15), $DE_{Full}^{CC} = 0.1171 \times 2.2 = 0.2577$. Finally from equation (13.16), the sample size is $N_{SWD}^{CC} = 0.2577 \times 868 = 223.69$ or 225.

References

Technical

Day S (2007). *Dictionary for Clinical Trials*. (2nd edn). Wiley, Chichester

Hemming K and Taljaard M (2017). Sample size calculations for stepped wedge and cluster randomised trials: a unified approach. *Journal of Clinical Epidemiology*, **69**, 137–146.

Hooper R, Teerenstra S, de Hoop E and Eldridge S (2016). Sample size calculation for stepped wedge and other longitudinal cluster randomized trials. *Statistics in Medicine*, **35**, 4718–4728.

Woertman W, de Hoop E, Moerbeek M, Zuidema SU, Gerritsen DL and Teerenstra S (2013). Stepped wedge designs could reduce the required sample size in cluster randomized trials. *Journal of Clinical Epidemiology*, **66**, 752–758.

Examples

Mhurchu CN, Gorton D, Turley M, Jiang Y, Michie J, Maddison R and Hattie J (2013). Effects of a free school breakfast programme on children's attendance, academic achievement and short-term hunger: results from a stepped-wedge, cluster randomised controlled trial. *J Epidemiology & Community Health*, **67**, 257–264.

Poldervaart JM, Reitsma JB, Koffijberg H, Backus BE, Six AJ, Doevendans PA and Hoes AW (2013). The impact of the HEART risk score in the early assessment of patients with acute chest pain: design of a stepped wedge, cluster randomised trial. *BMC Cardiovascular Disorders*, **13**, 77.

Table 13.1 The Design Effect (DE_{Full}^{CS}), with the cluster-correlation $\omega = 1$, for a full cross-sectional SWD and the corresponding multiplier required for sample size inflation when compared to an independent two-group parallel trial [Equations 13.2 to 13.6 and part of 13.7].

ρ	S	m	DE_{Full}^{CS}	$(S+1)DE_{Full}^{CS}$
0.01	2	10	1.073	3.220
0.05	2	10	1.194	3.581
0.10	2	10	1.210	3.631
0.01	3	10	0.624	2.497
0.05	3	10	0.717	2.866
0.10	3	10	0.730	2.918
0.01	4	10	0.457	2.287
0.05	4	10	0.535	2.676
0.10	4	10	0.545	2.723
0.01	5	10	0.367	2.203
0.05	5	10	0.434	2.606
0.10	5	10	0.441	2.646
0.01	2	25	1.156	3.468
0.05	2	25	1.294	3.883
0.10	2	25	1.281	3.844
0.01	3	25	0.686	2.745
0.05	3	25	0.780	3.121
0.10	3	25	0.772	3.087
0.01	4	25	0.510	2.549
0.05	4	25	0.582	2.911
0.10	4	25	0.574	2.871
0.01	5	25	0.413	2.478
0.05	5	25	0.471	2.827
0.10	5	25	0.463	2.780
0.01	2	50	1.239	3.716
0.05	2	50	1.349	4.047
0.10	2	50	1.313	3.939
0.01	3	50	0.743	2.973
0.05	3	50	0.813	3.251
0.10	3	50	0.790	3.158
0.01	4	50	0.555	2.775
0.05	4	50	0.605	3.024
0.10	4	50	0.586	2.932
0.01	5	50	0.451	2.703
0.05	5	50	0.488	2.929
0.10	5	50	0.472	2.834

Table 13.2 Design Effect(DE_{Full}^{CC}) required for sample size adjustment for a full Closed-Cohort SWD for differing intra-class correlation (ρ) cluster and individual auto-correlations (w and π), S and m, as compared to the case of an independent two-group comparative trial. [Equations 13.14 to 13.15].

			Cluster-autocorrelation, ω			
			0.05		0.10	
			Individual autocorrelation, π			
ρ	S	m	0.8	0.9	0.8	0.9
0.01	2	10	0.356	0.218	0.287	0.146
0.05	2	10	0.621	0.494	0.278	0.141
0.10	2	10	0.946	0.831	0.266	0.134
0.01	3	10	0.214	0.131	0.173	0.088
0.05	3	10	0.374	0.298	0.167	0.085
0.10	3	10	0.570	0.501	0.160	0.080
0.01	4	10	0.159	0.097	0.128	0.065
0.05	4	10	0.278	0.221	0.124	0.063
0.10	4	10	0.425	0.373	0.118	0.060
0.01	5	10	0.129	0.078	0.103	0.052
0.05	5	10	0.225	0.179	0.100	0.050
0.10	5	10	0.343	0.301	0.095	0.048
0.01	2	25	0.460	0.325	0.288	0.146
0.05	2	25	1.130	1.010	0.281	0.141
0.10	2	25	1.955	1.846	0.268	0.134
0.01	3	25	0.277	0.195	0.173	0.088
0.05	3	25	0.681	0.608	0.169	0.085
0.10	3	25	1.178	1.113	0.161	0.081
0.01	4	25	0.206	0.145	0.129	0.065
0.05	4	25	0.508	0.453	0.125	0.063
0.10	4	25	0.879	0.830	0.119	0.060
0.01	5	25	0.166	0.117	0.104	0.053
0.05	5	25	0.410	0.366	0.101	0.051
0.10	5	25	0.711	0.671	0.096	0.048
0.01	2	50	0.632	0.500	0.290	0.147
0.05	2	50	1.970	1.855	0.282	0.142
0.10	2	50	3.626	3.521	0.269	0.135
0.01	3	50	0.381	0.301	0.174	0.088
0.05	3	50	1.188	1.118	0.170	0.085
0.10	3	50	2.186	2.123	0.161	0.081
0.01	4	50	0.284	0.224	0.129	0.065
0.05	4	50	0.886	0.834	0.126	0.063
0.10	4	50	1.631	1.584	0.120	0.060
0.01	5	50	0.229	0.181	0.104	0.053
0.05	5	50	0.717	0.674	0.101	0.051
0.10	5	50	1.321	1.282	0.096	0.048

14

More than Two Groups Designs

SUMMARY
In this chapter extensions of the basic parallel two-group randomised trial are considered. These include parallel designs of three or more groups, with no structure in the groups to be compared, those comprising different doses of a drug under investigation, and those comparing each of several interventions with a standard which may be a placebo. The specific situation of the factorial design in which more than one type of intervention comparison can be included in the same trial is also described.   Some of the methods outlined in this chapter need to be combined with those of earlier chapters to obtain the required sample size.

14.1   More than Two Groups

The majority of clinical trials involve a simple comparison between two interventions or treatments. When there are more than two treatments, the situation is much more complicated. This is because there is no longer one clear alternative hypothesis. Thus, for example, with three groups and a continuous endpoint, although the null hypothesis is that the population means are all equal, there are several potential alternative hypotheses. In other circumstances the investigators may simply wish to compare all three groups, leading to three pairwise comparisons not all of which may be equally important.

One problem arising at the time of analysis is that such situations may lead to multiple significance tests, resulting in misleading p-values. Various solutions have been proposed, each resulting in different analysis strategies and therefore different design and sample size considerations. One approach is to conduct an analysis of variance (ANOVA) or a similar global statistical test, with pairwise or other comparisons of means only being made if the global test is significant. Another approach is to use conventional significance tests but with an adjusted significance level obtained from the Bonferroni correction—essentially reducing the conventional test size (say, 0.05) by dividing this by the number of comparisons to be made. However, the simplest strategy is to adopt the approach which regards, for example, a three-treatment groups comparison as little different from carrying out a series of three independent trials, and to use conventional significance tests without adjustment as argued by Saville (1990). As a consequence, and assuming equal numbers of subjects per treatment arm, the sample size is first estimated for the three distinct trial comparisons. Then for each treatment group simply take the maximum of these as the sample size required.

Sample Sizes for Clinical, Laboratory and Epidemiology Studies, Fourth Edition. David Machin, Michael J. Campbell, Say Beng Tan and Sze Huey Tan.
© 2018 John Wiley & Sons Ltd. Published 2018 by John Wiley & Sons Ltd.

Unstructured Groups

In an unstructured design of $g > 2$ groups, the interventions to be compared may be unrelated; for example, perhaps they are using totally different approaches to the treatment of a disease or condition and also for which no standard approach has been established. In this case, assuming the outcome will be summarised by the mean value for each group, then the null hypothesis is $H_0: \mu_1 = \mu_2 = \ldots = \mu_g$. However, there is now a whole range of possible alternative hypotheses. For example, for $g = 3$ these are $H_{A1}: \mu_1 = \mu_2 \neq \mu_3$, $H_{A2}: \mu_1 \neq \mu_2 = \mu_3$, $H_{A3}: \mu_1 = \mu_3 \neq \mu_2$, and $H_{A4}: \mu_1 \neq \mu_2 \neq \mu_3$. This multiplicity raises problems with respect to determining an appropriate study size.

Although such situations imply multiple significance tests arising from these comparisons, with distorted *p*-values potentially resulting, the simplest strategy is to ignore this difficulty. Thus, for example, a three group (*A*, *B*, *C*) comparison study is then regarded as little different from carrying out a series of three independent two-group studies. One is designed to compare *A* v *B*, the second *B* v *C* and the third *A* v *C*. Once the study data is available then conventional significance tests of each are made.

Assuming equal numbers of subjects per group, pre-specified 2-sided α and β, this approach implies that sample size is first estimated for the three distinct comparisons ($N_{A\,v\,B}$, $N_{B\,v\,C}$, $N_{C\,v\,A}$). The maximum of these, N_{Max}, is then determined. The final sample size for each group is then set as $n_3 = N_{Max}/2$, so that the total study size becomes $N = 3n_3 = 3N_{Max}/2$

An alternative is to reduce the Type-I error using the Bonferroni correction of equation (2.7) to give for this example, $\alpha_{Bonferroni} = \alpha/3$. This will considerably inflate the N_{Max} of the preceding paragraph.

Dose Response Designs

As indicated in **Chapter 2**, studies with g (>2) groups may compare different doses of the same therapy or some other type of ordered treatment groups. Thus, although the null hypothesis would still be that all population means are equal, the alternative will now be $H_{Ordered}$, which is either $\mu_{Pop1} < \mu_{Pop1} < \ldots < \mu_{Popg}$ or $\mu_{Pop1} > \mu_{Pop1} > \ldots > \mu_{Popg}$. In the simplest case, if there are g doses of the same drug concerned, these can be labelled $d_0, d_1, d_2, \ldots, d_{g-1}$. When the outcome is continuous and, if the response to the drug can be regarded as linear (possibly on a logarithmic scale), then the underlying dose-response relationship can be described by a modified equation (2.3) as

$$y_i = \beta_0 + \beta_{Dose} d_i. \tag{14.1}$$

The object of the trial will be to calculate, from the subsequent data, b_{Dose} to provide an estimate of β_{Dose}.

To assess an appropriate sample size, the fundamental equation (1.7) has to be modified by replacing in equations (1.4) and (1.6) δ by β_{Plan} and $SE(\bar{x}_1 - \bar{x}_2) = \sigma\sqrt{\dfrac{2}{n}}$ by

$$SE(b_{Dose}) = \frac{\sigma}{\sqrt{nD}}. \tag{14.2}$$

Here the same number, n, of subjects is included at each dose and

$$D = \sum_{i=0}^{g-1}(d_i - \bar{d})^2. \tag{14.3}$$

From these, for the pre-specified g dose levels and values for β_{Plan}, σ_{Plan}, D, α and β, the total sample size required is

$$N = gn = g \times \frac{1}{D}\left(\frac{\sigma^2_{Plan}}{\beta^2_{Plan}}\right) \times \left(z_{1-\alpha/2} + z_{1-\beta}\right)^2. \tag{14.4}$$

In the absence of more precise information, a planning value for the regression slope, β_{Plan}, might be estimated by the difference between the expected mean values of the endpoint measure at the highest dose and that at the lowest dose, that is $(\mu_{g-1} - \mu_0)$, divided by the range, $(d_{g-1} - d_0)$, of the doses to be included in the design.

In the special case where the doses are equally spaced, they can then be coded as, $0, 1, 2, ..., g - 1$, so that equation (14.3) becomes

$$D = g\left(g^2 - 1\right)/12. \tag{14.5}$$

The corresponding sample size is then estimated by

$$N = gn = \left(\frac{12}{g^2-1}\right)\frac{\sigma^2_{Plan}}{\beta^2_{Plan}} \times \left(z_{1-\alpha/2} + z_{1-\beta}\right)^2. \tag{14.6}$$

As one would expect, for the case $g = 2$, equation (14.6) becomes the fundamental equation (1.7) as then, $\dfrac{12}{\left(g^2-1\right)} = 4$.

Several Comparisons with a Reference

In certain clinical trial situations, there may be several potentially active treatment options under consideration each of which it would be desirable to test against a reference (*Ref*) that could be, for example, a placebo. The test treatments considered may be entirely different formulations and one is merely trying to determine which, if any, are active relative to *Ref*. Thus, no formal statistical comparison between the new formulations is intended. In such cases a common minimum effect size, δ_{Min}, above or below the *Ref* as appropriate will be set by the clinical team for all the comparisons. Any treatment that demonstrates this minimum level would then be considered as potentially 'more efficacious' and perhaps then evaluated further in subsequent trials.

Equally in some situations, there may be several interventions proposed which are linked in such a way that they can be ranked in terms of the increasing degree of the intervention yet cannot be placed on a numerical scale. In such cases, the δ_{Min} can be set at a value for a threshold of worthwhile clinical benefit.

In either if these situations, the conventional parallel group design would be to randomise these $(g - 1)$ interventions and *Ref* options to equal numbers of subjects, perhaps in blocks of size, $b = g$ or $2g$. However, it is statistically more efficient to have a larger number of subjects receiving *Ref* than each of the other interventions. This is because every one of the $g - 1$ comparisons is made against *Ref* so that the estimated endpoint summary statistic of the *Ref* group needs to be well established. To achieve this, the *Ref* group is organised to have $\sqrt{(g-1)}$ patients for every patient in the other options. For example, if $g = 5$, then $\sqrt{(g-1)} = \sqrt{4} = 2$, thus the recommended randomisation ratios are 2:1:1:1:1. This can then be implemented in blocks of size $b = 6$ or 12. However, if $g = 6$ for example, then $\sqrt{6} = 2.45$ which is not an integer. However, with convenient rounding, this leads to a randomisation ratio of 2.5:1:1:1:1:1 or equivalently 5:2:2:2:2:2. These options can then be randomised in blocks of size, $b = 15$ or 30.

If the endpoint is binary, and $g - 1$ proportions are being compared with π_{Ref} and π_{Min} represents the anticipated minimal response of interest from any of the $g - 1$ comparator interventions, then the number of subjects required for a two group comparison, N_2, is first calculated with $\delta_{Min} = \pi_{Ref} - \pi_{Min}$ by

$$N_2 = \left(\frac{1+\varphi}{\varphi}\right)\frac{\left\{z_{1-\alpha}\sqrt{\left[(1+\varphi)\bar{\pi}(1-\bar{\pi})\right]} + z_{1-\beta}\sqrt{\left[\varphi\pi_{Ref}\left(1-\pi_{Ref}\right) + \pi_{Min}\left(1-\pi_{Min}\right)\right]}\right\}^2}{\delta_{Min}^2}, \qquad (14.7)$$

where $\bar{\pi} = \left(\pi_{Ref} + \varphi\pi_{Min}\right)/(1+\varphi)$ and $\varphi = \dfrac{1}{\sqrt{g-1}}$. This is the same form as equation (3.2) but using 1-sided test size α.

If the variable being measured is continuous and can be assumed to have a Normal distribution, then the number of subjects required for a two group comparison, N_2, is first calculated with $\delta_{Min} = \mu_{Ref} - \mu_{Min}$ by

$$N_2 = \frac{(1+\varphi)^2}{\varphi}\frac{\left(z_{1-\alpha} + z_{1-\beta}\right)^2}{\left(\delta_{Min}/\sigma_{Plan}\right)^2} + \frac{z_{1-\alpha}^2}{2}, \qquad (14.8)$$

and $\varphi = \dfrac{1}{\sqrt{g-1}}$. This is essentially the same form as equation (5.4) but using a 1-sided test size α.

For both the calculations of (14.7) and (14.8), the number of subjects in the reference group is

$$m_{Ref} = \frac{N_2 \times \sqrt{g-1}}{1 + \sqrt{g-1}} \qquad (14.9)$$

and for the $g - 1$ comparator groups is

$$m = \frac{N_2}{1 + \sqrt{g-1}}. \qquad (14.10)$$

Finally, the total trial size is given by

$$N_{Total} = m_{Ref} + (g-1)m = N_2/\varphi = N_2 \times \sqrt{g-1}. \qquad (14.11)$$

Similar adjustments can be made in the cases of ordered categorical and time-to-event outcomes.

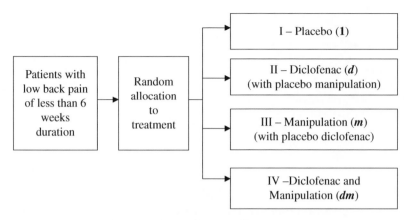

Figure 14.1 Randomised 2×2 factorial trial of diclofenac and manipulation as adjunct to advice and paracetamol in patients with low back pain (after Hancock, Maher, Latimer *et al*, 2007).

Factorial Designs

Suppose a 2×2 factorial trial compares two factors, **D** and **M**, as in the trial conducted by Hancock, Maher, Latimer, *et al* (2007) in patients with low back pain. As shown in **Figure 14.1**, these patients were randomised to receive one of the following: neither diclofenac nor manipulation (double-placebo) (**1**); diclofenac (with placebo manipulation) (**d**); manipulation (with placebo diclofenac) (**m**); or both diclofenac and manipulation (**dm**). Thus, the two questions posed simultaneously are the effects of diclofenac (termed the main effect of **D**) and of manipulative therapy (main effect of **M**).

In such a 2×2 factorial trial, and when the endpoint is continuous, there are four means to be estimated, each from m subjects within the respective intervention. However, when estimating the influence of each factor (the main effect), two means are compared each based on $n = 2m$ observations. These two analyses (since there are 2 factors) make the assumption that there is no interaction between them, that is, the effect of factor **D** (say) is the same irrespective of which level of factor **M** is also given to the patient.

In planning the size of the trial, the first step might be to consider the sample size, N_D, for **D** and the second to calculate N_M for **M**. This latter calculation may involve an effect size, test size and power that are different from those of the **D** comparison. Clearly, if N_D and N_M are similar in magnitude, then there is no difficulty in choosing the larger, N_{Max}, as the required sample size. If the sample sizes are disparate, then a discussion would ensue as to the most important comparison and perhaps a reasonable compromise be reached. In any event once the sample size, N_{Final}, is determined, the trial will plan to randomise $m = N_{Final}/4$ patients to each of the four options.

14.2 Bibliography

In the situation when several options are compared against a reference group (possibly a placebo), Fleiss (1986, pp 95-96 and 116) has shown that it is statistically more efficient to have a larger number of patients receiving the reference group than those of the other groups. The corresponding sample sizes for binary and continuous endpoints are given by equations (14.7) and (14.8) combined with (14.9), (14.10) and (14.11).

14.3 Examples

Table 1.2
For one-sided test size, $\alpha = 0.05$, $z_{0.95} = 1.6449$. For two-sided test size, $\alpha = 0.05$ and 0.0167, $z_{0.975} = 1.96$ and $z_{0.9833} = 2.3932$. For one-sided, $1 - \beta = 0.8$ and 0.9, $z_{0.8} = 0.8416$ and $z_{0.9} = 1.2816$.

Equation 3.2

Example 14.1   Three groups with partial structure - type 2 diabetes
Weng, Li, Xu, *et al* (2008) conducted a randomised trial in newly diagnosed patients treated with type 2 diabetes to compare multiple daily insulin injections (M), subcutaneous insulin infusion (I), and an oral hypoglycaemic agent (O). The observed remission rates at 1-year in those who achieved glycaemic control were 51.1% (68/133) with I, 44.9% (53/118) with M and 26.7% (27/101) with O. How large should a repeat trial be if patients are to be randomised equally to the three options and assuming planning values suggested by the results of the earlier trial?

The endpoint is binary, so that sample size calculations associated with **Chapter 3** are required.

If the planning responses assumed are $\pi_M = 0.50$, $\pi_I = 0.45$ and $\pi_O = 0.25$, then the corresponding effect sizes are M v $I = 0.50 - 0.45 = 0.05$, I v $O = 0.45 - 0.25 = 0.20$ and O v $M = 0.25 - 0.50 = -0.25$. If the investigators further assume 2-sided $\alpha = 0.05$ and $\beta = 0.2$, then successive uses of equation (3.2) with $\varphi = 1$ gives the following from ^SS_S for the $k = 3$ comparisons: $N_{M\,v\,I} = 3{,}130$, $N_{I\,v\,O} = 178$ and $N_{O\,v\,M} = 116$. From these $N_{Max} = 3{,}130$, and this plan would then involve $N = (3 \times 3{,}130)/2 = 4{,}595$ patients in all who would then be randomised equally to the three treatment groups.

Had the planning team adjusted the Type I error using the Bonferroni correction of equation (3.7), then $\alpha_{Bonferroni} = 0.05/3 = 0.0167$. Calculations using ^SS_S then give $N_{M\,v\,I} = 4{,}174$, $N_{I\,v\,O} = 236$ and $N_{O\,v\,M} = 156$. From these $N_{Max} = 4{,}174$, and this revised plan would then require $N = 3 \times (4{,}174/2) = 6{,}261$ patients.

It is clear from these calculations that such a trial is unlikely to be a viable option. Perhaps the investigators then suggest a two-treatment trial comparing (say) O and M with 116 patients. This is now a proposed trial of $g = 2$ groups and so requires no Bonferroni correction.

The trial of Weng, Li, Xu, *et al* (2008) recruited 352 patients. Suppose the new investigating team were also restricted to this number. This implies $352/3 = 117.3$ or approximately 120 patients per group. Using 2-sided $\alpha = 0.05$ and $\beta = 0.2$ once more, equation (3.2) with (say) $\pi_{Plan} = \pi_O = 0.25$, they can investigate a range of effect sizes, δ_{Plan}, by means of ^SS_S until one is found which gives $N = 240$. This investigation would then establish the minimum effect size that could be detected with this limitation on patient numbers. In fact if $\delta_{Min} = 0.17$, then an increase over $\pi_O = 0.25$ to 0.42 for the comparison group could be detected with this sample size. However, if we set $\pi_{Plan} = \pi_I = 0.45$ and then $\pi_{Plan} = \pi_M = 0.5$, the corresponding δ_{Min} become 0.18 and 0.178. This suggests that 120 patients in each group will only enable differences greater than about 0.18 to be detected by such a trial irrespective of the base value for π_{Plan} that is set.

Equations 14.3, 14.4 and 14.5

Example 14.2 Dose–response - tocilizumab in rheumatoid arthritis

Smolen, Beaulieu, Rubbert-Roth, *et al* (2008) compared Tocilizumab in two doses of 4 (*T4*) and 8 (*T8*) mg/kg against placebo (*T0*) to test the therapeutic effect of blocking interleukin in patients with rheumatoid arthritis. They randomised a total of 623 patients to the three arms. The patients were assessed at the point of randomisation and then following treatment at 24 months using the American College of Rheumatology (ACR) criteria. The final outcome was summarised as the proportion achieving a 20% improvement (denoted ACR20) over the baseline score. The trial results suggest a dose response in favour of *T* with the following response rates: *T0*: 54/204 (26%); *T4*: 102/214 (48%); and *T8*: 120/205 (59%).

The $g = 3$ doses correspond to $d_0 = 0$, $d_1 = 1$ and $d_2 = 2$. Thus $\bar{d} = \dfrac{0+1+2}{3} = 1$ and, from equation (14.3), $D = \sum_{i=0}^{2}\left(d_i - \bar{d}\right)^2 = (0-1)^2 + (1-1)^2 + (2-1)^2 = 2$. As the doses are equally spaced, this quantity can be calculated more directly from equation (14.5) by $D = g(g^2 - 1)/12 = 3 \times (3^2 - 1)/12 = 2$.

However, if we now assume that the actual ACR score was used as the endpoint of concern and can be considered as continuous, then, with the dose levels determined, the investigators would have to stipulate β_{Plan} and σ_{Plan} or at least their ratio. If we assume only the ratio $\Delta = \beta_{Plan}/\sigma_{Plan} = 0.45$ is provided, rather than the individual components, then for 2-sided $\alpha = 0.05$ and $\beta = 0.1$, equation (14.4) gives $N = 3 \times \dfrac{1}{2} \times \dfrac{1}{0.45^2} \times (1.96 + 1.2816)^2 = 77.83$ or 78. This implies that 26 patients will be randomly allocated to each of the three dose groups.

Equations 14.3 and 14.4

Example 14.3 Dose Response - plaque Psoriasis

Papp, Bissonnette, Rosoph, *et al* (2008) compared ISA247, a novel calcineurin inhibitor, in three doses of 0.2, 0.3 and 0.4 mg/kg against placebo (0 mg/kg) in patients with moderate to severe psoriasis. They concluded that the highest dose provided the best efficacy.

Suppose we wish to repeat this trial with the Psoriasis Area and Severity Index (PASI) score assumed as a continuous variable and we wish to detect a 'moderate' standardised effect change comparing 0 to 0.4 mg/kg of $\Delta = 0.5$. Then, in terms of the regression slope this implies $\Delta_{Plan} = 0.5/(0.4 - 0) = 1.25$.

As the doses are not equally spaced, equation (14.3) is used to calculate $D = \sum_{i=0}^{3}\left(d_i - \bar{d}\right)^2 = 0.0875$. Finally, with a 2-sided test size of $\alpha = 0.05$ and power $1 - \beta = 0.9$, use of equation (14.4) gives $N = 4 \times \dfrac{1}{0.0875} \times \dfrac{1}{1.25^2} \times (1.96 + 1.2816)^2 = 307.43$ or approximately 77 patients per dose. Although not directly comparable, this is fewer than the 451 recruited to the published trial.

Equation 14.7

Example 14.4 Several comparisons with a standard – binary endpoint - first-episode schizophrenia

Kahn, Fleischhacker, Boter, *et al* (2008) describe a randomised trial comparing four second generation antipsychotic drugs: Amisulpride (*A*), Olanzapine (*O*), Quetiapine (*Q*), and Ziprasidone (*Z*), with the first generation drug Haloperidol (H) in patients with first-episode schizophrenia and schizophreni-form disorder. In this example, the comparison is not with a placebo but with the first generation drug, H. A total of 498 patients were randomised with a $1:1:1:1:1$ allocation ratio. The endpoint was the time from randomisation to discontinuation of the treatment allocated (the event) and the Kaplan-Meier estimates of the 12-month discontinuation rates were A 40%, O 33%, Q 53%, Z 45% respectively compared to that of the reference drug H 72%.

If a repeat trial is planned but taking into account the fact that all new generation drugs are to be compared with H, what minimal affect size, δ_{Min}, would imply a trial of $N=500$ patients would be appropriate? The endpoint is whether or not the patient is still using the prescribed drug 1-year post-randomisation.

In this planned trial there are $g=5$ drugs concerned, so the randomisation ratios will be $\sqrt{(5-1)}=2:1:1:1:1$. This suggests randomisation using blocks of $b=6$ or 12 in which case a revised trial size of 504 patients would be required if $b=12$ is chosen. Further we assume $\pi_{Ref}=\pi_H=0.72$ and knowledge from the previous trial which demonstrated that all the second generation drugs led to a reduced discontinuation rate.

In this new design, if $N_{Total}=504$ is stipulated, then this implies that $m_{Ref}=(504/6)\times 2=168$ and the size for each of the other 4 groups is $m=504/6=84$. Use can then be made of equation (14.7) with $N_2=m_{Ref}+m=168+84=252$ and $\pi_{Ref}=0.72$ (assuming 1-sided, $\alpha=0.05$ and $\beta=0.2$) to search for the corresponding π_{Min}. This search establishes $\pi_{Min}=0.562$ so that $\delta_{Min}=0.158$ or approximately 0.16 is obtained.

Equations 14.7, 14.8 and 14.11

Example 14.5 Several comparisons with a placebo – binary endpoint - myocardial infarction
Wallentin, Wilcox, Weaver *et al* (2003) included, in a randomised trial, Placebo and 4 doses of a thrombin inhibitor Ximelagatran (X) to test for its possible use for secondary prophylaxis after myocardial infarction. Patients were randomly allocated to Placebo or 24, 36, 48 and 60 mg twice daily of X for 6 months on a 2: 1: 1: 1: 1 basis.

Suppose we intend to run a trial with a similar design, but with a continuous outcome such as a liver enzyme concentration. Assuming liver enzyme concentration has an approximately Normal distribution at each dose, how large should the trial be?

For this trial $g=5$, and suppose the minimal standardised effect size of clinical interest has been set at $\Delta_{Plan}=\delta_{Plan}/\sigma_{Plan}=0.5$, then with 1-sided test size $\alpha=0.05$ and power $1-\beta=0.8$, $^S S_S$ or equation (14.8) with $\varphi=1/\sqrt{5-1}=0.5$ gives $N_2=\dfrac{(1+0.5)^2}{0.5}\dfrac{(1.6449+0.8416)^2}{0.5^2}+\dfrac{1.6449^2}{2}=112.64$.

Thus $m_{Placebo}=112.64\times\dfrac{\sqrt{5-1}}{1+\sqrt{5-1}}=75.09$ or 76 and so each of the other $g-1$ treatments will be given to $m=m_{Placebo}/\sqrt{(g-1)}=76/2=38$ patients. The trial could then be conducted with $N_{Total}=N_2\times\sqrt{(5-1)}=228$ patients either in $r=38$ replicate randomised blocks of size $b=6$ or with $r=19$ of $b=12$.

Wallentin, Wilcox, Weaver, *et al* (2003) expected a myocardial infarction rate of about 20% with placebo in their trial and expected the biggest reduction with active treatment to give an infarction rate of about 14%.

Using $^S S_S$, or equation (14.7) directly, for $g=5$, hence $\varphi=1/\sqrt{5-1}=0.5$, $\pi_{Placebo}=0.14$ and $\pi_{Min}=0.20$, with 1-sided test size $\alpha=0.05$ and power $1-\beta=0.8$, gives $N_2=1071$. Thus $m_{Placebo}=1071\times\dfrac{\sqrt{5-1}}{1+\sqrt{5-1}}=714$

and this implies that each of the other $g-1$ treatments will be given to $m = m_{Placebo} \sqrt{(5-1)} = 714/2 = 357$ patients. Thus, from equation (14.11), $N_{Total} = 714 + (5-1) \times 357 = 2{,}142$ patients would seem appropriate. If this is increased to 2148, the trial could then be conducted in $r = 180$ replicate randomised blocks each of size $b = 12$ patients.

The important feature here is that each dose is considered in isolation whereas Walletin Wilcox, Weaver *et al* (2003) considered a more sensitive dose response design and estimated they needed 1,800 subjects in all.

Equation 5.4

Example 14.6 2×2 factorial - chronic obstructive pulmonary disease
Calverley, Pauwels, Vestbo, *et al* (2003) used a 2×2 factorial design to investigate the combination of salmeterol and flucticasone for patients with chronic obstructive pulmonary disease in a structure similar to that of Hancock, Maher, Latimer, *et al* (2007) illustrated in **Figure 14.1**.

The four treatment groups were placebo (**1**), salmeterol (*s*), flucticasone (*f*) and the combination salmeterol and flucticasone (*sf*). The trial was double-blind and the endpoint was FEV_1 assessed 1-year from randomisation. The authors report mean values for (**1**), (*s*), (*f*) and (*sf*) as 1.264, 1.323 1.302 and 1.396 L, based on information on approximately 250 patients per group. From these, those who receive the high level of factor *F* have mean $(1.302 + 1.396)/2 = 1.349$ L, while for those from the low level it is $(1.264 + 1.323)/2 = 1.294$ L, with a difference between these means of 0.045 L. The corresponding difference for *S* is similar at 0.077 L. From the reported confidence intervals, it can be deduced that the standard deviation (*SD*) is approximately 0.265 L.

However, when planning the trial Calverley, Pauwels, Vestbo, *et al* (2003) postulated a larger difference, $\delta_{Plan} = 0.1$ L and $SD_{Plan} = 0.35$ L, for each of the two factors, *F* and *S*, under investigation. For a 2-sided test size of 5% and power 90%, direct use of equation (5.4) or $\boxed{S_{S}}$ gives 518 patients. However, this is not divisible by 4, so is increased to 520 to allow 130 patients to be allocated to each of the four treatment groups.

The strength of the interaction term is assessed in Calverley, Pauwels, Vestbo, *et al* (2003) by contrasting the (**1**) and (*sf*) groups with the (*s*) and (*f*) groups, hence $I = (1.264 + 1.396)/2 - (1.323 + 1.302)/2 = 0.0175$ L. This is very small hence it is unlikely to be of clinical relevance.

In practice, interactions are often smaller in magnitude than the main effects so that conducting trials to examine interactions in more detail would necessarily entail large factorial trials.

References

Technical
Fleiss JL (1986). *The Design and Analysis of Clinical Experiments*. Wiley, New York.
Saville DJ (1990). Multiple comparison procedures: The practical solution. *The American Statistician*, **44**, 174–180.

Examples
Calverley P, Pauwels R, Vestbo J, Jones P, Pride N, Gulsvik A, Anderson J and Maden C (2003). Combined salmeterol and flucticasone in the treatment of chronic obstructive pulmonary disease: a randomised controlled trial. *Lancet*, **361**, 449–456.

Hancock MJ, Maher CG, Latimer J, McLachlan AJ, Cooper CW, Day RO, Spindler MF and McAuley JH (2007). Assessment of diclofenac or spinal manipulative therapy, or both, in addition to recommended first-line treatment for acute low back pain: a randomised controlled trial. *Lancet*, **370**, 1638–1643.

Kahn RS, Fleischhacker WW, Boter H, Davidson M, Vergouwe Y, Keet IPM, Gheorghe MD, Rybakowski JZ, Galderisi S, Libiger J, Hummer M, Dollfus S, López-Ibor JJ, Hranov KG, Gaebel W, Peuskins J, Lindfors N, Riecher-Rössler A and Grobbee DE (2008). Effectiveness of antipsychotic drugs in first-episode schizophrenia and schizophreniform disorder: an open randomised clinical trial. *Lancet*, **371**, 1085–1097.

Papp K, Bissonnette R, Rosoph L, Wasel N, Lynde CW, Searles G, Shear NH, Huizinga RB and Maksymowych WP (2008). Efficacy of ISA247 in plaque psoriasis: a randomised multicentre, double-blind, placebo-controlled phase III study. *Lancet*, **371**, 1337–1342.

Smolen JS, Beaulieu A, Rubbert-Roth A, Ramos-Remus C, Rovensky J, Alecock E, Woodworth T and Alten R (2008). Effect of interleukin-6 receptor inhibition with tocilizumab in patients with rheumatoid arthritis (Option study): a double-blind, placebo-controlled, randomised trial. *Lancet*, **371**, 987–997.

Wallentin L, Wilcox RG, Weaver WD, Emanuelsson H, Goodvin A, Nyström P and Bylock A (2003). Oral ximelagatran for secondary prophylaxis after myocardial infarction: the ESTEEM randomised controlled trial. *Lancet*, **362**, 789–797.

Weng J, Li Y, Xu W, Shi L, Zhang Q, Zhu D, Hu Y, Zhou Z, Yan X, Tian H, Ran X, Luo Z, Xian J, Yan L, Li F, Zeng L, Chen Y, Yang L, Yan S, Liu J, Li M, Fu Z and Cheng H (2008). Effect of intensive insulin therapy on β-cell function and glycaemic control in patients with newly diagnosed type 2 diabetes: a multicentre randomised parallel-group trial. *Lancet*, **371**, 1753–1760.

15

Genomic Targets and Dose-Finding

SUMMARY

The purpose of this chapter is to give an overview of the sample size approaches for two types of clinical trials—those involving drugs for a specific genomic target and those determining an appropriate dose of a new drug to be given in the first trials involving patients. The intent is not to provide a detailed discussion of the sample size approaches required for trials with genomic targets but rather to give an overview of the rationale for such studies and the general approach that can be used to determine the sample size. For dose-finding studies, step-by-step increasing dose designs as well as an accelerated approach are described.

15.1   Introduction

Many of the sample size approaches discussed can be applied to a wide variety of studies. These include epidemiological studies, laboratory experiments, pre-clinical studies and clinical trials. Each of these types serves a particular purpose and the choice of design depends on the nature of the research question to be answered and the feasibility of obtaining the data required. In particular, clinical trials represent the gold standard for answering many research questions of interest. Within clinical trials, different designs are available. For some designs, the sample size can be computed using one of the generic sample size approaches discussed in earlier chapters. However, for others, more specialised designs are required.

15.2   Genomic Targets

For many clinical trials, even though the eligibility criteria is carefully defined, the patients eventually recruited into the trial may be very heterogeneous in terms of their potential response to the treatment. There is thus a risk that patients may be exposed to potentially toxic treatments for which they do not benefit due to their particular genetic make-up. This leads to the concept of a *predictive classifier*, which is defined as: A measurement made before treatment to select patients who are most likely to respond to and thus benefit from the treatment. With this in mind, many drugs, particularly in oncology, are increasingly developed for specific molecular targets. This gives rise to the need for clinical trial designs for such 'targeted therapies'.

Sample Sizes for Clinical, Laboratory and Epidemiology Studies, Fourth Edition. David Machin, Michael J. Campbell, Say Beng Tan and Sze Huey Tan.
© 2018 John Wiley & Sons Ltd. Published 2018 by John Wiley & Sons Ltd.

(i) Development of a predictive classifier (based on a molecular target) using preclinical and early phase clinical studies.
(ii) Development of a validated test for the measurement of that classifier.
(iii) Use of the classifier and validated test to design, conduct and analyse a new clinical trial to evaluate the effectiveness of that drug and how the effectiveness relates to the classifier.

Figure 15.1 Approach for drug development involving molecular targets (from Simon, 2005).

Single Classifier

As described by Simon (2005), the approach for drug development for targeted therapies should ideally involve the steps outlined in **Figure 15.1**.

In the enrichment and biomarker stratified designs described below, the process of discovering and developing a predictive classifier and the corresponding diagnostic test for its presence in a patient is performed prior to the clinical trial being planned, that is steps (i) and (ii) of the process described in **Figure 15.1**. The assumption is thus that a single classifier and validated test is already available for use in the trial.

Enrichment Design

An enrichment design is appropriate when there is compelling *prior* evidence that patients who test negative for the classifier will not benefit from the treatment. Thus in the enrichment design of **Figure 15.2**, a diagnostic test is used to restrict the eligibility for a randomised clinical trial comparing a new drug (*Test, T*) with a standard (*Standard, S*). The conclusion from using the enrichment design would be whether the treatment is effective for diagnosis positive (*D+*) patients. If it is, then future application would be restricted only to such patients.

The efficiency of the enrichment design depends on the prevalence of *D+* patients and on the lack of effectiveness of *T* in diagnosis negative (*D–*) patients. When a small proportion of the patients are *D+* and *T* is relatively ineffective in *D–* patients, the number of randomised patients required for an enrichment design is much smaller than the number required for a conventional (non-enrichment) design in which all patients are randomised to *S* or *T*. This is because the sample size calculation for this design

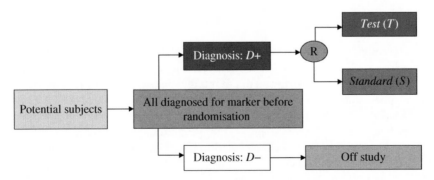

Figure 15.2 An Enrichment Design in which subjects are selected for randomisation provided they are diagnosis positive (*D+*) for a specific molecular target. (*See insert for color representation of the figure.*)

essentially involves using one of the standard approaches described elsewhere in this book but with a much larger expected difference (effect size) to be detected between the two arms (since we are restricting the trial to only the $D+$ patients for whom we are expecting to respond better to the treatment.)

The enrichment design is thus appropriate for the situation where there is such a strong biological basis for believing that $D-$ patients will not benefit from T so that including them in the trial could raise important ethical concerns. Clearly, the design does not provide data on the effectiveness of T compared with S for $D-$ patients. Consequently, unless there is compelling biological or clinical data that T is indeed ineffective in $D-$ patients, it may not be the ideal design to use.

Biomarker Stratified Design

In the situation when there is no compelling prior evidence from biological or clinical data that patients who test $D-$ for the predictive classifier will not benefit from T, a biomarker stratified design can be used. In this case, all potential and consenting subjects are diagnosed as $D+$ or $D-$ using the predictive marker of (as yet) uncertain utility. It is generally best to include both $D+$ and $D-$ patients in the randomised clinical trials comparing T to S as shown in **Figure 15.3**. With the biomarker stratified design, the purpose of the clinical trial is to evaluate T overall and in the subsets determined by the classifier (note that the purpose is not to modify or optimize the classifier).

For studies using this design, it is essential that an appropriate analysis plan is predefined in the protocol for how the predictive classifier will be used in the analysis.

Analysis plan A

In the case where we do not expect T to be effective in the $D-$ patients unless it is effective in the $D+$ patients, we might first compare T versus S in $D+$ patients using a threshold of significance of (say) 5%. Only if the T versus S comparison is significant at this level in $D+$ patients will the T be compared with S among $D-$ patients, again using a threshold of statistical significance of 5%. This sequential approach controls the overall Type I error at 5%. With this design, the number of $D+$ patients required is the same as for the enrichment design. If this is denoted as N, the total number of patients required for the trial would be N / γ where γ denotes the proportion of patients who are $D+$. When γ is small,

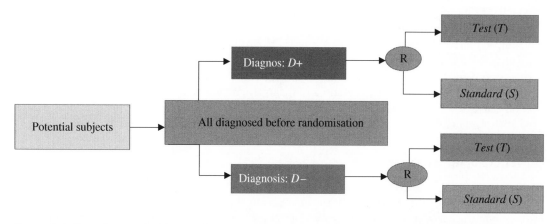

Figure 15.3 Biomarker stratified design (after Simon, 2008a, b). (*See insert for color representation of the figure.*)

a large number of $D-$ patients will be randomised, treated, and followed in the study rather than excluded as for the enrichment design. This will be problematic if one does not, *a priori*, expect T to be effective for $D-$ patients. In this case it will be important to establish an interim monitoring plan to terminate the accrual of $D-$ patients when interim results and prior evidence of lack of effectiveness makes it no longer appropriate to enter them.

Analysis plan B

In the situation where there is greater uncertainty associated with the predictive marker, Simon and Wang (2006) and Jiang, Freidlin and Simon (2007) discussed an analysis plan in which T is first compared with S overall. If that difference is not significant at a reduced significance level such as 0.03, then T is compared with S just for $D+$ patients. The latter comparison uses a threshold significance of 0.02 or whatever portion of the traditional 0.05 is not used by the initial test. In terms of the sample size, this again involves the use of standard approaches for sample size calculation, but with a lower Type 1 error (that is, 0.03 in the situation we are describing). This would result in a generally larger sample size being required.

Adaptive Threshold Design

In some situations, a classifier may be available, but it is less well understood and in particular a threshold value has yet to be determined for which the predictive classifier will be deemed to be test positive. For these circumstances, Jiang, Freidlin and Simon (2007) describe the 'adaptive threshold design'. With this design, tumour specimens are collected from all patients at trial entry and the classifier assessed but no diagnostic decision made on this basis. Thus the value of the predictive test is not used as an eligibility criterion for entry to the trial; rather all patients tested, irrespective of the outcome, are randomised to either S or T.

In terms of the analysis, this begins with comparing the outcomes for all patients receiving T with all S patients. If this difference is significant at a pre-specified significance level (α_1), T is considered effective for the eligible population as a whole and the analysis terminates without investigation of the value of the (potential) classifier.

If the first test is not significant, then it is presumed that the classifier may be important and so an investigation to find a cut-point to define 'good' (those in which T brings benefit over S) and 'poor' (those in which T brings no benefit over S) patients is undertaken. This second stage test involves finding the cut-point b^* for which the difference in outcome of T *versus* S (the treatment effect) is maximized when the comparison is restricted to patients with predictive test scores above that cut-point. The second-stage test is performed using a smaller significance threshold of $\alpha_2 = 0.05 - \alpha_1$. The statistical significance of that maximized treatment effect is determined by generating the null distribution of the maximized treatment effect under random permutations of the treatment labels. If the maximized treatment effect is significant at level α_2 of this null distribution, T is considered effective for the subset of patients with a predictive classifier value above the cut-point at which the maximum treatment effect occurred.

Other Developments

For the Biomarker Stratified Design, Wang, O'Neill and Hung (2007) build on the work of Simon and Wang (2006) to show that the power of the analysis approach described can be improved by taking into account the correlation between the overall significance test and the significance test comparing treatment groups in the subset of $D+$ patients.

We have not discussed the situation where there is clearly uncertainty about the identity of the target(s). In such situations, one might argue that it is no different from the situation in which no target(s) is known, and the 'standard designs' discussed elsewhere in the book should be utilised. However, there are also more specialized designs that have been proposed, and readers are referred to Freidlin and Simon (2005), Freidlin, Jiang and Simon (2010) and Simon (2010, 2012) for discussion of these.

15.3 Dose-Finding

In the early stages of, for example, drug development, the step from the laboratory to the clinic is a major one. At this stage safety is the first priority and so initially use of even very low doses might be anticipated. However, low doses may imply low efficacy, so dose escalation to a more realistic and hence therapeutic range is ultimately desirable.

Taking cancer as an example, the objective of chemotherapy is to reduce (ideally eradicate) the tumour. However, it is recognised that any attack on a tumour by the chemotherapeutic agent may bring collateral damage to normal tissue and vital organs. The usual strategy is to attempt to balance the two by first establishing the concept of dose limiting toxicity (DLT), which then helps identify the Maximum Tolerated Dose (MTD) of the drug concerned.

Thus the aim of a dose-finding study is to establish the MTD of a particular compound or treatment modality so that it can then be tested at that dose in a subsequent trial to assess activity. In contrast to many other situations, for dose-finding designs, the number of patients to be recruited is dependent on the accumulating results from the study, with a maximum number of patients often stated in advance.

To design a dose-finding study, the investigators first identify the range of the doses to consider and all the specific dose levels within this range to test. In particular, the minimum dose to investigate, d_{MIN}, is determined, as is the maximum dose, d_{MAX}, for the study. Assuming there are k dose levels in the range of doses to be considered, we can label these as $d_1 = d_{MIN}$, d_2, d_3, ..., $d_k = d_{MAX}$. In many cases, there is often very little knowledge about the MTD, and one could only suggest a starting dose, d_{START}, based on animal studies. Thus d_{START} will be one of d_1, d_2, d_3, ..., d_k as will be the ultimately identified MTD.

Step-by-Step Designs

The basic design consists of giving one or more subjects a specific starting dose and then, depending on the number of DLTs observed amongst them, stepping up to the next higher pre-specified dose level or stepping down to the nearest lower level. At this new dose level, the process is then repeated. Standard design options often include 1, 3 or 5 patients at each dose.

Storer—precursor design

This design usually starts at d_{MIN}, gives successive (single) patients increasing doses of the compound under investigation, and monitors whether or not they experience DLT with each dose. The dose given depends on the experience of the immediately preceding patient; an absence of DLT will increase the dose for the next patient, while the presence of a DLT will suggest that the immediate prior (and lower) dose will be the MTD. In fact, this is not usually regarded as establishing the MTD but rather as the suggested d_{START} for commencing a second stage design comprising one of the full C33D, Best-of-5 or CRM designs described below. The strategy is essentially to enable the start of the alternative designs to begin at a more informative dose than d_{MIN}. Clearly if a DLT occurs at d_{MIN}, the investigators would have to reconsider their whole dose level choice strategy. Such a review would also follow if no DLT is observed at all the doses up to and including d_{MAX}.

Although we have termed Storer as a 'precursor' design, as its objective is to determine a starting dose for other designs, it may be used as a 'stand-alone' design, examining a different dose range (perhaps wider or with intermediate steps) than might have been considered if one of the 'full' designs had been initiated. Conducted in this way, it may be used to guide the ultimate choice of the doses to be investigated in the more detailed study planned for the next stage of the investigation.

C33D

A common dose-finding design is termed the 'three-subjects-per-cohort design', or 'Cumulative 3 + 3 Dose' (C33D). This design chooses a 'low' starting dose perhaps with $d_{START} = d_{MIN}$ (or one suggested by the Storer precursor) and has 3 replicates at each dose. The choice of the next dose, d_{NEXT}, then depends on the number of patients (0, 1, 2 or 3) experiencing DLT. Clearly if no patients experience DLT then the subsequent dose to investigate will be higher than the one just tested. This process continues until either the stopping level of DLT is attained in the successive groups of 3 patients or d_{MAX} has been tested. In circumstances where the first 2 patients both experience DLT at a particular dose, it is not usual to give the third patient this same dose but to change the dose chosen to a lower one from the pre-specified dose range.

Although this process will (in general) establish the MTD, a pragmatic consideration then dictates that a dose-finding study should have tested at least 6 patients at d_{MTD}. This usually implies that, once the MTD is first identified, extra patients are then recruited and tested at this provisional d_{MTD} until 6 patients in total have experienced this dose. It is also based on the premise that an acceptable probability of DLT will be somewhere between 1 in 6 (17%) and 1 in 3 (33%) of patients.

However, practical issues often constrain the size of dose-finding studies and a maximum size in the region of 24 (8×3) is often chosen. This implies that if pre-determined doses are to be used, and the final dose chosen will have 3 extra patients tested, then $k = 7$ dose options are the maximum that can be chosen for the design as $(k \times 3) + 3 = 24$ patients, although the precise numbers included will be dependent on the DLT experience observed.

The full strategy is described by Storer (2001) and is implemented by following the rules of **Figure 15.4** to determine whether dose-escalation should or should not occur.

Best-of-5

This follows the same format as C33D except that 5 replicates are used rather than 3. The process is summarised in **Figure 15.5**.

The C33D and Best-of-5 designs, with or without the Storer (2001) modification, have no real statistical basis, and more efficient alternatives have been sought. Efficiency here can be thought of as achieving the right MTD and with as few patients as possible. However, the designs are easy to implement and require little (statistical) manipulation—only keeping a count of the number of patients experiencing DLT at each dose tested.

Commencing with dose h:

(**A**) Evaluate 3 patients at d_h:

   (**A1**) If 0 of 3 experience DLT, then escalate to d_{h+1}, and go to (**A**).

   (**A2**) If 1 of 3 experience DLT, then go to (**B**)

   (**A3**) If at least 2 of 3 experience DLT, then go to (**C**).

(**B**) Evaluate an additional 3 patients at d_h:

   (**B1**) If 1 of 6 experience DLT, then escalate to d_{h+1}, and go to (**A**).

   (**B2**) If at least 2 of 6 experience DLT, then go to (**C**).

(**C**) Discontinue dose escalation.

Figure 15.4 Establishing the MTD in a C33D for a Phase I trial (after Storer, 2001).

Commencing with dose, h:

(**A**) Evaluate 3 patients at d_h:

   (**A1**) If 0 of 3 experience DLT, then escalate to d_{h+1}, and go to (**A**).

   (**A2**) If 1 or 2 of 3 experience DLT, then go to (**B**).

   (**A3**) If 3 of 3 experience DLT, then go to (**D**).

(**B**) Evaluate an additional 1 patient at d_h:

   (**B1**) If then 1 of now 4 experience DLT, then escalate to d_{h+1}, and go to (**A**).

   (**B2**) If then 2 of now 4 experience DLT, then go to (**C**).

   (**B3**) If then 3 of now 4 experience DLT, then go to (**D**).

(**C**) Evaluate an additional 1 patient at d_h:

   (**C1**) If then 2 of now 5 experience DLT, then escalate to d_{h+1}, and go to (**A**).

   (**C2**) If then 3 of now 5 experience DLT, then go to (**D**).

(**D**) Discontinue dose escalation.

Figure 15.5 Establishing the MTD in a 'Best-of-5' design for a Phase I trial (after Storer, 2001).

Continual Reassessment Method

This design gives successive groups of patients differing doses of the compound under investigation and monitors the number who experience DLT with each dose. The dose given to the next patient at any one time depends on the experience of *all* the preceding patients. In general an unacceptable level of DLT in the preceding group will lower the next dose utilised, while an acceptable level will increase the next dose.

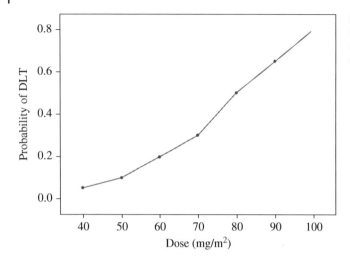

Figure 15.6 Empirical dose-response curve based on prior probabilities of DLT against a dose (data from Flinn, Goodman, Post *et al*, 2000).

The same process of selecting the range and actual doses for the step-by-step designs is necessary for the CRM design. In addition, however, it is also necessary to attach to each of these doses (based on investigator's opinion and/or other information) the anticipated probability of patients experiencing DLT at that dose. We label these *prior* probabilities θ_1, θ_2, θ_3, ..., θ_k. Once these prior probabilities are attached to each dose that has been selected for investigation, they provide an initial dose-response plot such as that of **Figure 15.6**.

It is implicit in the method of selecting these probabilities that, once they are assigned, then a 'reasonable' starting dose, d_{START}, would correspond to the dose that gives a value of θ_{START} close to some predefined 'acceptable' value, termed the target value and denoted, θ_0. This probability is often chosen as less than 1/7 (0.14). The chosen d_{START} would not usually correspond to the extremes d_{MIN} or d_{MAX} of the dose range cited.

CRM assumes a continuous dose-toxicity model like **Figure 15.7**, with a specified mathematical model, such that as the dose increases the probability of DLT also increases. The CRM process thus essentially involves starting with a dose close to the target DLT (although this is not essential) and then escalating or de-escalating following the result observed at that dose in a single patient (or more generally, in a pre-specified cohort of patients). Once the results from a second patient (or cohort) are obtained, the θ_i values are updated using either a Bayesian or combined Bayesian/Maximum Likelihood approach, and the recommended dose for the third patient decided on the basis of which is the dose level with (updated) θ_i now closest to the target θ_0. This process continues until it converges on the dose level with the probability of DLT closest to θ_0. This is the MTD.

Details of the CRM, including the possible mathematical models that can be used as well as the full updating process, can be found in O'Quigley, Pepe and Fisher (1990) and O'Quigley (2001).

Which Design?

Although the CRM method is more efficient than the C33D and Best-of-5 designs, it is considerably more difficult to implement, as the (statistical) manipulation required to determine the next dose to use is technically complex and requires specialist computer statistical software.

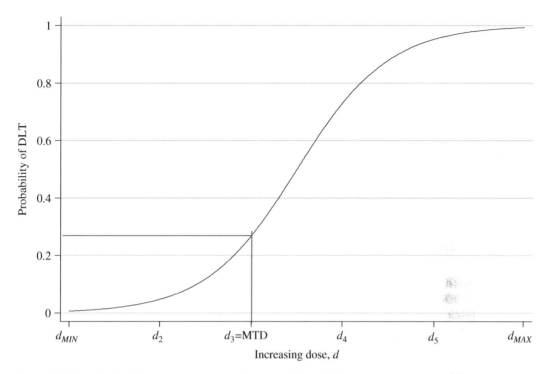

Figure 15.7 Hypothetical dose-response curve of the probability of DLT against a received dose. (*See insert for color representation of the figure.*)

The CRM design reduces the number of patients receiving the (very) low dose options. O'Quigley, Pepe and Fisher (1990) argue this avoids patients receiving doses at which there is little prospect of them deriving benefit, but the design has been criticised by Korn, Midthune, Chen, *et al* (1994) for exposing patients to the risk of receiving potentially very toxic doses. However, the use of the Storer (2001) precursor prior to the original design allows both these difficulties (too low or too high) to be overcome. Other modifications proposed by Goodman, Zahurak and Piantadosi (1995) also help deal with these difficulties.

15.4 Examples

Example 15.1 Enrichment design – lapatanib vs hormone therapy in renal cell carcinoma
Ravaud, Hawkins, Gardner, *et al* (2008) conducted a phase III clinical trial comparing lapatanib with hormone therapy for the treatment of patients with advanced renal cell carcinoma who express the epidermal growth factor receptor (EGFR) and/or the human epidermal growth factor receptor 2 (HER-2). The primary endpoint of interest was time-to-progression (TTP) of the disease, with overall survival (OS) being a secondary endpoint. The trial was designed on the basis that a comparison would be made on all patients regardless of whether they were EGFR positive, HER-2 positive or both.

The sample size was computed using the approach of equations (7.7) and (7.8) assuming a 50% increase in median TTP (from 4 to 6 months), with 1-sided 5% significance level and 80% power. Allowing for a loss of follow up of 10%, 400 patients were needed for the trial and 416 were actually recruited.

For the purpose of our discussion, we will group the patients into two categories, EGFR+ (comprising patients who were only EGFR positive or both EGFR and HER-2 positive) and EGFR– (all other patients in the trial). The primary analysis of the trial showed no difference in TTP between the two arms ($HR = 0.94$, p-value = 0.6) and no difference in OS ($HR = 0.88$, $p = 0.29$).

However, in a subset analysis of the 241 EGFR+ patients, the results suggested that there was a statistically significant difference in OS ($HR = 0.69$, $p = 0.02$), although there remained weak evidence of a difference in TTP ($HR = 0.76$, $p = 0.06$). As this was a secondary subset analysis, the findings relating to the efficacy of lapatanib compared to hormone therapy for EGFR+ patients was not regarded as confirmatory.

However, assume the investigators knew in advance that EGFR was an important predictive classifier for the effectiveness of lapatanib. The investigators could then have designed the study using an enrichment design with EGFR as the predictive classifier of interest. With this design, they would only randomise EGFR+ patients to the trial and would have carried out their primary analysis on that group of patients alone. Their sample size calculations would have been based on the difference they expected to see between the two arms for EGFR+ patients alone and could use the same log-rank test approach adopted by the investigators (but likely with a much larger anticipated difference in TTP between the two arms). Note that this sample size would correspond to the number of EGFR+ patients to be recruited, as EGFR– patients would not be included in the trial.

Example 15.2 Biomarker stratified design – lapatanib vs hormone therapy in renal cell carcinoma
Alternatively, suppose the investigators in *Example 15.1* were less certain prior to the start of the trial as to the usefulness of EGFR as a predictive classifier. Then, rather than using an enrichment design, they could have used a biomarker stratified design and adopted the approach of *Analysis Plan A*. With this design, they would randomise all patients (that is, both EGFR+ and EGFR–) to the trial. For the analysis, they would then first compare the two treatments among EGFR+ patients. If that suggested a difference between the two arms, they would then do a comparison of the two arms among patients who were EGFR–.

To compute the total sample size for the trial, they would have done the same calculation as for the enrichment design, to obtain the target number of EGFR+ patients. They would then need to estimate the proportion of EGFR+ patients relative to EGFR– in the population of interest, and from there estimate the number of EGFR– patients required, and hence the total sample size.

Example 15.3 C33D - stroke survivors
Dite, Langford, Cumming, *et al* (2015) conducted a study in stroke survivors with impaired walking which was designed to test increasing doses of multimodal exercise in successive cohorts using the C33D design. The 'dose' was defined as the ability to reach a fixed maximal level of exercise (type, duration, and intensity) per week without experiencing dose-limiting tolerance (DLT). DLT thresholds were: (1) failure to complete more than 20% of a prescribed weekly exercise dose due to pain, fatigue, or effort required, and (2) being unable to perform activities of daily living (ADL).

In the first '3' cohort, 1 patient experienced DLT (hamstring soreness), and in the second '3' cohort, 1 also experienced DLT (fatigue). As a consequence the dose was not escalated and a third cohort was not recruited. Nevertheless, four participants were able to tolerate up to 1.5 h/week of exercise which included 283 min of endurance, 182 min of task practice, 138 min of strengthening, and 128 min resting. The authors claim: 'The maximal dose of exercise identified was dramatically higher than the dose typically delivered to stoke survivors ...' .

Example 15.4 CRM - capecitabine in metastatic colorectal cancer
Farid, Chowbay, Chen, *et al* (2012) used CRM to guide dose escalation and determined the MTD, which was defined as the dose lower than the dose achieving a DLT of 20%. The escalating dose levels of Capecitabine were set from 2,500 to 5,000 mg in steps of 500 mg. The doses given and number of patients concerned were 2,500 (3), 3,000 (3) 3,500 (3), 4,000 (4) and 4,500 (6). No DLTs were observed and so the MTD was taken to be 4,500 mg.

References

Genomic targets

Freidlin B, Jiang W and Simon R (2010). The cross-validated adaptive signature design for predictive analysis of clinical trials. *Clinical Cancer Research*, **16**, 691–698.

Freidlin B and Simon R (2005). Adaptive signature design: An adaptive clinical trial design for generating and prospectively testing a gene expression signature for sensitive patients. *Clinical Cancer Research*, **11**, 7872–7878.

Jiang W, Freidlin B and Simon R (2007). Biomarker adaptive threshold design: A procedure for evaluating treatment with possible biomarker-defined subset effect. *Journal of the National Cancer Institute*, **99**, 1036–1043.

Simon R (2005). A roadmap for developing and validating therapeutically relevant genomic classifiers. *Journal of Clinical Oncology*, **23**, 7332–7341.

Simon R (2008a). Using genomics in clinical trial design. *Clinical Cancer Research*, **14**, 5984–5993.

Simon R (2008b). Designs and adaptive analysis plans for pivotal clinical trials of therapeutics and companion diagnostics. *Expert Opinion of Molecular Diagnostics*, **2**, 721–729.

Simon R (2010). Clinical trial designs for evaluating the medical utility of prognostic and predictive biomarkers in oncology. *Personalized Medicine*, 7, 33–47.

Simon R (2012). Clinical trials for predictive medicine. *Statistics in Medicine*, **31**, 3031–3040.

Simon R and Wang SJ (2006). Use of genomic signatures in therapeutics development. *The Pharmacogenomics Journal*, **6**, 167–173.

Wang SJ, O'Neill RT and Hung HMJ (2007). Approaches to evaluation of treatment effect in randomised clinical trials with genomic subset. *Pharmaceutical Statistics*, **6**, 227–244.

Dose-finding

Flinn IW, Goodman SN, Post L, Jamison J, Miller CB, Gore S, Diehl L, Willis C, Ambinder RF and Byrd JC (2000). A dose-finding study of liposomal daunorubicin with CVP (COP-X) in advanced NHL. *Annals of Oncology*, **11**, 691–695.

Goodman SN, Zahurak ML and Piantadosi S (1995). Some practical improvements in the continual reassessment method for phase I studies. *Statistics in Medicine*, **14**, 1149–1161.

Korn EL, Midthune D, Chen TT, Rubinstein LV, Christian MC and Simon RM (1994). A comparison of two Phase I trial designs. *Statistics in Medicine*, **13**, 1799–1806.

O'Quigley J (2001). Dose-finding designs using continual reassessment method. In: Crowley J (ed) *Handbook of Statistics in Clinical Oncology*, Marcel Dekker Inc, New York, pp 35–72.

O'Quigley J, Pepe M and Fisher L (1990). Continual reassessment method: a practical design for phase I clinical trials in cancer. *Biometrics*, **46**, 33–48.

Storer BE (2001). Choosing a Phase I design. In: Crowley J (ed) *Handbook of Statistics in Clinical Oncology*, Marcel Dekker Inc, New York, pp 73–91.

Examples

Dite W, Langford ZN, Cumming TB, Churilov L, Blennerhassett JM and Bernhardt J (2015). A Phase 1 exercise dose escalation study for stroke survivors with impaired walking. *International Journal of Stroke*, **10**, 1051–1056.

Farid M, Chowbay B, Chen X, Tan S-H, Ramasamy S, Koo W-H, Toh H-C, Choo S-P and Ong SY-K (2012). Phase I pharmacokinetic study of chronomodulated dose-intensified combination of capecitabine and oxaliplatin (XELOX) in metastatic colorectal cancer. *Cancer Chemotherapy and Pharmacology*, **70**, 141–150.

Ravaud A, Hawkins R, Gardner JP, von der Maase H, Zantl N, Harper P, Rolland F, Audhuy B, Machiels JP, Pétavy F, Gore M, Schöffski P and El-Hariry I (2008). Lapatinib versus hormone therapy in patients with advanced renal cell carcinoma: a randomized phase III clinical trial. *Journal of Clinical Oncology*, **26**, 2285–2291.

16

Feasibility and Pilot Studies

SUMMARY

This chapter describes the general nature of feasibility studies and, amongst these, what distinguishes pilot studies. Two specific types of pilot study are described. One type is an Internal-Pilot, which is designed mainly to enable a reassessment of the sample size within an ongoing (Main) study and in which the data of the pilot is to be regarded as an integral part of the Main study analysis and interpretation. In contrast an External-Pilot study provides information upon which a definitive (Main) study will be designed but the pilot data do not form part of the analysis of this Main study once it is concluded. Issues of determining the size of a Pilot study are discussed and, in the case of an External-Pilot, methods of determining the optimum total (Pilot plus Main) study size are included.

16.1   Introduction

The term 'feasibility study' encompasses a wide range of possibilities for the actual type of study but in general refers to any study which is conducted as a precursor (or in some cases as adjunct) to an eventual Main study. Thus feasibility may be reserved for a certain type of early study or may equally describe, for example, a pilot or a proof-of-concept study.

Although feasibility studies are relevant to many intended study types, we use the randomised control trials (RCTs) to illustrate the issues. In practice RCTs often fail to complete, not because of lack of efficacy of the intervention but, for example, because patients refuse consent, clinicians refuse to refer patients, or there are far fewer patients with a particular condition than initially believed. Thus as a preliminary step to designing an RCT, or a study of whatever type, there will usually be a protracted period in which the research question is identified, associated work reviewed, preliminary options for the chosen design investigated, sample sizes determined and the protocol written and reviewed before the definitive study can commence. If, for example, information is sparse on one or more of the planning features then it may be appropriate to use this planning interval to firm up on some of these aspects. This might include conducting a preliminary investigation to refine details on, for example, the precise nature of the interventions to be compared or more mundane but important logistical issues. This chapter first describes some types of preliminary studies and then focusses on the more 'statistical' uncertainties that arise in these early stages.

Sample Sizes for Clinical, Laboratory and Epidemiology Studies, Fourth Edition. David Machin, Michael J. Campbell, Say Beng Tan and Sze Huey Tan.
© 2018 John Wiley & Sons Ltd. Published 2018 by John Wiley & Sons Ltd.

16.2 Feasibility or Pilot?

Eldridge, Lancaster, Campbell, *et al* (2016) describe the conceptual framework of **Figure 16.1** in which 'feasibility' is an over-arching concept which may concern refining qualitative and quantitative aspects pertinent to design and operation in order to facilitate the planning of a future (Main) study. Thus 'Pilot' studies, as well as 'Other feasibility' studies, are included within this framework. An 'Other feasibility' study asks whether something can be done, should we proceed with it, and if so, how, and generally applies to more logistical aspects of study design. In contrast, a pilot study, although it asks essentially the same questions, is conducted on a smaller scale than the proposed Main study. Consequently Whitehead, Sully and Campbell (2014) suggest that the term 'pilot' could be reserved for a study that mimics the definitive Main trial design in that it may include control groups and randomisation but whose explicit objective is *not* to compare groups but rather to ensure the Main trial once conducted delivers maximum information.

Feasibility Studies

Feasibility studies (that are not pilot studies) are those in which investigators attempt to answer a question about whether some element of the future Main trial can be done but do not implement the

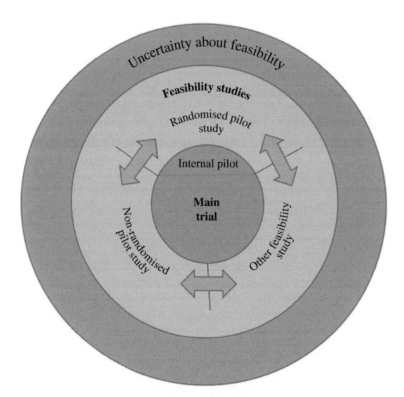

Figure 16.1 Conceptual framework for feasibility and pilot studies (from Eldridge, Lancaster, Campbell, *et al*, 2016, Figure 7). (*See insert for color representation of the figure.*)

intervention to be evaluated or other processes to be undertaken in a future trial, though they may be addressing intervention development in some way.

Examples of feasibility studies might include reviews of patient records to determine patient availability or interviews with clinicians to determine their willingness to contribute patients to a proposed trial.

Pilot Studies

Randomised pilot studies are those studies in which the future RCT, or parts of it, including the randomisation of participants, is conducted on a smaller scale (piloted) to see if it can be done. Thus randomised pilot studies can include studies that for the most part reflect the design of a future definitive trial but, if necessary due to remaining uncertainty, may involve trying out alternative strategies, for example, collecting an outcome variable via telephone for some participants and online for others.

Non-randomised pilot studies are similar to randomised pilot studies; they are studies in which all or part of the intervention to be evaluated and other processes to be undertaken in a future trial is/are carried out (piloted) but without randomisation of participants. These studies cover a wide range from those that are very similar to randomised pilot studies except that the intervention and control groups have not been randomised, to those in which only the test intervention itself is piloted. In other circumstances, it may be relevant to conduct a single arm pilot study of the control arm of the intended Main trial in order to establish a reasonable estimate of the standard deviation (*SD*) for the planned (continuous data) endpoint measure.

External- and Internal-Pilot Studies

For an External-Pilot, the Main trial has not started and the data obtained from the pilot do not contribute to an efficacy evaluation of the interventions concerned. When the design of the Main trial is settled upon, and the trial started, then early participants could form part of an Internal-Pilot. In which case, the assumption is that at some stage during the course of the Main trial an assessment will be made. At this point a decision may be made as to whether the Main trial continues or stops, or if it continues whether the initially planned sample size should be increased. The Main trial may stop if recruitment is too slow, or external and convincing evidence becomes available about the efficacy of the intervention. In any event, the data from the Internal-Pilot participants form part of the final Main trial analysis.

Proof-of-Concept Study

An alternative type of preliminary study often associated with pharmaceutical studies is the proof-of-concept study. This is an attempt to show that a product might have the desired clinical effect. This is often done in Phase II studies by using biological markers or surrogate markers. If an effect is seen on the marker, then it suggests that the product might have a therapeutic effect. Although 'proof-of-concept' studies may be thought of as feasibility studies, the term is usually confined to the therapeutic exploratory studies discussed in **Chapters 17 and 18**.

16.3 Design Criteria

In planning an RCT, (although much of what follows also relates to other types of comparative studies), the interventions to compare and the overall statistical design are selected by the research team. Once determined, the sample size has to be estimated and the corresponding test size and power will be set as well as a clinically important difference (on an appropriate scale) identified. Although there may be other considerations, together these provide the essential components for sample size determination. For a continuous endpoint variable, the anticipated difference is expressed in the form of the standardised effect size defined as

$$\Delta_{Plan} = \frac{\delta_{Plan}}{\sigma_{Plan}}. \qquad (16.1)$$

Here δ_{Plan} is the anticipated difference in means (the effect size) between the two interventions considered and σ_{Plan} the corresponding *SD*, which is often anticipated to be the same within each intervention group.

Clinical experience, the research literature and other information may provide a reasonable value for δ_{Plan} while in many circumstances an appropriate value for σ_{Plan} is more problematic. However, as indicated in **Chapter 5**, investigators may have a better feel for Δ_{Plan} rather than its individual component values. In practical terms, Cohen (1998) suggested a realistic range of values for Δ_{Plan} is from 0.1 to 1.0. He further defined a 'small' effect, that is a stringent planning criterion, might be $\Delta_{Plan} = 0.2$, a 'moderate' one $\Delta_{Plan} = 0.5$ and a 'large' effect, that is a liberal criterion, $\Delta_{Plan} = 0.8$.

An inappropriate value of σ_{Plan} used in setting Δ_{Plan} can have a serious effect on sample size for a given power required of the trial. If the anticipated σ_{Plan} is set too high, the trial will contain more subjects than necessary. If too low, the number of subjects will be too small and hence the trial will be underpowered. To overcome some of the uncertainty associated with a suitable choice for σ_{Plan}, strategies for conducting a pilot study can be adopted.

16.4 External-Pilot

Although an External-Pilot randomised trial is one which mimics the design of the Main trial, it does not aim to prove the superiority of one intervention over another but rather to try out aspects of the proposed Main trial. Also one would usually expect a 1:1 randomisation although this may not be necessarily envisaged for the eventual Main trial. Information from the External-Pilot is not expected to lead to many changes between it and the Main trial. However, the data from the External-Pilot and that of the eventual Main trial are *not* combined.

As an External-Pilot does not have the same objectives as the intended Main trial, setting the sample size in the same way is not likely to be appropriate. Nevertheless, it is still necessary to provide a sample size justification even if the reasons for choosing a particular size are made on pragmatic grounds.

The External-Pilot should contain participants who are representative of the intended Main trial to follow. However, it may happen that pilots are conducted in specialist centres, where the participants are tightly controlled and so less variation is present than in a more general medical setting anticipated for the Main trial. In this case, there may be some difficulty in assessing appropriate values for the component parameters of Δ_{Plan}.

Once complete, the data from an External-Pilot is used to estimate the *SD*, denoted s_{Pilot}, which is then used as the basis for determining the value of σ_{Plan} to be used in equation (16.1) and for subsequent sample size calculations for the intended Main trial. Thus the Main trial commences sometime after the closure of the External-Pilot.

Sample Size Issues

There are two situations to consider.

1) The results of a Pilot study, perhaps conducted by a different investigating team, are available and one wishes to use these results to plan the intended Main trial.
2) The team wishes to plan the size of a Pilot study with the objective to provide reliable information on which to plan the Main trial.

Using the Results of a Pilot to Plan the Main Study

Commonly, an External-Pilot will give estimates of the mean and *SD* of the outcome variable of interest for the Main study. On occasion the Pilot study may also provide an estimate of the effect size. It is not recommended that this is used as the sole source of information when considering the effect size that goes into a sample size calculation for the Main trial. The chosen effect size should be a synthesis of information from (many) potential sources including patients as well as the clinical team. For example, in diabetes a reduction of 0.5% in HbA1c is generally considered worthwhile, and this would lead to noticeable benefits in patients' health.

The estimate of the effect from a pilot study will have considerable uncertainty. However if the upper limit of the resulting confidence interval (CI) obtained from the External-Pilot is less than any difference considered clinically worthwhile, one may then question whether the intended Main trial is likely to be worth conducting. Similarly, if the lower limit of the CI is greater than a worthwhile difference, one may wonder if the effectiveness of the test treatment has been proven and whether a subsequent Main trial remains ethical.

Apart from the potential effect size, a very useful component of the External-Pilot is the associated estimate of the *SD* of the outcome variable it provides.

Accounting for Imprecision in the Standard Deviation

The usually relatively small sample size of the External-Pilot, N_{Pilot}, will necessarily affect the accuracy of the resulting *SD*, s_{Pilot}, obtained through the corresponding number of degrees of freedom, f. The small f introduces a type of imprecision that should be allowed for when determining the corresponding planning value, σ_{Plan}, which is then to be used as a key component when estimating the sample size of the Main trial, N_{Main}.

Two different methods, the Upper Confidence Limit (UCL) and the Non-central t (NCT) approach, have been developed to deal with the issue of imprecise *SD* estimates. Both methods allow for the imprecision of s_{Pilot} by automatically inflating its observed value. It is this inflated estimate, σ_{Main}, which is then used for the Main trial sample size calculation.

Upper Confidence Limit (UCL)

When determining the Main trial sample size, s_{Pilot} is replaced by the corresponding $\gamma\%$ Upper Confidence Limit (UCL) given by

$$\sigma_{Main} = UCL\left(\gamma, f\right) = \sqrt{\frac{f}{\chi^2\left(1-\gamma, f\right)}} \times s_{Pilot} = \kappa s_{Pilot}. \tag{16.2}$$

Here $\chi^2(1-\gamma, f)$ represents the $1-\gamma$ percentile of the Chi-squared distribution with f degrees of freedom which, for a parallel two-group External-Pilot design, are $f = N_{Pilot} - 2$. Values of the multiplier κ are given for differing f and γ in **Table 16.1**.

Thus, the Main trial size is then estimated using equation (5.4) of **Chapter 5** but replacing σ_{Plan} by σ_{Main} from equation (16.2). Thus, for a 2-sided test size α and power $1 - \beta$, the number of subjects required is

$$N_{Main} = \frac{(\varphi+1)^2}{\varphi} \frac{\left(z_{1-\beta} + z_{1-\alpha/2}\right)^2}{\left(\delta_{Plan}/\sigma_{Main}\right)^2} + \left[\frac{z_{1-\alpha/2}^2}{2}\right], \tag{16.3}$$

where φ is the corresponding allocation ratio. Values for $z_{1-\alpha/2}$ and $z_{1-\beta}$ can be obtained from **Table 1.2**. The number of subjects required in each intervention are $n_S = N/(1+\varphi)$ and $n_T = \varphi N/(1+\varphi)$ respectively.

Non-central *t*-distribution (NCT)

The NCT approach sets $\sigma_{Plan} = s_{Pilot}$ based on $f_{Pilot} = N_{Pilot} - 2$ degrees of freedom, but it replaces the $(z_{1-\alpha/2} + z_{1-\beta})$ component from the Normal distribution in the numerator of equation (5.4) by

$$\theta = NCT\left\{1-\beta, f_{Pilot}, t_{1-\alpha/2, N_{Main}-2}\right\} \tag{16.4}$$

from the NCT distribution which is discussed briefly in **Chapter 1.5**.

Thus the anticipated sample size for the Main trial is

$$N_{Main} = \frac{(\varphi+1)^2}{\varphi} \frac{\theta^2}{\left(\delta_{Plan}/s_{Pilot}\right)^2}, \tag{16.5}$$

The influence of the test size, α, is taken account of within the non-centrality parameter, $\psi = t_{1-\alpha/2, N_{Main}-2}$. However, the quantity N_{Main} on the left of (16.5) is also a component of ψ, on the right of this expression. Thus, to find a solution for the sample size, an iterative process is required. A starting point for the iterations is obtained by first replacing in θ the quantity, $t_{1-\alpha/2, N_{Main}-2}$, of the t-distribution by $z_{1-\alpha/2}$ of the Normal distribution to give $\theta_0 = NCT\{1-\beta, f_{Pilot}, z_{1-\alpha/2}\}$. The right hand side of equation (16.5) now no longer depends on N_{Main} and becomes

$$N_0 = \frac{(\varphi+1)^2}{\varphi} \frac{\theta_0^2}{\left(\delta_{Plan}/s_{Pilot}\right)^2}. \tag{16.6}$$

This provides an initial sample size N_0, which then enables $t_{1-\alpha/2;N_0-2}$ to be found and substituted in equation (16.5) to obtain θ_1; after which a revised sample size N_1 is calculated. This value then results in values for $t_{1-\alpha/2;N_1-2}$, θ_2 and a second revised sample size, N_2. This iterative process continues until successive values of N_i remain essentially unchanged and so establish N_{Main}.

Sample Size of an External-pilot

Although the previous sections state how one might use the results of an External-Pilot to better determine the size of the Main trial, clearly the size of the External-Pilot has to be specified before such a calculation can be implemented. Unlike the situations described in most of this book, the required size of an External-Pilot is not based on a power calculation but is simply a justification to show that the aims of the pilot can be met successfully.

Flat Rule-of-thumb

In the very preliminary stages of planning Main trials, the actual value of SD, σ_{Plan}, to be used ultimately for the specification may be uncertain before an External-Pilot is conducted. Thus, with this uncertainty in mind, sample size possibilities, N_{Pilot}, for a two equal-group comparative External-Pilot study have been suggested to obtain an estimate of σ_{Plan}. These are summarised in **Table 16.2** and indicate a wide range of values from 20 to more than 70 subjects. The term 'Flat' indicates that the ultimate standardised effect size, Δ_{Plan}, has not been taken account of by these suggestions. Thus, the External-Pilot sample size is fixed no matter how large the subsequent Main trial is intended to be.

Stepped Rule-of-thumb

If the planning team know something of the magnitude of Δ_{Plan} intended for the Main trial then they can use this knowledge in determining the planned External-Pilot sample size. Thus **Table 16.3** suggests a range of total sample sizes for an External-Pilot, based on whether (at this preliminary stage) $\Delta_{Initial}$ for the Main trial is thought likely to be in one of the four regions: < 0.1 (extra small), centred on 0.2 (small), 0.5 (medium) and 0.8 (large). The term 'Stepped' indicates that the provisional standardised effect size for the Main trial has been taken into account in these suggestions. However, once the External-Pilot is completed, the team will have s_{Pilot} and hence a better value for σ_{Plan} and a possibly revised Δ_{Plan}. They will then be able to review the previously proposed estimate for the Main trial sample size, N_{Main}.

16.5   Considerations Across External-Pilot and Main Trials

If one of the adjustment methods described above is used as a basis for using the estimate of the SD provided by the External-Pilot then the size of that pilot ultimately affects the sample size of the Main trial. That is, since the adjustment methods depend on the *degrees of freedom* with which s_{Pilot} is estimated, so ultimately does the size of the Main trial. Thus, there is a trade-off between having a small External-Pilot (large κ) and the likelihood of a larger Main trial, or a larger External-Pilot (smaller κ) and a likely smaller Main trial.

Optimising Overall Sample Size

Here we think of the External-Pilot and the Main trial as comprising one Overall study programme. This leads to the idea of minimising the sum of External-Pilot and the Main trial together to produce an optimal 'Overall' study sample size based on an 'optimal' External-Pilot sample size.

Once the required Main trial size, N_{Main}, assuming equal numbers per group, has been determined, the Overall study sample size then becomes

$$N_{Overall} = N_{Pilot} + N_{Main}. \qquad (16.7)$$

Table 16.4 gives optimal sample sizes of the External-Pilot, N_{Pilot}, the Main trial, N_{Main}, and their collective total, $N_{Overall}$, for the UCL80%, UCL95% and NCT approaches to their calculation. The NCT approach gives total sample sizes less than those for UCL80% and UCL95%.

16.6   Internal-Pilot Studies

The idea of an Internal-Pilot study is to plan the Main study on the basis of the best (current) available information, but to regard the first block of patients entered as the Internal-Pilot. This contrasts with a planned *interim* analysis which may be an integral part of the data and safety monitoring of a Main trial whose specific purpose is to stop or modify the trial if necessary for (mainly) safety considerations or, in some circumstances, to close the trial early should sufficient information be accrued from the current trial data (and before the full recruitment target is fully complete) to establish convincing evidence of whether or not the test intervention is effective.

Some grant review bodies, such as the UK National Institute for Health Research (NIHR), request a review after a Main trial has run for a period of time to assess, for example, whether recruitment rates are on target. Thus, in the Putting Life in Years (PLINY) trial of Mountain, Hind, Gossage-Worrall, *et al* (2014), there was a pre-specified target for collecting valid primary outcome data for 80% of those recruited at the 6-month follow-up during the Internal-Pilot stage.

An Internal-Pilot can also be used to revise the initial sample size, $N_{Initial}$, of the Main trial which had been estimated using $\sigma_{Initial}$ as the anticipated *SD*. Once N_{Pilot} ($< N_{Initial}$) subjects have been recruited to the Main Trial (and these are considered as the Internal-Pilot) and the corresponding endpoints recorded, the *SD* is calculated as $\sigma_{Internal}$ and then compared to $\sigma_{Initial}$. Two vital features which accompany this approach are summarised in **Figure 16.2**.

This first point of **Figure 16.2** is crucial and implies no note of the observed difference (the effect size) between groups is purposely made at the end of the Internal-Pilot stage. Thus the initially assumed δ_{Plan} remains unchanged in any revised calculations of sample size.

---

1. Only use the Internal-Pilot information in order to improve the design features which are independent of the measure that is used to establish any difference between the comparison groups concerned

2. The final sample size should only ever be adjusted upwards from the Initial, never down

---

Figure 16.2 Vital features of an Internal-Pilot study.

If the two randomised groups are to be compared using a t-test, then a basic ingredient of the initial sample size calculation is, as we have indicated, $\sigma_{Initial}$. This value may need to be amended following estimation of its value using the Internal-Pilot data. If $\sigma_{Internal}$ is larger than $\sigma_{Initial}$, then this is used to revise upwards the final sample size from $N_{Initial}$ to N_{Final}.

On the other hand should $\sigma_{Internal}$ be smaller than σ_{Plan}, then $N_{Initial}$ is retained as the final sample size.

The advantage of an Internal-Pilot for determining the SD is that it can be relatively large—perhaps one-third to a half of the initially anticipated subjects. It provides an insurance against misjudgement regarding the baseline planning assumptions. It is, nevertheless, important that the intention to conduct an Internal-Pilot is recorded at the outset with full details provided in the study protocol and the eventual published report.

16.7 Bibliography

Whitehead, Sully and Campbell (2014) provide a definition of an External-Pilot randomised trial, while Eldridge, Lancaster, Campbell, *et al* (2016) give a conceptual framework linking pilot and feasibility studies. Browne (1995) advocated the use of an External-Pilot study, proposed the use of equation (16.2) to modify the planning SD and suggested using an 80% UCL. In contrast Sim and Lewis (2011) suggested using a 95% UCL. Julious and Owen (2006) describe the Non-central t-distribution (NCT) approach of equation (16.4) leading to equation (16.5).

Lancaster, Dodd and Williamson (2004), Thabane, Ma, Chu, *et al* (2010) and Arain, Campbell, Cooper, *et al* (2010) point out that for an External-Pilot trial, the objective is not to prove superiority of the treatment, but to test trial procedures and processes and to get estimates of parameters for the Main trial sample size calculation. Kraemer, Mintz, Nosa, *et al* (2006) recommend that the effect size obtained from an External-Pilot should *not* be used as the effect size for the Main study.

The method of setting the External-Pilot trial sample size in order to minimise the Overall sample size of the External-Pilot and the Main trial together was described by Kieser and Wassmer (1996) and was also investigated by Sim and Lewis (2011). Whitehead, Julious, Cooper, *et al*, (2015) suggest the method which relates the size of the External-Pilot to the effect size planned for the Main trial, while Avery, Williamson, Gamble, *et al* (2015) discuss the use of 'progression criteria' to determine whether the Internal-Pilot should continue into the Main trial.

The revised CONSORT statement described by Eldridge, Chan, Campbell, *et al* (2016) and bodies such as the UK NIHR state that pilot studies do not necessarily need a power-based sample size calculation, but they do all need a sample size justification.

16.8 Examples

Table 16.2

Example 16.1   Single group feasibility - reflexology in managing secondary lymphoedema
Whatley, Street, Kay and Harris (2016) describe what they term a feasibility study aimed to examine the use of reflexology lymphatic drainage (RLD) in the treatment of breast-cancer related lymphoedema (BCRL) as a preliminary to possible further research. Following design suggestions by White

and Ernst (2001) and guidelines suggested by, for example, Lancaster, Dodd and Williamson (2004), they planned a single arm study of 30 patients. This is the number suggested for a single group study by Browne (1995) of **Table 16.2**.

In the event, the investigators recruited 26 women for whom they compared the affected and non-affected arms of each woman at baseline and post RLD and recorded the respective arm volumes in their Table 3. They noted 'a significant reduction in the volume of the affected arm ... compared to baseline'. They also commented: ' ... although the results could not be attributed to the reflexology intervention because of research design limitations'. Their final conclusion was: ' ... there was sufficient evidence for further research using a randomized trial.'

This study clearly demonstrates the feasibility of, for example, delivering the reflexology and estimating the arm volume changes, as well as providing some indication which may help to establish planning values for any subsequent comparative trial.

Tables 16.1 and 16.2 and Equations 5.4, 16.1 and 16.2

Example 16.2   External Pilot to determine the planning SD - intradialytic oral nutritional supplement during dialysis

The NOURISH pilot study of Jackson, Cohen, Sully and Julious (2015) aimed to examine the feasibility of conducting a trial to assess the impact of an intradialytic oral nutritional supplement in addition to nutritional advice from a renal dietitian in patients on dialysis. The two parallel-group External-Pilot aimed to recruit 30 patients to ensure 24 evaluable patients as suggested by Julious (2005b) in **Table 16.2**. The outcome was a change in handgrip strength (HGS) assessed in kg. In fact, only 20 patients were recruited to the pilot, from which the authors estimated the *SD* for HGS to be 10.7 kg. For the intended Main trial, a minimum clinically important difference of $\delta_{Plan} = 4$ kg was anticipated, which suggested from equation (16.1), $\Delta_{Plan} = 4/10.7 = 0.374$. Use of equation (5.4) or $^{\S}S_S$ requires 304 participants with equal numbers per arm for a 90% power and 2-sided 5% significance.

However, the *SD* has considerable uncertainty, so that with a pilot of size 20, $df = 18$ and equation (16.2), evaluated in **Table 16.1**, suggests with $\gamma = 0.9$ that one should inflate the planning SD, σ_{Plan}, by $\kappa = 1.287$. Hence the initial sample size is inflated by $1.287^2 = 1.656$ to be confident of maintaining 90% power in the Main study. This suggests the Main NOURISH trial should recruit $N_{Main} = 304 \times 1.656 = 503.42$ or approximately 500 patients in total.

Table 16.2 and Equations 8.1, 8.2, 8.3 and 8.4

Example 16.3   Single arm pilot - severe pelvic endometriosis

In planning a randomised trial in women with bilateral endometriosis who would receive standard surgical treatment with the difference that, at the end of surgery, one ovary was randomised to ovarian suspension (OS) and the other to non-suspension (ONS), Hoo, Stavroulis, Pateman, *et al* (2014) describe what they term as a pilot study.

This study comprised a sample of 32 ovaries in 16 women to determine the prevalence of ovarian adhesions on transvaginal ultrasound 3 months after routine laparoscopic treatment for severe pelvic endometriosis (without ovarian suspension). Although the number of ovaries is within the range of smaller sample sizes of **Table 16.2** this ignores any association between the two ovaries of each woman.

The investigators found 4 women had unilateral adhesions and 7 had adhesions in both ovaries. From which they calculated the adhesion rate per ovary with ONS as 18/32 (56.3%) with 95% CI 31.9 to 80.6%, albeit this was calculated ignoring the association between ovaries within the same woman.

From these results they then assumed, when determining the sample size for the randomised trial, an adhesion proportion for ONS of 0.6 and defined a clinically significant improvement with OS as a 50% reduction in this prevalence to 0.3. Expressed in terms of the anticipated odds ratio, this gives $\psi_{Plan} = \dfrac{0.6/0.4}{0.3/0.7} = 3.5$. They further assumed the proportion of discordant pairs to be $\pi_{Dis} = 0.54$, giving from equation (8.4) $\pi_{01} = 0.53/(1 + 3.5) = 0.12$. Then with a 2-sided 5% significance level and power 80%, use of equation (8.1) or $\boxed{S_{SS}}$ gives the number of women with bilateral endometriosis to recruit as $N_{Women} = 45$. Alternatively using the approach of equations (8.2) and (8.3) gives $N_{Women} = 43$.

The investigators then anticipated a possible 10% dropout during the follow-up period and so planned to recruit at least 50 patients to the Main trial.

Table 16.2

Example 16.4   Three-group randomised pilot - major depressive disorder
Atiwannapat, Thaipisuttikul, Poopityastaporn and Katekaew (2016) reported a three intervention-group randomised trial in patients with major depressive disorder (MDD) of Active Music (AM) therapy which began with group singing, Receptive Music (RM) therapy which began with music listening and Sham-operated control (SC) with group therapy without music. The primary outcome was the change from baseline in the MADRS Thai depression total score. The investigators screened 22 patients for eligibility and recruited 14 who were randomised to AM (5), RM (5) and SC (4). At one month post randomisation, the mean score changes from baseline were reported as −11.75, −10.5 and −6 for AM, RM and SC respectively. Despite this being clearly a pilot study (as indicated by the article's title), several statistical significance tests using ANOVA were reported. Amongst the limitations described by the authors is: '..., our sample size was small ... which limited the study statistical power'.

In short, there is nothing intrinsically wrong in conducting and reporting this study provided sensible interpretation without statistical testing is conducted. Given the size of the study, it is inevitable that the statistical tests reported are non-significant, but one should not conclude from these that the intervention failed. Nevertheless, one would expect the size of a three-group intervention pilot to involve at least 3/2 times the recommendations of **Table 16.2** or, in this case, approximately 45 patients to be randomised.

Table 16.2 and Equation 5.4

Example 16.5   Randomised pilot - ventilator-dependent extremely preterm infants
A small randomised trial of hydrocortisone against placebo in 64 ventilator-dependent extremely preterm infants exposed to the risk of bronchopulmonary dysplasia (BPD) was conducted by Parikh, Kennedy, Lasky, *et al* (2013). It was designed using conventional methods corresponding to the use of equation (5.4), assuming a patient loss of 25% and a primary outcome of total brain tissue volume at 38 weeks postmenstrual age, as follows: 'Assuming an alpha error of 0.05, a 25% mortality, and a total brain tissue volume of $357 \pm 50\,\text{cm}^3$ for infants with BPD, 32 infants per group provided 80% power to detect a $43\,\text{cm}^3$ absolute improvement in the primary outcome.

This difference equates to a 2-week growth in brain size.' The chosen sample size is larger than the minimum recommended by Sim and Lewis (2011) and close to that of Teare, Dimairo, Shephard, *et al* (2014) referred to in **Table 16.2**.

The study is described in the title as a 'Pilot' and in the corresponding discussion section of the paper as an 'exploratory pilot', suggesting that this would not be regarded as a definitive study. However, the authors make a formal statistical comparison suggesting this is really a small Main randomised controlled trial. To be an External-Pilot, the information generated by the study should only help to make more informed decisions on key design aspects of the Main randomised trial. Indeed, the authors state: 'Our findings ... have implications for the design and conduct of future hydrocortisone trials, particularly for the selection of patient population and drug regimen.' Unfortunately, they do not describe plans to do this themselves.

Tables 16.3 and 16.4

Example 16.6   External-pilot and main trial
A two-armed parallel group (Main) randomised controlled clinical trial is being planned with a 2-sided $\alpha = 0.05$ and power $1 - \beta = 0.9$. The primary outcome is a continuous variable with an approximate Normal distribution. As the investigators are unsure about design aspects of the Main trial such as what the *SD* of the outcome measure is anticipated to be, the likely recruitment and the dropout rates, they decide to run an External-Pilot trial.

Suppose the standardised effect size to be used in the Main trial, which is the minimum that is clinically worthwhile, is $\Delta_{Plan} = 0.2$. Then the stepped rule-of-thumb sample size options for comparative External-Pilot suggested by **Table 16.3** for UCL 80%, UCL 90% and NCT are 40, 60 and 50. However, if the optimal approach of **Table 16.4** is chosen, the corresponding size of the External Pilot would be much larger, with suggested values of 92, 144 and 56. The associated Main trial sizes are 1,206, 1,294 and 1,104 respectively, implying the corresponding potential Overall sample sizes of the External-Pilot plus the Main trial of 1,298, 1,438 and 1,160 participants.

Equation 5.4

Example 16.7   Internal-pilot - children with non-anaemic iron deficiency
Abdullah, Thorpe, Mamak, *et al* (2015) conducted an Internal-Pilot within their randomised trial comparing oral iron plus nutritional guidance (ING) over placebo plus nutritional guidance (PNG) in improving the development, hematological and behavioural outcomes in children with non-anaemic iron deficiency (NAID). The primary outcome measure was the Early Learning Composite (ELC) score at 4 months post-randomisation. The Main trial planning values used comprised of the *SD* for the ELC score as $\sigma_{Plan} = 15$ and differences between the interventions, δ_{Plan}, ranging from 6 to 8. Then with a 2-sided $\alpha = 0.05$ and $1 - \beta = 0.8$, the use of equation (5.4) or $^S S_S$ gives, with equal allocation, $\varphi = 1$, sample sizes ranging from 114 to 200.

The corresponding Internal-Pilot was designed to include the first 30 children randomised, although for 3 of these children the ELC assessment was not made. The blinded results (coded as *A* and *B*) gave $n_A = 14$, $s_A = 21.17$ and $n_B = 13$, $s_B = 12.05$ from which a pooled estimate, $s_{Pilot} = 17.4$ was obtained. As this value was greater than the initial $\sigma_{Plan} = 15$, the revised sample sizes from $^S S_S$ range from 152 to 266.

References

Technical

Arain M, Campbell MJ, Cooper CL and Lancaster GA (2010). What is a pilot or feasibility study? A review of current practice and editorial policy. *BMC Medical Research Methodology*, **10**, 67.

Avery KNL, Williamson P, Gamble C, O'Connell E, Metcalfe C, Davidson P and Williams H (2015). Informing efficient randomised controlled trials: exploration of challenges in developing progression criteria for internal pilot studies. *Trials*, **16**(Suppl 2), P10.

Birkett MA and Day SJ (1994). Internal pilot studies for estimating sample size. *Statistics in Medicine*, **13**, 2455–2463.

Browne RH (1995). On the use of a pilot study for sample size determination. *Statistics in Medicine*, **14**, 1933–1940.

Cohen J (1988). *Statistical Power Analysis for the Behavioral Sciences*, (2nd edn) Lawrence Earlbaum, New Jersey.

Eldridge SM, Chan CL, Campbell MJ, Bond CM, Hopewell S, Thabane L, Lancaster GA on behalf of the PAFS Consensus group (2016). CONSORT 2010 statement: extension to randomised pilot and feasibility trials. *British Medical Journal*, **355**:i5239 | doi: 10.1136/bmj.i5239.

Eldridge SM, Lancaster GA, Campbell MJ, Thabane L, Hopewell S, Coleman CL and Bond CM (2016). Defining feasibility and pilot studies in preparation for randomised controlled trials: development of a conceptual framework. *PLoS One*, **11**: doi:19.1371/journal.pone.0150205.

Julious SA (2005b). Sample size of 12 per group rule of thumb for a pilot study. *Pharmaceutical Statistics*, **4**, 287–291.

Julious SA and Owen NRJ (2006). Sample size calculations for clinical studies allowing for uncertainty about the variance. *Pharmaceutical Statistics*, **5**, 29–37.

Kieser M and Wassmer G (1996). On the use of the upper confidence limit for the variance from a pilot sample for sample size determination. *Biometrical Journal*, **8**, 941–949.

Kraemer HC, Mintz J, Nosa A, Tinklenberg J and Yesavage JA (2006). Caution regarding the use of pilot studies to guide power calculations for study purposes. *Archives of General Psychiatry*, **63**, 484–489.

Lancaster GA, Dodd S and Williamson PR (2004). Design and analysis of pilot studies: recommendations for good practice. *Journal of Evaluation in Clinical Practice*, **10**, 307–312.

Mountain GA, Hind D, Gossage-Worrall R, Walters SJ, Duncan R, Newbould L, Rex S, Jones C, Bowling A, Cattan M, Cairns A, Cooper C, Tudor Edwards R and Goyder EC (2014). 'Putting Life in Years' (PLINY) telephone friendship groups research study: pilot randomised controlled trial. *Trials*, **15**, 141–152.

Sim J and Lewis M (2011). The size of a pilot study for a clinical trial should be calculated in relation to considerations of precision and efficiency. *Journal of Clinical Epidemiology*, **65**, 301–308.

Teare MD, Dimairo M, Shephard N, Hayman A, Whitehead A and Walters SJ (2014). Sample size requirements to estimate key design parameters from external pilot randomised controlled trials: A simulation study. *Trials*, **15**, 264.

Thabane L, Ma J, Chu R, Cheng J, Ismaila A, Rios LP, Robson R, Thabane M, Giangregorio L and Goldsmith CH (2010). A tutorial on pilot studies: The what, why and how. *BMC Medical Research Methodology*, **10**, 1.

White A and Ernst E (2001). The case for uncontrolled clinical trials: A starting point for the evidence base for CAM. *Complementary Therapies in Medicine*, **9**, 111–115.

Whitehead AL, Julious SA, Cooper CL and Campbell MJ (2015). Estimating the sample size for a pilot randomised trial to minimise the overall trial sample size for the external pilot and main trial for a continuous outcome variable. *Statistical Methods in Medical Research*, **25**, 1057–1073.

Whitehead AL, Sully BGO and Campbell MJ (2014). Pilot and feasibility studies: Is there a difference from each other and from a randomised controlled trial? *Contemporary Clinical Trials*, **38**, 130–133.

Examples

Abdullah K, Thorpe KE, Mamak E, Maguire JL, Birken CS, Fehlings D, Hanley AJ, Macarthur C, Zlotkin SH and Parkin PC (2015). An internal pilot study for a randomized trial aimed at evaluating the effectiveness of iron interventions in children with non-anemic iron deficiency: the OptEC trial. *Trials*, **16**, 303.

Atiwannapat P, Thaipisuttikul P, Poopityastaporn P and Katekaew W (2016). Active versus receptive group music therapy for major depressive disorder – A pilot study. *Complementary Therapies in Medicine*, **26**, 141–145.

Hoo WL, Stavroulis A, Pateman K, Saridogan E, Cutner A, Pandis G, Tong ENC and Jurkovic D (2014). Does ovarian suspension following laparoscopic surgery for endometriosis reduce postoperative adhesions? An RCT. *Human Reproduction*, **29**, 670–676.

Jackson L, Cohen J, Sully B and Julious SA (2015). NOURISH, Nutritional OUtcomes from a Randomised Investigation of Intradialytic oral nutritional Supplements in patients receiving Haemodialysis: a pilot randomised controlled trial. *Pilot and Feasibility Studies*, **1**, 11.

Parikh NA, Kennedy KA, Lasky RE, McDavid GE and Tyson JE (2013). Pilot randomized trial of hydrocortisone in ventilator-dependent extremely preterm infants: Effects on regional brain volumes. *The Journal of Pediatrics*, **162**, 685–690.

Whatley J, Street R, Kay S and Harris PE (2016). Use of reflexology in managing secondary lymphoedema for patients affected by treatments for breast cancer: A feasibility study. *Complementary Therapies in Clinical Practice*, **23**, 1–8.

White A and Ernst E (2001). The case for uncontrolled clinical trials: A starting point for the evidence base for CAM. *Complementary Therapeutics in Medicine*, **9**, 111–115.

Table 16.1 The multiplier κ of the estimated standard deviation, s, to obtain the estimated $\gamma\%$ upper confidence limit (UCL) for the actual standard deviation σ [Equation 16.2].

Degrees of freedom f	$\gamma=0.8$	$\gamma=0.9$	$\gamma=0.95$	Degrees of freedom f	$\gamma=0.8$	$\gamma=0.9$	$\gamma=0.95$
1	3.947	7.958	15.947	31	1.131	1.203	1.268
2	2.117	3.081	4.415	32	1.128	1.199	1.263
3	1.728	2.266	2.920	33	1.126	1.195	1.258
4	1.558	1.939	2.372	34	1.123	1.191	1.253
5	1.461	1.762	2.089	35	1.121	1.188	1.248
6	1.398	1.650	1.915	36	1.119	1.185	1.244
7	1.353	1.572	1.797	37	1.117	1.182	1.240
8	1.320	1.514	1.711	38	1.116	1.179	1.236
9	1.293	1.469	1.645	39	1.114	1.176	1.232
10	1.272	1.434	1.593	40	1.112	1.173	1.228
11	1.255	1.404	1.551	50	1.098	1.152	1.199
12	1.240	1.380	1.515				
13	1.227	1.359	1.485	60	1.088	1.136	1.179
14	1.216	1.341	1.460				
15	1.206	1.325	1.437	70	1.081	1.125	1.163
16	1.198	1.311	1.418				
17	1.190	1.298	1.400	80	1.075	1.116	1.151
18	1.183	1.287	1.384				
19	1.177	1.277	1.370	90	1.070	1.108	1.141
20	1.171	1.268	1.358				
21	1.166	1.259	1.346	100	1.066	1.102	1.133
22	1.161	1.252	1.335				
23	1.157	1.245	1.326	125	1.059	1.090	1.117
24	1.153	1.238	1.316				
25	1.149	1.232	1.308	150	1.053	1.081	1.106
26	1.145	1.226	1.300				
27	1.142	1.221	1.293	175	1.049	1.075	1.097
28	1.139	1.216	1.286				
29	1.136	1.211	1.280	200	1.045	1.070	1.090
30	1.133	1.207	1.274				

Table 16.2 Flat rule-of-thumb for the total sample size of a two equal-group comparative External-Pilot trial (partly based on Whitehead, Julious, Cooper and Campbell, 2015, Table 4).

Reference	N_{Pilot}
Birkett and Day (1994)	20
Julious (2005)	24
Kieser and Wassmer (1996)	20 to 40
Sim and Lewis (2011)	≥55
Browne (1995)	60*
Teare, Dimairo, Shephard, *et al* (2014)	≥ 70

*Actually recommended 30 for a single-arm study

Table 16.3 Stepped rule-of-thumb total sample size for an External-Pilot trial for varying standardised differences, Δ, and power of the potential two equal-group comparative Main trial using the UCL and NCT approaches (partly based on Whitehead, Julious, Cooper and Campbell, 2015, Table 8).

Power of the Main Trial			80%			90%		
			UCL			UCL		
	Inflation Method		80%	95%	NCT	80%	95%	NCT
Anticipated	Extra small	$\Delta < 0.1$	150	225	100	175	275	150
Standardised	Small	$0.1 \leq \Delta < 0.3$	35	50	40	40	60	50
Difference,	Medium	$0.3 \leq \Delta < 0.7$	20	30	20	15	30	30
Δ	Large	$\Delta \geq 0.7$	10	15	20	10	15	20

Table 16.4 Optimal values of Pilot, Main and hence Overall two equal-group comparative trial size for UCL80%, UCL90% and NCT inflation methods for a given standardised difference, Δ [From a combined iterative solution of Equations 16.4 and 16.5 to minimise 16.7] (based on Whitehead, Julious, Cooper and Campbell, 2015, Table 6).

Standardised	Inflation Method								
Difference	UCL 80%			UCL 95%			NCT		
$\Delta_{Plan} = \delta_{Plan}/\sigma_{Plan}$	Pilot	Main	Overall	Pilot	Main	Overall	Pilot	Main	Overall
Main Trial Power 80%									
0.05	420	13,342	13,762	662	13,784	14,446	188	12,706	12,854
0.10	176	3,456	3,632	278	3,634	3,912	76	3,214	3,290
0.20	78	914	992	122	986	1,108	40	824	864
0.30	48	426	474	76	468	544	28	376	404
0.40	36	250	286	56	278	334	22	216	238
0.50	28	166	194	44	188	232	20	140	160
0.60	24	120	144	36	138	174	20	98	118
0.70	20	90	110	32	106	138	20	72	92
0.80	20	70	90	28	84	112	20	56	76
0.90	20	58	74	26	70	96	20	44	64
1.00	20	22	64	22	58	80	20	36	56
Main Trial Power 90%									
0.05	506	17,760	18,266	796	18,298	19,094	212	17,022	17,234
0.10	212	4,584	4,796	334	4,800	5,134	108	4,308	4,416
0.20	92	1,206	1,298	144	1,294	1,438	56	1,104	1,160
0.30	58	558	616	90	610	700	38	504	542
0.40	42	326	368	66	362	428	30	290	320
0.50	32	216	248	52	244	296	24	190	214
0.60	28	156	184	42	178	220	22	136	158
0.70	24	118	142	36	136	172	20	100	120
0.80	20	92	112	32	108	140	20	78	98
0.90	20	76	94	28	88	116	20	62	82
1.00	20	60	80	26	74	100	20	50	70

17

Therapeutic Exploratory Trials: Single Arm with Binary Outcomes

SUMMARY
In this chapter we describe single- and two-stage designs for Therapeutic Exploratory (often described as Phase II) clinical trials involving a single arm and where the outcome of interest is binary in nature, for example, whether the tumour responds or not. We discuss the single-stage Fleming-A'Hern design as well as two-stage designs such as the Simon-Optimal and the Simon-Minimax designs. The designs by Tan-Machin and Mayo-Gajewski are based on Bayesian methods and have two options: single or dual threshold designs.

17.1   Introduction

Before embarking on large-scale randomised Phase III clinical trials, investigators will often first conduct a Phase II trial, sometimes also known as a 'Therapeutic Exploratory (TE) trial', to investigate the activity of the compound under consideration. The primary goal is to decide if it warrants further investigation. With the advancement of medical research, including the advent of genomic medicine and molecular targeted therapies, questions have been raised regarding the continued relevance of such clinical trials as part of the drug development process, with the alternative being to go directly from Phase I trials to Phase III. This issue has been reviewed by groups such as the NDDO Research Foundation's Task Force on Methodology for the Development of Innovative Cancer Therapies, which concluded in Booth, Calvert, Giaccone, *et al* (2008) that 'an appropriately designed phase II study remains an important mechanism for screening out ineffective agents'.

There are a large number of designs for TE trials. In a review by Brown, Gregory, Twelves, *et al* (2011) just covering cancer clinical trials alone, the group found over 100 statistical designs. These include single-stage designs, in which a predetermined number of patients are recruited, and two-stage designs, in which patients are recruited in two stages with the move to Stage 2 being consequential on the results observed in Stage 1. A key advantage of a two-stage design is that the trial may stop, after relatively few patients have been recruited, should the response rate appear to be unacceptably low. Brown, Gregory, Twelves *et al* (2011) found that two-stage designs and in particular the Simon optimal and minimax designs were the most common designs used. Designs with more than two stages have also been proposed, but the practicalities of having several decision points have limited their use. **Figure 17.1** provides an overview of the different considerations of a TE clinical trial design.

Sample Sizes for Clinical, Laboratory and Epidemiology Studies, Fourth Edition. David Machin, Michael J. Campbell, Say Beng Tan and Sze Huey Tan.
© 2018 John Wiley & Sons Ltd. Published 2018 by John Wiley & Sons Ltd.

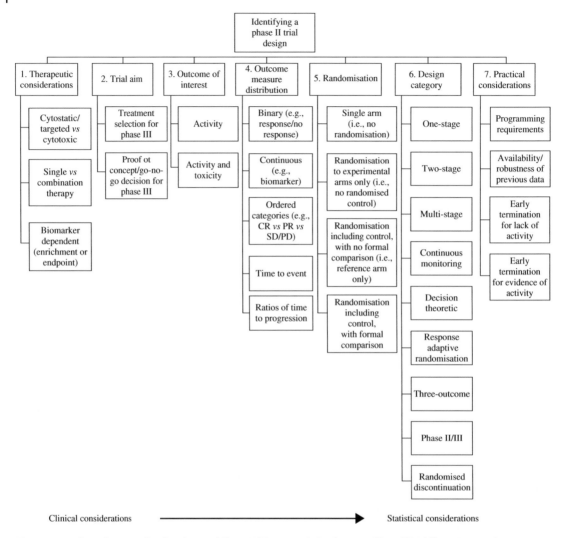

Figure 17.1 Considerations for the choice of Phase II/Therapeutic Exploratory Clinical Trial (from Brown, Gregory, Twelves, *et al*, 2011, Figure 4).

17.2 Theory and Formulae

A common feature of many of the TE designs is the requirement that the investigators set the largest response proportion as π_0 which, if true, would clearly imply that the treatment does not warrant further investigation. The investigators then judge what is the smallest response proportion, π_{New}, that would imply that the treatment clearly warrants further investigation. This implies that the 1-sided hypotheses to be tested are: H_0: $\pi \leq \pi_0$ versus H_A: $\pi \geq \pi_{New}$, where π is the actual probability of response which is to be estimated.

It is typically also necessary to specify α, the probability of rejecting H_0 when it is true, together with β, the probability of rejecting H_A when that is true.

In practice, for a two-stage design, the appropriate number of patients is recruited to Stage 1 and once (not necessarily all) their responses are observed, a decision of whether or not to proceed to Stage 2 is made. If Stage 2 is implemented, then once recruitment is complete and all assessments made, the response rate (and corresponding confidence interval, *CI*) is calculated. A decision with respect to efficacy is then made. If Stage 2 is not activated, the response rate (and *CI*) can still be calculated for the Stage 1 patients despite failure to demonstrate sufficient activity.

Single-Stage Design

Fleming-A'Hern

The Fleming (1982) single-stage design for TE trials recruits a predetermined number of patients and a decision about activity is obtained from their responses.

If $N_{Fleming}$ patients are recruited then the observed number of patient responses r will have a Binomial distribution with parameter π. If $N_{Fleming}$ is reasonably large and π not too small, the sample size required for the single-stage procedure is approximately

$$N_{Fleming} = \frac{\left\{ z_{1-\alpha} \sqrt{\left[\pi_0 \left(1 - \pi_0 \right) \right]} + z_{1-\beta} \sqrt{\left[\pi_{New} \left(1 - \pi_{New} \right) \right]} \right\}^2}{\left(\pi_{New} - \pi_0 \right)^2}, \tag{17.1}$$

where $z_{1-\alpha}$ and $z_{1-\beta}$ are the standardised Normal deviates of **Table 2.1**. However, A'Hern (2001) has used the exact Binomial probabilities to calculate the sample size (denoted $N_{A'Hern}$ and which is calculated in $^S S_S$). In general, these are marginally greater than those given by (17.1).

The design would reject the null hypothesis $\pi \le \pi_0$ and thereby conclude that $\pi \ge \pi_{New}$, if the observed number of responses R is $\ge C_{A'Hern}$ where

$$C_{A'Hern} = N_{A'Hern} \times \left\{ \pi_0 + \left[\frac{z_{1-\alpha}}{z_{1-\alpha} + z_{1-\beta}} \right] \left(\pi_{New} - \pi_0 \right) \right\}. \tag{17.2}$$

Two-Stage Designs

Simon-Optimal and Simon-Minimax

As with Fleming-A'Hern, for the Simon (1989) design, the investigators set π_0 and π_{New} as we have described previously. The trial proceeds by recruiting n_{S1} patients in Stage 1 from which r_{S1} responses are observed. A decision is then made to recruit n_{S2} patients to Stage 2 if $r_{S1} > R_{S1}$. Otherwise, the trial is closed at the end of Stage 1. At the end of the second stage, the drug is rejected for further use if a predetermined $R_{Simon} = (R_{S1} + R_{S2})$ or fewer responses are observed.

In such a design, even if $\pi > \pi_0$ there is a possibility that the trial once conducted will *not* go into Stage 2. The probability that the trial is terminated after Stage 1, that is there are R_{S1} or fewer responses observed, is

$$P_{Early} = B \left(R_{S1}; \pi, n_{S1} \right), \tag{17.3}$$

where $B(.)$ is the cumulative Binomial distribution of equation (1.11) with $R = R_{S1}$ and $n = n_{S1}$. The expected sample size is

$$N_{Expected} = n_{S1} + \left(1 - P_{Early}\right)n_{S2}. \tag{17.4}$$

In this context, *expected* means the average sample size that would turn out to have been used had a whole series of studies been conducted with the same design parameters in situations where the true activity is also the same.

Optimal design

The Simon-Optimal design seeks to minimise $N_{Expected}$ in the event that $\pi = \pi_0$.

A computer search is necessary to determine the sample size. Essentially for each potential (Stage 1 plus Stage 2) sample size N_{Simon} and each value of n_{S1} in the range $(1, N_{Simon} - 1)$, values of R_{S1} and R_{S2} are found corresponding to the specified values of π_0, π_{New}, α and β, and which minimise the expected sample size of equation (17.4) when $\pi = \pi_0$.

Minimax design

Although the Simon-Optimal design seeks to minimise the expected sample size in the event that the drug does not appear effective, it could result in an unnecessarily large total sample size (that is, Stage 1 and Stage 2 together). In the Simon-Minimax design, the total size of the trial, that is the sum of patients required for Stage 1 and Stage 2 together, is chosen to minimise the maximum trial size.

Again a computer search is necessary to determine sample size. The search strategy is the same as for the optimal design, except that the values of n_{S1} n_{S2}, R_{S1} and R_{S2} that result in the smallest total sample size are determined.

Bayesian Designs

In the TE designs discussed so far, the final response rate is estimated by R/N, where R is the total number of responses observed from the total number of patients recruited, N (whether obtained from a single-stage design or one or both stages of a 2-stage design). This response rate, together with the corresponding 95% *CI*, provides the basic information for the investigators to decide if a subsequent Phase III trial is warranted. However, as TE trials are usually of modest size, the resulting *CIs* will usually be rather wide—encompassing a wide range of options for π. Moreover, the definition of a 95% *CI* may not provide the investigator with the information he requires, for example the range of values for which he is 95% certain that π falls. With a relatively small sample size, the role of external or prior information also becomes more important. These considerations and others have motivated the development of Bayesian designs for TE trials.

Bayesian designs for TE trials can be broadly divided into those that are based on posterior credible intervals or those that are based on Bayesian hypothesis tests.

Designs based on Bayesian posterior credible intervals

The posterior credible interval refers to an interval within the posterior distribution for which we can compute the probability for which π falls. Tan and Machin (2002) proposed two variants of Bayesian 2-stage designs where the focus of the design is typically to estimate the posterior probability that $\pi > \pi_{New}$, denoted $Prob(\pi > \pi_{New})$. If this probability is high (a threshold level is set by the design) at the end of the trial, the investigators can be reasonably confident in recommending the compound for a Phase III trial.

Single Threshold Design

In the 2-stage Single Threshold Design (STD), the investigator first sets the minimum interest response rate π_{New} as for other designs but now specifies π_{Prior} (not π_0) as the *anticipated* response rate of the drug under test. Further, in place of α and β, λ_1, the required threshold probability following Stage 1 that $\pi > \pi_{New}$, denoted $\text{Prob}_{Stage-1}(\pi > \pi_{New})$, and the required threshold $\text{Prob}_{End}(\pi > \pi_{New})$ after completion of Stage 2 are specified. Here λ_2 is set to be greater than λ_1. Once Stage 1 of the trial is completed, the estimated value of λ_1, that is u_1, is computed and a decision is made to proceed to Stage 2 if $u_1 \geq \lambda_1$. Should the trial continue to Stage 2 then, on trial completion, u_2 is computed and a recommendation to proceed to Phase III is made if $u_2 \geq \lambda_2$.

The design then determines the sample sizes for the trial based on the following principle. Suppose also that the (hypothetical) response proportion is just larger than the pre-specified π_{New}, say $\pi_{New} + \varepsilon$, with $\varepsilon > 0$ being small. We then want the smallest overall sample size, N_{T-M}, that will enable $\text{Prob}_{End}(\pi > \pi_{New})$ to be at least λ_2. At the same time, we also want the smallest possible Stage 1 sample size n_{T-M1} which is just large enough so that $\text{Prob}_{Stage-1}(\pi > \pi_{New})$ is at least λ_1.

Dual Threshold Design

The Dual Threshold Design (DTD) is identical to the STD except that the Stage 1 sample size is determined not on the basis of the probability of exceeding π_{New} but on the probability that π will be less than the 'no further interest' proportion, π_0. Thus π_0 functions as a lower threshold on the response rate. The rationale behind this aspect of the DTD is that we want our Stage 1 sample size to be large enough so that, if the trial data really does suggest a response rate that is below π_0, the posterior probability of π being below π_0 is at least λ_1. The design determines the smallest Stage 1 sample size that satisfies this criterion.

The DTD requires the investigators to set π_{Prior} as the anticipated value of π for the drug being tested. A convenient choice may be $(\pi_0 + \pi_{New})/2$, but this is not a requirement. Further, λ_1 is set as the required threshold probability following Stage 1, that $\pi < \pi_0$, while λ_2 is the required threshold probability, that, after the completion of Stage 2, $\pi > \pi_{New}$. Note that unlike STD, it is no longer a requirement that $\lambda_1 < \lambda_2$. Once Stage 1 of the trial is completed, u_1 is computed, and should the trial continue to Stage 2, then on its completion u_2 is computed. The latter is then used to help decide whether or not a Phase III trial is suggested.

Prior distributions

In the original version of the designs proposed by Tan and Machin (2002), the designs work on the basis of having a 'vague' prior distribution. Mayo and Gajewski (2004) extended the designs to allow for the inclusion of informative prior distributions. In $\boxed{S_S}$ users have the option of using such informative prior distributions (which could also be set to be equivalent to the vague priors used by Tan and Machin). Moreover, Tan and Machin imposed some practical constraints on their designs so as to encourage the adoption of the designs into practice. In particular, they constrained the total study size, N_{T-M}, to be a minimum of 10 and a maximum of 90, with Stage 1 size, n_{T-M1}, having a minimum size of 5 and a maximum of $N_{T-M} - 5$. These constraints are not applied in $\boxed{S_S}$.

Design based on Bayesian hypothesis tests

Johnson and Cook (2009) describe a Bayesian hypothesis test-based approach for TE clinical trials with binary outcomes. In a Bayesian hypothesis test, the posterior odds in favour of the alternative hypothesis is a multiplication of the prior odds in favour of the alternative hypothesis and the Bayes factor. This is represented by

$$\frac{Prob(H_1 \mid x)}{Prob(H_0 \mid x)} = \frac{\alpha}{1-\alpha} \times \frac{m_1(x)}{m_0(x)}. \tag{17.5}$$

Here α is the prior probability assigned to the alternative hypothesis and $\alpha/(1 - \alpha)$ is the prior odds in favour of the alternative hypothesis. Often the null and alternative hypotheses are assumed to be equally likely at the beginning of a clinical trial, which means that $\alpha = 0.5$ and $\alpha/(1 - \alpha) = 1$.

The quantities $m_1(x)$ and $m_0(x)$ denote the marginal densities of the data defined under the alternative and null hypotheses respectively, and their ratio is called the Bayes factor. The marginal density under the null hypothesis $m_0(x)$ is defined to be

$$m_0(x) = \int_\theta f(x \mid \theta) \pi_0(\theta) d\theta. \tag{17.6}$$

This is a weighted average of the sample density $f(x|\theta)$ of the parameter of interest with respect to the prior density $\pi_0(\theta)$. A similar expression can be used to define the marginal density, $m_1(x)$, of the data under the alternative hypothesis.

In the binary case, the number of r responses (successes) out of n treated subjects follows a Binomial distribution. Hence

$$f(x \mid \theta) = b(r; \theta, n), \tag{17.7}$$

where $b(.)$ is the sampling density of the Binomial distribution of equation (1.10) with $\pi = \theta$.

A class of non-local prior densities called inverse moment (iMOM) densities, as proposed by Johnson and Rossell (2010), is used for the alternative hypothesis. This takes the form

$$\pi_I(\theta; \theta_0, k, \upsilon, \tau) = \frac{k\tau^{\upsilon/2}}{\Gamma(\upsilon/2k)} \left[(\theta - \theta_0)^2 \right]^{-\frac{\upsilon+1}{2}} exp\left\{ -\left[\frac{(\theta - \theta_0)^2}{\tau} \right]^{-k} \right\}, \tag{17.8}$$

where k, υ, $\tau > 0$ and $\Gamma(.)$ is the gamma function. Johnson and Cook (2009) suggest $k = 1$ and $\upsilon = 2$ as default values to use.

Using the design

The approach involves performing simulations to test a single arm binary endpoint based on a null hypothesis (H_0) such as 'H_0: The response rate using the treatment is 20%' versus an alternative hypothesis (H_1) such as 'H_1: The response rate using the treatment is 30%'.

The trial stops for inferiority if $Prob(H_1|x) < C_I$ (the cut-off for inferiority stopping) or for superiority if $Prob(H_1|x) > C_S$ (the cut-off for superiority stopping). It is recommended that $0 < C_I < 0.5$ and $0.5 < C_S < 1$.

To use the design, besides specifying the null and alternative hypothesis response rates and the values of C_I and C_S, there is also a need to specify the maximum number of patients to be recruited into the trial, the minimum number to be enrolled before applying the stopping rules as well as the cohort size. The trial will enrol patients with a cohort of this many patients at each enrolment, and consequently, the stopping rules will be applied for a complete cohort of patients. The maximum number of patients must be a multiple of the cohort size.

17.3   Bibliography

Fleming (1982) and A'Hern (2001) provide further details of the single-stage design discussed. Simon (1989) describes two designs, one which minimizes the expected sample size in the event that the drug appears ineffective after for Stage I and the other which minimises the maximum sample size. He provides tables for sample size and compares the two approaches. For the Bayesian designs, Tan and Machin (2002) discuss the original versions of the Bayesian Single and Dual Threshold Designs and compare these with the Simon (1989) designs. Several other papers discuss the properties and expand on the ideas of Tan and Machin, including Mayo and Gajewski (2004), Tan, Wong and Machin (2004), Wang, Leung, Li and Tan (2005) and Gajewski and Mayo (2006). Thall and Simon (1994) discuss an alternative design also based on Bayesian posterior credible intervals. More generally, Biswas, Liu, Lee and Berry (2009) share some of their experience in the practical use of Bayesian designs in clinical trials.

17.4   Examples

Table 17.1

Example 17.1   Fleming-A'Hern - sequential hormonal therapy in advanced and metastatic breast cancer

Iaffaioli, Formato, Tortoriello, *et al* (2005) used A'Hern's design for two Phase II studies of sequential hormonal therapy with first-line Anastrozole (Study 1) and second-line Exemestane (Study 2) in advanced and metastatic breast cancer.

For Study 1 they set $\alpha = 0.05$, $1 - \beta = 0.9$, $\pi_0 = 0.5$ and $\pi_{New} = 0.65$. With these inputs, **Table 17.1** and $^S S_S$ give for the A'Hern design a sample size of 93, with 55 being the minimum number of responses required for a conclusion of 'efficacy'.

In the event, 100 patients were recruited amongst whom 8 complete responses and 19 partial responses were observed. These give an estimated response rate of 27% with 95% *CI* 19.3 to 36.4% calculated using equation (1.19). This is much lower than the desired minimum of 65%.

For Study 2, the investigators set $\alpha = 0.05$, $1 - \beta = 0.9$, $\pi_0 = 0.2$ and $\pi_{New} = 0.4$, giving rise to a sample size of 47 with a minimum of 15 responses required.

In the event, 50 patients were recruited amongst whom 1 complete response and 3 partial responses were observed. These give an estimated response rate of 8% (95% *CI* 3.2 to 18.8%). Again this is much lower than the desired minimum of 40%.

Table 17.2

Example 17.2   Simon-optimal and Simon-minimax designs - gemicitabine in metastatic nasopharyngeal carcinoma

In a trial of Gemicitabine in previously untreated patients with metastatic nasopharyngeal carcinoma (NPC), Foo, Tan, Leong, *et al* (2002) utilised the Simon-Minimax design. The trial design assumed a desired overall response rate (complete and partial) of at least 30% and no further interest in Gemicitabine if the response was as low as 10%.

Thus, for $\alpha = 0.05$, $1 - \beta = 0.8$, $\pi_0 = 0.1$ and $\pi_{New} = 0.3$, $^S S_S$ gives:

Stage 1:   A sample size of 15 patients; if responses are less than 2, stop the trial and claim Gemicitabine lacks efficacy.

Stage 2: An overall sample size of 25 patients for both stages, hence 10 more patients are to be recruited; if the total responses for the two stages combined are less than 6, stop the trial as soon as this is evident and claim Gemicitabine lacks efficacy.

Once the Phase II trial was conducted, the investigators observed $r_{S1} = 3$ and $r_{S2} = 4$ responses, giving $p = (3 + 4)/25$ or 28% (95% *CI* 14 to 48%).

Had the above trial been designed using the optimal design but with the same characteristics, namely, $\alpha = 0.05$, $1 - \beta = 0.8$, $\pi_0 = 0.1$ and $\pi_{New} = 0.3$, then $\boxed{SS_s}$ gives the following results:

Stage 1: A sample size of 10 patients; if responses are less than 2, stop the trial and claim Gemicitabine lacks efficacy.

Stage 2: An overall sample size of 29 patients for both stages, hence 19 more patients are to be recruited; if the total responses for two stages combined are less than 6, stop the trial as soon as this is evident and claim Gemicitabine lacks efficacy.

In this case, for the same design parameters, the optimal design has 5 fewer patients in Stage 1 of the design, but 4 more patients if the trial goes on to complete Stage 2, than the corresponding minimax design. However, the numbers of responses to be observed are the same in each stage for both designs.

Tables 17.3 and 17.4

Example 17.3 Bayesian STD and DTD - combination therapy for nasopharyngeal cancer
A Phase II trial using a triplet combination of Paclitaxel, Carboplatin and Gemcitabine in metastatic nasopharyngeal carcinoma was conducted by Leong, Tay, Toh, *et al* (2005).

The trial was expected to yield a minimum interest response rate of 80% and a no further interest response of 60%. The anticipated response rate was assumed to be equal to the minimum interest response rate and the overall threshold probability at the start and end of the trial is set to be 0.65 and 0.7 respectively. The sample size of the trial was calculated using the DTD.

Entering the no interest response rate $\pi_0 = 0.6$, minimum interest response rate $\pi_{New} = 0.8$; anticipated response rate $\pi_{Prior} = 0.8$, minimum desired threshold probability at the start of the trial $\lambda_1 = 0.65$, minimum desired threshold probability at the end of the trial $\lambda_2 = 0.7$, along with the default settings of $\varepsilon = 0.05$ and $n_{Prior} = 3$ (corresponding to a vague prior), $\boxed{SS_s}$ gives the following design:

Stage 1: A sample size of 19 patients; if responses are less than 15, stop the trial as soon as this becomes apparent and declare lack of efficacy. Otherwise complete Stage 1 and commence to Stage 2.

Stage 2: An overall sample size of 32 patients for both stages, hence 13 Stage 2 patients are to be recruited; if the total responses for the two stages combined are less than 28, stop the trial as soon as this becomes apparent and declare lack of efficacy. Otherwise complete the trial.

Had, for example, the investigators chosen the first STD design of **Table 17.3**, that is with $\pi_{Prior} = 0.1$ and a much lower $\pi_{New} = 0.3$, then the first row corresponding to $\lambda_1 = 0.6$ and $\lambda_2 = 0.7$ suggests recruiting 5 patients for Stage 1 and, if 2 or more responses are observed, recruiting another $(24 - 5) = 19$ patients. Alternatively, the corresponding DTD of **Table 17.4** for these same design specifications and with $\pi_0 = 0.1$ also suggests 18 patients for Stage 1 and 6 for Stage II to give the same total of 24. Only 3 responses would be sufficient to move into Stage II, but should such a low figure in practice occur, then all the 6 of the 9 Stage II patients would have to respond to claim efficacy.

References

Technical

A'Hern RP (2001). Sample size tables for exact single stage phase II designs. *Statistics in Medicine*, **20**, 859–866.

Biswas S, Liu DD, Lee JJ and Berry DA (2009). Bayesian clinical trials at the University of Texas M. D. Anderson Cancer Centre. *Clinical Trials*, **6**, 205–216.

Booth CM, Calvert AH, Giaccone G, Lobbezoo MW, Eisenhauer EA and Seymour LK (2008). Design and conduct of phase II studies of targeted anticancer therapy: Recommendations from the task force on methodology for the development of innovative cancer therapies (MDICT). *European Journal of Cancer*, **44**, 25–29.

Brown SR, Gregory WM, Twelves CJ, Buyse M, Collinson F, Parmar M, Seymour MT and Brown JM (2011). Designing phase II trials in cancer: a systematic review and guidance. *British Journal of Cancer*, **105**, 194–199.

Fleming TR (1982). One-sample multiple testing procedure for Phase II clinical trials. *Biometrics*, **38**, 143–151.

Gajewski BJ and Mayo MS (2006). Bayesian sample size calculations in phase II clinical trials using a mixture of informative priors. *Statistics in Medicine*, **25**, 2554–2566.

Johnson VE and Cook JD (2009). Bayesian design of single-arm phase II clinical trials with continuous monitoring. *Clinical Trials*, **6**, 217–226.

Johnson VE and Rossell D (2010). On the use of non-local prior densities in Bayesian hypothesis tests. *Journal of the Royal Statistical Society B*, **72**, 143–170.

Mayo MS and Gajewski BJ (2004). Bayesian sample size calculations in phase II clinical trials using informative conjugate priors. *Controlled Clinical Trials*, **25**, 157–167.

Simon R (1989). Optimal two-stage designs for phase II clinical trials. *Controlled Clinical Trials*, **10**, 1–14.

Tan SB and Machin D (2002). Bayesian two-stage designs for phase II clinical trials. *Statistics in Medicine*, **21**, 1991–2012.

Tan SB, Wong EH and Machin D (2004). Bayesian two-stage design for phase II clinical trials. In Encyclopedia of Biopharmaceutical Statistics, 2nd edn (online) (Ed: Chow SC), http://www.dekker.com/servlet/product/DOI/101081EEBS120023507. Marcel Dekker, New York.

Thall P and Simon R (1994). A Bayesian approach to establishing sample size and monitoring criteria for phase II clinical trials. *Controlled Clinical Trials*, **15**, 463–481.

Wang YG, Leung DHY, Li M and Tan SB (2005). Bayesian designs for frequentist and Bayesian error rate considerations. *Statistical Methods in Medical Research*, **14**, 445–456.

Examples

Foo K-F, Tan E-H, Leong S-S, Wee JTS, Tan T, Fong K-W, Koh L, Tai B-C, Lian L-G and Machin D (2002). Gemcitabine in metastatic nasopharyngeal carcinoma of the undifferentiated type. *Annals of Oncology*, **13**, 150–156.

Iaffaioli RV, Formato R, Tortoriello A, Del Prete S, Caraglia M, Pappagallo G, Pisano A, Fanelli F, Ianniello G, Cigolari S, Pizza C, Marano O, Pezzella G, Pedicini T, Febbraro A, Incoronato P, Manzione L, Ferrari E, Marzano N, Quattrin S, Pisconti S, Nasti G, Giotta G, Colucci G and other Goim authors (2005). Phase II study of sequential hormonal therapy with anastrozole/exemestane in advanced and metastatic breast cancer. *British Journal of Cancer*, **92**, 1621–1625.

Leong SS, Wee J, Tay MH, Toh CK, Tan SB, Thng CH, Foo KF, Lim WT, Tan T and Tan EH (2005). Paclitaxel, carboplatin and gemcitabine in metastatic nasopharyngeal carcinoma: A phase II trial using a triplet combination. *Cancer*, **103**, 569–575.

Table 17.1 Fleming-A'Hern Single-Stage Design.
Sample size, $N_{A'H}$, and minimum number of successes required, $C_{A'H}$, to conclude that the drug is effective [Based on exact calculations for which equation (17.1) Is an approximation].

		$\alpha=0.05$		$\alpha=0.01$	
		$1-\beta$		$1-\beta$	
		0.8	0.9	0.8	0.9
π_0	π_{New}	$C_{A'H}/N_{A'H}$	$C_{A'H}/N_{A'H}$	$C_{A'H}/N_{A'H}$	$C_{A'H}/N_{A'H}$
0.10	0.25	8 / 40	10 / 55	13 / 62	15 / 78
	0.30	6 / 25	7 / 33	9 / 37	11 / 49
	0.35	5 / 18	6 / 25	7 / 25	9 / 35
	0.40	4 / 13	5 / 18	6 / 19	7 / 24
	0.45	4 / 11	4 / 13	5 / 14	6 / 19
	0.50	3 / 8	4 / 12	5 / 12	5 / 14
	0.55	3 / 7	3 / 8	4 / 9	5 / 13
	0.60	3 / 6	3 / 7	4 / 8	4 / 9
0.20	0.35	17 / 56	22 / 77	27 / 87	34 / 115
	0.40	12 / 35	15 / 47	18 / 52	22 / 67
	0.45	8 / 21	10 / 29	14 / 36	16 / 44
	0.50	7 / 17	8 / 21	11 / 26	13 / 33
	0.55	6 / 13	7 / 17	9 / 19	10 / 23
	0.60	5 / 10	6 / 13	8 / 16	9 / 19
	0.65	4 / 7	5 / 10	7 / 13	8 / 16
	0.70	4 / 7	5 / 9	6 / 10	7 / 13
0.30	0.45	27 / 67	36 / 93	43 / 104	53 / 133
	0.50	17 / 39	22 / 53	27 / 60	34 / 79
	0.55	12 / 25	16 / 36	20 / 41	25 / 53
	0.60	9 / 17	12 / 25	14 / 26	18 / 36
	0.65	8 / 14	9 / 17	12 / 21	14 / 26
	0.70	6 / 10	8 / 14	10 / 16	12 / 21
0.40	0.55	36 / 71	46 / 94	58 / 113	72 / 144
	0.60	23 / 42	29 / 56	35 / 63	45 / 84
	0.65	16 / 28	19 / 34	25 / 42	31 / 54
	0.70	12 / 19	15 / 25	18 / 28	22 / 36
	0.75	10 / 15	12 / 19	15 / 22	17 / 26
	0.80	8 / 11	9 / 13	11 / 15	14 / 20
0.50	0.65	42 / 69	55 / 93	69 / 112	86 / 143
	0.70	24 / 37	33 / 53	42 / 64	51 / 80
	0.75	16 / 23	22 / 33	28 / 40	34 / 50
	0.80	13 / 18	16 / 23	20 / 27	25 / 35
	0.85	10 / 13	12 / 16	15 / 19	17 / 22
	0.90	7 / 8	9 / 11	12 / 14	14 / 17
0.60	0.75	44 / 62	59 / 85	74 / 103	92 / 131
	0.80	27 / 36	33 / 45	42 / 55	52 / 70
	0.85	17 / 21	21 / 27	26 / 32	33 / 42
	0.90	12 / 14	14 / 17	19 / 22	21 / 25
0.70	0.85	40 / 49	55 / 69	65 / 79	84 / 104
	0.90	24 / 28	31 / 37	38 / 44	45 / 53

Table 17.2 Simon Optimal and Minimax Designs.
Stage I sample size, N_{S1}, and the minimum number of successes required, R_{S1}, to conclude that the drug should be tested in Stage II, and the overall sample size (Stage I plus Stage II), N_S, and minimum overall number of successes required, R_S, to conclude that the drug is effective [Based on exact calculations].

$\alpha=0.05$			Optimal		Minimax	
π_0	π_{New}	$1-\beta$	Stage 1	Overall	Stage 1	Overall
	$\pi_{New}-\pi_0=0.15$		R_{S1}/N_{S1}	R_S/N_S	R_{S1}/N_{S1}	R_S/N_S
0.05	0.20	0.8	0/10	3/29	0/13	3/27
		0.9	1/21	4/41	1/29	4/38
0.10	0.25	0.8	2/18	7/43	2/22	7/40
		0.9	2/21	10/66	3/31	9/55
0.20	0.35	0.8	5/22	19/72	6/31	15/53
		0.9	8/37	22/83	8/42	21/77
0.30	0.45	0.8	9/27	30/81	16/46	25/65
		0.9	13/40	40/110	27/77	33/88
0.40	0.55	0.8	11/26	40/84	28/59	34/70
		0.9	19/45	49/104	24/62	45/94
0.50	0.65	0.8	15/28	48/83	39/66	40/68
		0.9	22/42	60/105	28/57	54/93
0.60	0.75	0.8	17/27	46/67	18/30	43/62
		0.9	21/34	64/95	48/72	57/84
0.70	0.85	0.8	14/19	46/59	16/23	39/49
		0.9	18/25	61/79	33/44	53/68
0.80	0.95	0.8	7/9	26/29	7/9	26/29
		0.9	16/19	37/42	31/35	35/40
	$\pi_{New}-\pi_0=0.20$					
0.05	0.25	0.8	0/9	2/17	0/12	2/16
		0.9	0/9	3/30	0/15	3/25
0.10	0.30	0.8	1/10	5/29	1/15	5/25
		0.9	2/18	6/35	2/22	6/33
0.20	0.40	0.8	3/13	12/43	4/18	10/33
		0.9	4/19	15/54	5/24	13/45
0.30	0.50	0.8	5/15	18/46	6/19	16/39
		0.9	8/24	24/63	7/24	21/53
0.40	0.60	0.8	7/16	23/46	17/34	20/39
		0.9	11/25	32/66	12/29	27/54
0.50	0.70	0.8	8/15	26/43	12/23	23/37
		0.9	13/24	36/61	14/27	32/53
0.60	0.80	0.8	7/11	30/43	8/13	25/35
		0.9	12/19	37/53	15/26	32/45
0.70	0.90	0.8	4/6	22/27	19/23	21/26
		0.9	11/15	29/36	13/18	26/32

Table 17.3 Bayesian Single Threshold Design (STD).
Sample sizes and cut-off values for Stage 1 and Overall trial size for π_{Prior} and π_{New}. The two rows correspond to designs for the pairs (λ_1, λ_2) of (0.6, 0.7) and (0.6, 0.8) respectively. *A* implies designs for which $N_{T-M} < 10$; and *B* those with $N_{T-M} \geq 10$ but $n_{T-M1} < 5$. [Based on exact calculations].

π_{Prior}	0.1		0.3		0.5		0.7		0.9	
π_{New}	Stage 1	Overall	Stage 1	Overall	Stage 1	Overall	Stage 1	Overall	Stage 1	Overall
0.30	2 / 5	9 / 24	*B*		*A*		*A*		*A*	
	2 / 5	22 / 61	*B*		*B*		*B*		*B*	
0.35	4 / 10	12 / 30	*B*		*B*		*A*		*A*	
	4 / 10	28 / 70	*B*		*B*		*B*		*B*	
0.40	7 / 14	16 / 35	4 / 7	13 / 28	*B*		*A*		*A*	
	7 / 14	36 / 78	4 / 7	32 / 70	*B*		*B*		*B*	
0.45	9 / 17	20 / 40	6 / 11	17 / 33	*B*		*B*		*A*	
	9 / 17	42 / 84	6 / 11	38 / 76	*B*		*B*		*B*	
0.50	11 / 20	25 / 44	9 / 15	21 / 37	5 / 9	17 / 30	*B*		*B*	
	11 / 20	49 / 88	9 / 15	45 / 81	5 / 9	41 / 73	*B*		*B*	
0.55	14 / 23	29 / 47	11 / 18	25 / 41	8 / 12	21 / 34	4 / 6	16 / 26	*B*	
	C		11 / 18	51 / 84	8 / 12	47 / 77	4 / 6	42 / 69	*B*	
0.60	17 / 26	33 / 50	14 / 21	29 / 44	10 / 15	25 / 37	6 / 9	20 / 30	*B*	
	C		14 / 21	56 / 86	10 / 15	51 / 78	6 / 9	47 / 71	*B*	
0.65	21 / 29	37 / 52	17 / 24	33 / 46	13 / 18	28 / 39	10 / 13	23 / 32	5 / 6	18 / 25
	C		17 / 24	61 / 86	13 / 18	56 / 79	10 / 13	50 / 71	5 / 6	45 / 64
0.70	24 / 31	40 / 53	20 / 26	36 / 47	16 / 21	31 / 41	12 / 15	26 / 34	8 / 10	21 / 27
	C		20 / 26	63 / 84	16 / 21	58 / 77	12 / 15	53 / 70	8 / 10	48 / 63
0.75	27 / 33	43 / 53	23 / 28	39 / 48	19 / 23	34 / 42	15 / 18	28 / 35	10 / 12	24 / 29
	27 / 33	71 / 88	23 / 28	65 / 81	19 / 23	60 / 75	15 / 18	55 / 68	10 / 12	48 / 60
0.80	30 / 35	46 / 53	26 / 30	40 / 47	22 / 25	35 / 41	17 / 20	31 / 36	13 / 15	25 / 29
	30 / 35	71 / 83	26 / 30	66 / 77	22 / 25	60 / 70	17 / 20	54 / 63	13 / 15	48 / 56
0.85	33 / 36	46 / 51	28 / 31	42 / 46	24 / 26	36 / 40	19 / 21	32 / 35	15 / 16	27 / 29
	33 / 36	69 / 76	28 / 31	63 / 70	24 / 26	58 / 64	19 / 21	52 / 57	15 / 16	45 / 50
0.90	35 / 36	47 / 49	31 / 32	42 / 44	26 / 27	37 / 38	22 / 23	32 / 33	18 / 18	26 / 27
	35 / 36	64 / 67	31 / 32	58 / 61	26 / 27	53 / 55	22 / 23	47 / 49	18 / 18	41 / 43
0.95	36 / 36	44 / 44	32 / 32	39 / 39	27 / 27	34 / 34	23 / 23	30 / 30	19 / 19	25 / 25
	36 / 36	55 / 55	32 / 32	49 / 49	27 / 27	44 / 44	23 / 23	38 / 38	19 / 19	33 / 33

Table 17.4 Bayesian Dual Threshold Design (DTD): Sample sizes, and cut-off values, for Stage 1 and Overall trial size for π_{Prior}, π_0 and π_{New}. [Based on exact calculations].
B those with $N_{T-M} \geq 10$ but $n_{T-M1} < 5$; and C those with $N_{T-M} > 90$ or $n_{t-m1} > 85$.

| | | | π_{Prior} 0.1 | | 0.3 | | 0.5 | | 0.7 | | 0.9 | |
| | | | Stage 1 | Overall | Stage 1 | Overall | Stage 1 | Overall | Stage 1 | Overall | Stage 1 | Overall |
π_0	π_{New}	λ_1,λ_2	n_{T-M1}	N_{T-M}	n_{T-M1}	N_{T-M}	n_{T-M1}	N_{T-M}	n_{T-M1}	N_{T-M}	n_{T-M1}	N_{T-M}
0.1	0.20	0.6, 0.7	1/18	6/23	2/23	7/28	2/27	7/32	3/32	8/37	4/36	9/41
		0.6, 0.8	1/18	10/38	2/23	8/29	3/27	8/32	4/32	9/37	5/36	10/41
	0.25	0.6, 0.7	2/18	7/23	3/23	8/28	4/27	9/32	5/32	10/37	6/36	11/41
		0.6, 0.8	1/18	16/51	2/23	13/42	5/27	10/32	6/32	11/37	7/36	12/41
	0.30	0.6, 0.7	3/18	9/24	5/23	10/28	6/27	11/32	7/32	12/37	9/36	14/41
		0.6, 0.8	1/18	22/61	2/23	19/53	2/27	16/44	8/32	13/37	10/36	15/41
0.2	0.30	0.6, 0.7	3/15	9/24	4/20	9/25	5/25	10/30	7/30	12/35	8/35	13/40
		0.6, 0.8	3/15	22/61	4/20	19/53	4/25	16/44	8/30	13/35	9/35	14/40
	0.35	0.6, 0.7	3/15	12/30	5/20	10/25	7/25	12/30	9/30	14/35	10/35	15/40
		0.6, 0.8	3/15	28/70	4/20	25/62	4/25	22/54	5/30	18/45	11/35	16/40
	0.40	0.6, 0.7	3/15	16/35	5/20	13/28	9/25	14/30	11/30	16/35	13/35	18/40
		0.6, 0.8	3/15	36/78	4/20	32/70	4/25	28/62	5/30	24/53	11/35	20/44
0.3	0.40	0.6, 0.7	3/10	16/35	4/15	13/28	7/21	12/26	9/26	14/31	11/31	16/36
		0.6, 0.8	3/10	36/78	4/15	32/70	6/21	28/62	7/26	24/53	8/31	20/44
	0.45	0.6, 0.7	3/10	20/40	4/15	17/33	8/21	13/26	11/26	16/31	13/31	18/36
		0.6, 0.8	3/10	42/84	4/15	38/76	6/21	34/68	7/26	30/60	8/31	26/51
	0.50	0.6, 0.7	3/10	25/44	4/15	21/37	8/21	17/30	12/26	17/31	15/31	20/36
		0.6, 0.8	3/10	49/88	4/15	45/81	6/21	41/73	7/26	36/65	8/31	32/57
0.4	0.50	0.6, 0.7	B		4/9	21/37	6/15	17/30	10/21	15/26	12/26	17/31
		0.6, 0.8	B		4/9	45/81	6/15	41/73	8/21	36/65	10/26	32/57
	0.55	0.6, 0.7	B		4/9	25/41	6/15	21/34	11/21	16/26	14/26	19/31
		0.6, 0.8	C		4/9	51/84	6/15	47/77	8/21	42/69	10/26	37/61
	0.60	0.6, 0.7	B		4/9	29/44	6/15	25/37	11/21	20/30	15/26	20/31
		0.6, 0.8	C		4/9	56/86	6/15	51/78	8/21	47/71	10/26	41/63

(Continued)

Table 17.4 (Continued)

| | | | 0.1 | | 0.3 | | 0.5 | | 0.7 | | 0.9 | |
| | | | Stage 1 | Overall | Stage 1 | Overall | Stage 1 | Overall | Stage 1 | Overall | Stage 1 | Overall |
π_0	π_{New}	λ_1, λ_2	n_{T-M1}	N_{T-M}	n_{T-M1}	N_{T-M}	n_{T-M1}	N_{T-M}	n_{T-M1}	N_{T-M}	n_{T-M1}	N_{T-M}
0.5	0.60	0.6, 0.7	B		B		5/9	25/37	7/15	20/30	12/20	17/25
		0.6, 0.8	C		B		5/9	51/78	7/15	47/71	10/20	41/63
	0.65	0.6, 0.7	B		B		5/9	28/39	7/15	23/32	13/20	18/25
		0.6, 0.8	C		B		5/9	56/79	7/15	50/71	10/20	45/64
	0.70	0.6, 0.7	B		B		5/9	31/41	7/15	26/34	14/20	21/27
		0.6, 0.8	C		B		5/9	58/77	7/15	53/70	10/20	48/63
0.6	0.70	0.6, 0.7	B		B		B		4/7	26/34	8/14	21/27
		0.6, 0.8	C		B		B		4/7	53/70	8/14	48/63
	0.75	0.6, 0.7	B		B		B		4/7	28/35	9/14	24/29
		0.6, 0.8	C		B		B		4/7	55/68	8/14	48/60
	0.80	0.6, 0.7	B		B		B		4/7	31/36	10/14	25/29
		0.6, 0.8	C		B		B		4/7	54/63	8/14	48/56
0.7	0.80	0.6, 0.7	B		B		B		B		4/5	25/29
		0.6, 0.8	B		B		B		B		4/5	48/56
	0.85	0.6, 0.7	B		B		B		B		4/5	27/29
		0.6, 0.8	C		B		B		B		4/5	45/50
	0.90	0.6, 0.7	B		B		B		B		4/5	26/27
		0.6, 0.8	C		B		B		B		4/5	41/43

18

Therapeutic Exploratory Trials: Survival, Dual Endpoints, Randomised and Genomic Targets

SUMMARY
In this chapter, we discuss Therapeutic Exploratory trials which include the Case-Morgan design, which concerns survival time endpoints, and the Bryant-Day design, which involves the simultaneous consideration of the dual endpoints of response and toxicity. The randomised Simon-Wittes-Ellenberg design selects the best of several potential therapeutic options for further study in Phase III trials. Also included is how single arm and randomised comparative trials may be modified for the situation when genomic targets are involved. The overlap with topics such as pilot studies of **Chapter 16** and aspects concerning genomic targets of **Chapter 15** is indicated.

18.1   Time-to-Event (Survival) Endpoint

In many instances, survival times, more generally time-to-event (TE), or survival proportions at a fixed time may be viewed as a relevant outcome of interest for some TE trials, perhaps those in patients diagnosed with very advanced diseases whose subsequent survival is likely to be short.

Case-Morgan

In the Case and Morgan (2003) two-stage TE trial designs, 'survival' times are utilised, and these times usually correspond to the interval between commencement of treatment and when the 'event' of primary concern occurs, for example, recurrence of the disease, death or either of these. **Chapter 7** discusses sample sizes for survival time studies in situations where comparative studies, rather than single arm TE trials, are concerned. Thus some of the points made here have also been made in the earlier chapter.

To implement TE designs, it is important to distinguish between *chronological* time, that is the date (day, month, year) in which the trial recruits its first patient, the date of the planned interim analysis (end of Stage 1), the date the trial closes to recruitment (end of Stage 2) and the date all patient follow-up ends, from the time *interval* between start of therapy and the occurrence of the event for the individual patient. Trial conduct is concerned with *chronological* time while trial analysis is concerned with *interval* time.

Survival data are summarised by the Kaplan-Meier (*K-M*) survival curve, which takes into account censored observations. Censored survival time observations arise when a patient, although entered in the study and followed for a period of time, has not as yet experienced the 'event' defined as the

Sample Sizes for Clinical, Laboratory and Epidemiology Studies, Fourth Edition. David Machin, Michael J. Campbell, Say Beng Tan and Sze Huey Tan.
© 2018 John Wiley & Sons Ltd. Published 2018 by John Wiley & Sons Ltd.

outcome for the trial. For survival itself 'death' will be the 'event' of concern, whereas if event free survival was of concern, the 'event' may be recurrence of the disease.

Technical details

> **NOTE:**
>
> *The description that follows is not a precise summary of the technical details as set out by Case and Morgan (2003) but an attempt to summarise the rationale behind the designs. For example, Case and Morgan do not use the K-M estimate of survival in their description, and their estimate of the standard error differs from that indicated here.*

The *K-M* estimate of the proportion alive at any follow-up time, t, is denoted $S(t)$. For example, when $t = 1$ year, the *K-M* estimate at that time-point is denoted $S(1)$. In planning a trial, the investigators choose a convenient summary time-point, T_{Sum}, and postulate the value of the corresponding *K-M* at that time as $S(T_{Sum})$.

To implement the design, the investigators set the largest survival proportion as $S_0(T_{Sum})$ that, if true, would clearly imply that the treatment does not warrant further investigation. The investigators then judge what is the smallest survival proportion, $S_{New}(T_{Sum})$, that would imply the treatment warrants further investigation. (These are analogous to the π_0 and π_{New} of **Chapter 17.2** for binary endpoints.) This implies that the 1-sided hypotheses to be tested are $H_0: S(T_{Sum}) \leq S_0(T_{Sum})$ versus $H_{New}: S(T_{Sum}) \geq S_{New}(T_{Sum})$, where $S(T_{Sum})$ is the actual probability of survival which is to be estimated at the close of the trial. In addition, it is necessary to specify the test size, α, and the Type II error, β.

The Case-Morgan design assumes that the survival times follow the Exponential distribution of equation (1.15), which is

$$S(t) = exp(-\lambda t). \tag{18.1}$$

Here λ is termed the instantaneous event rate and is assumed to have the same constant value for all those entering the trial. It then follows from equation (18.1) that

$$CL(t) = log\left[-logS(t)\right] = log\,\lambda + log\,t. \tag{18.2}$$

This transformation results in $CL(t)$ having an approximately Normal distribution with standard error

$$SE\left[CL(t)\right] = SE\left[log\,\lambda\right] = 1/\sqrt{E}, \tag{18.3}$$

where E is the corresponding number of events observed by time t.

The assumption of Exponential survival times implies $S_0(T_{Sum}) = exp(-\lambda_0 T_{Sum})$ and $S_{New}(T_{Sum}) = exp(-\lambda_{New} T_{Sum})$ where λ_0 and λ_{New} are essentially the 'event' rates under the two hypotheses. This implies that the two 1-sided hypotheses discussed above can be alternatively expressed as $H_0: \lambda \leq \lambda_0$ and $H_{New}: \lambda \geq \lambda_{New}$.

Stage 1 and interim analysis

To implement a two-stage design, n_{C-M1} patients are recruited in Stage 1 whose duration D_{Stage1} ($= D_{Interim}$) is set to coincide with the interim analysis, which implies a standardised recruitment period of $R = D_{Stage1} / T_{Sum}$. The duration of Stage 1, and hence the date of the interim analysis, can potentially be at any time after a period equal to T_{Sum} has elapsed from the date the first patient is treated. At this analysis, E_{C-M1} ($\leq n_{C-M1}$) events will have been observed while other patients will have been on the trial for a time-period less than T_{Sum} without experiencing the event. These patients will be censored, as will those who have a 'survival' time greater than T_{Sum} but have not yet experienced the event. Thus, at chronological time $D_{Interim}$ for summary time-point T_{Sum}, the 1-sided hypothesis, H_0, can be tested by

$$z_{Interim} = \frac{CL_{Interim}\left(T_{Sum}\right) - CL_0\left(T_{Sum}\right)}{SE\left[CL_{Interim}\left(T_{Sum}\right)\right]}. \tag{18.4}$$

The components of this equation are obtained by use of equations (18.2) and (18.3).

This $z_{Interim}$ test has a standard Normal distribution with mean 0 and standard deviation 1 if H_0 is true. If $z_{Interim} < C_1$ (see below), then recruitment to the trial is stopped, that is, the hypothesis H_0: $S(T_{Sum}) \leq S_0(T_{Sum})$ is *accepted*.

Otherwise, if the decision is to recruit a further n_{C-M2} patients over a period D_{Stage2}, then the last of these patients so recruited will be followed for the minimum period of T_{Sum}. The final analysis will then be conducted at $D_{Final} = D_{Interim} + D_{Stage2} + T_{Sum} = D_{Accrual} + T_{Sum}$. By that time, and in addition to the events from some of the Stage 2 patients, there may be more events accumulated from the Stage 1 patients than were observed by $D_{Interim}$.

At chronological time D_{Final}, equation (18.4) is adapted to that involving the alternative hypothesis, H_{New}. Thus

$$z_{Final} = \frac{CL_{Final}\left(T_{Sum}\right) - CL_{New}\left(T_{Sum}\right)}{SE\left[CL_{Final}\left(T_{Sum}\right)\right]}. \tag{18.5}$$

This z_{Final} has a standard Normal distribution with mean 0 and standard deviation 1 if H_{New} is true. If $z_{Interim} > C_2$ (see below), then the alternative hypothesis H_{New}: $S(T_{Sum}) \geq S_{New}(T_{Sum})$ is *accepted* and activity is claimed.

When planning a two-stage trial, one cannot be certain that Stage 2 will be activated as this will depend on the patient outcomes from Stage 1, so Case and Morgan (2003) take the probability of stopping at the end of Stage 1 (P_{Early}) into their design considerations. This then leads to the Expected Duration of Accrual (*EDA*) as

$$EDA = D_{Stage1} + \left(1 - P_{Early}\right)D_{Stage2}, \tag{18.6}$$

where $D_{Accrual} = D_{Stage1} + D_{Stage2}$ and, using the notation of equation (1.2),

$$C_1 = \Phi^{-1}\left(P_{Early}\right). \tag{18.7}$$

In this context, *expected* means the average duration of accrual that would have occurred had a whole series of studies been conducted with the same design parameters. In a similar way, the Expected Total Study Length (duration) is

$$ETSL = D_{Stage1} + \left(1 - P_{Early}\right)\left(D_{Stage2} + T_{Sum}\right). \tag{18.8}$$

Assuming there is a constant (standardised) accrual rate, R, over the stages of the trial, then there are four unknowns, n_{C-M1} (or D_{Stage1}), n_{C-M2} (or D_{Stage2}), C_1 and C_2, but only two constraints, α and β. As a consequence there are more unknowns than constraints, hence those design options that minimise either the *EDA* of equation (18.6) or *ETSL* of equation (18.8) are chosen.

For either design, patients are recruited until chronological time D_{Stage1} to a total of n_{C-M1}. At this time the *K-M* estimate of $S(T_{Sum})$ and its *SE* are estimated. From these $z_{Interim}$ is calculated. If the decision is made to continue, repeat the process after a further n_{C-M2} patients have been recruited and a further additional T_{Sum} of time has elapsed since the last patient was entered into the study.

Determining C_1 and C_2

At the design stage of the trial, the values of the survival rates λ_0 and λ_{New} under each hypothesis are specified by the investigators, as are the corresponding error rates α and β. The values of C_1 and C_2 are determined as the solutions to the equations

$$1-\psi\left(C_1, C_2\right)=\alpha, \tag{18.9}$$

and

$$1-\psi\left(C_1-\rho u, C_2-u\right)=1-\beta, \tag{18.10}$$

which can only be found by computer search methods.

In these equations, $\psi\,(.,.)$ is the cumulative form of the bivariate Normal distribution while

$$u = \frac{CL_{New}\left(T_{Sum}\right)-CL_0\left(T_{Sum}\right)}{\sigma_{C-M}/\sqrt{N_{C-M}}} = \frac{\log\lambda_{New}-\log\lambda_0}{\sigma_{C-M}/\sqrt{N_{C-M}}}. \tag{18.11}$$

Case-Morgan Expected Duration of Accrual

To determine the Expected Duration of Accrual (*EDA*) design, the search process assumes that the Fleming-A'Hern single-stage design is to be implemented with response rates of $S_0(T_{Sum})$ and $S_{New}(T_{Sum})$. This gives a sample size, $N_{A'H}$, for which the investigator then specifies how long these would take to recruit, $D_{A'H}$; once specified this is related to T_{Sum}. The final (two-stage) solutions from the computer search depend on the ratio $D_{A'H}/T_{Sum}$. A search is then made for each total potential sample size N_{C-M} to find the Stage 1/Stage 2 split amongst these with the specific design parameters for survival rates of $S_0(T_{Sum})$ and $S_{New}(T_{Sum})$ and error constraints α and β that minimise the *EDA*.

The threshold Stage 1 and final thresholds, C_1 and C_2, for differing values of S_0, S_{New} and R are given for 1-sided $\alpha = 0.05$ and $1 - \beta$ of 0.8 and 0.9 in **Table 18.1**.

Case-Morgan Expected Total Study Length

To determine the Expected Total Study Length (*ETSL*) design, the same procedures are followed as for *EDA*, except that the final stage searches for designs that minimise *ETSL* rather than *EDA*. The threshold Stage 1 and final thresholds, C_1 and C_2, for differing values of S_0, S_{New} and R are given for 1-sided $\alpha = 0.05$ and $1 - \beta$ of 0.8 and 0.9 in **Table 18.2**.

18.2 Response and Toxicity Endpoints

Bryant-Day

Bryant and Day (1995) point out that a common situation when considering Phase I and Phase II/TE trials is that although the former primarily focuses on toxicity and the latter on efficacy, each in fact considers both. This provides the rationale for their TE design, which incorporates toxicity and activity considerations. Essentially, they combine a design for activity with a similar design for toxicity in which one is looking for both *acceptable* toxicity and *high* activity.

The Bryant and Day design implies that two 1-sided hypotheses are to be tested. These are that the true response rate π_R is either $\leq \pi_{R0}$, the maximum response rate of no interest, or $\geq \pi_{RNew}$, the minimum response rate of interest. Further, the probability of incorrectly rejecting the hypothesis $\pi_R \leq \pi_{R0}$ is set as α_R. Similarly, α_T is set for the hypothesis $\pi_T \leq \pi_{T0}$ where π_{T0} is an unacceptable rate of non-toxicity. In addition, the hypothesis $\pi_T \geq \pi_{TNew}$ has to be set, where π_{TNew} is the minimum acceptable (desirable) non-toxicity rate. (The terminology is a little clumsy here as it is more natural to talk in terms of 'acceptable toxicity' rates rather than 'acceptable non-toxicity' rates.) Further, the probability, β, of failing to recommend a treatment that is acceptable with respect to activity and acceptable to non-toxicity is required.

In the Bryant and Day design, toxicity monitoring is incorporated into the Simon (1989) design by requiring that the trial is terminated after Stage 1 if there is an inadequate number of observed responses or an excessive number of observed toxicities. The treatment under investigation is recommended at the end of Stage 2 only if there are both a sufficient number of responses and an acceptably small number of toxicities in total.

Since both toxicity and response are assessed in the same patient, the distributions of response and toxicity are not independent. These are linked by means of

$$\varphi = \frac{\eta_{00}\eta_{11}}{\eta_{01}\eta_{10}}. \tag{18.12}$$

Here, η_{00} is the true proportion of patients who both fail to respond and also experience unacceptable toxicity, η_{01} is the proportion of patients who fail to respond but have acceptable toxicity, η_{10} is the proportion of patients who respond but who have unacceptable toxicity, and finally η_{11} is the proportion of patients who respond and also have acceptable toxicity.

The design parameters chosen will establish a particular design with Stage 1 sample size, n_{B-D1}, with cut-off values for response and toxicity, C_{R1} and C_{T1}, in order to move from Stage 1 to Stage 2. The corresponding sample size for Stage 2, n_{B-D2}, is also established together with cut-off values, C_R and C_T, in order to declare sufficient activity with acceptable toxicity once the results from $N_{B-D} = n_{B-D1} + n_{B-D2}$ patients have been observed. These quantities are described collectively by

$$Q = \left\{ n_{B-D1}, C_{R1}, C_{T1}, n_{B-D2}, C_R, C_T \right\}. \tag{18.13}$$

The six components of Q are then determined by minimising the *expected* patient accrual under hypotheses of unacceptable treatment characteristics (inadequate response, excessive toxicity or both). In this context, *expected* refers to the average sample size that would turn out to have been used had a whole series of studies been conducted with the same design parameters in situations where the true activity, and true toxicity levels, remain constant.

In particular, suppose that the true response rate is indeed π_{R0} or more and the true non-toxicity rate is π_{T0} or more, then for the trial to proceed to Stage 2 both these response and toxicity criteria must be met. However, in such a two-stage design, even if both $\pi_R \le \pi_{R0}$ and $\pi_T \le \pi_{T0}$ are true, there is a possibility that the trial, once Stage 1 is completed, will go into the Stage 2 if (by chance) many responses and few toxicities have been observed.

The probability of *not* moving to Stage 2 based on the response criterion is $B(C_{R1}; \pi_{R0}, n_{B-D1})$, where $B(.)$ is the cumulative Binomial distribution of equation (1.11) with $R = C_{R1}$, $\pi = \pi_{R0}$ and $n = n_{B-D1}$. Similarly, based on the toxicity criterion, the probability of *not* moving to Stage 2 is $B(C_{T1}; \pi_{T0}, n_{B-D1})$. Thus, if we assume response and toxicity are not associated within patients, that is they are statistically *independent*, then the overall probability that the trial does *not* proceed to Stage 2 is given by

$$P_{00} = P_{Early} = 1 - \left[1 - B\left(C_{R1}; \pi_{R0}; n_{B-D1} \right) \right] \times \left[1 - B\left(C_{T1}; \pi_{T0}; n_{B-D1} \right) \right]. \tag{18.14}$$

This independence is equivalent to assuming that $\varphi = 1$ in equation (18.12).

The *expected* number of patients accrued given this situation is

$$N_{00} = N_{Expected} = n_{B-D1} + \left(1 - P_{00} \right) n_{B-D2}, \tag{18.15}$$

with similar expressions for N_{New0}, N_{0New} and N_{NewNew}.

The probability of recommending the treatment based on the response criterion is

$$\delta_{R0} = \sum_{y>C_{R1}} b\left(y; \pi_{R0}; n_{B-D1} \right) \left[1 - B\left(C_{R2} - y; \pi_{R0}, n_{B-D2} \right) \right], \tag{18.16}$$

where $b(y; \pi_{R0}, n_{B-D1})$ is equation (1.10) with $r = y$, $\pi = \pi_{R0}$ and $n = n_{B-D1}$. Similarly for the toxicity criterion,

$$\delta_{T0} = \sum_{y>C_{T1}} b\left(y; \pi_{T0}, n_{B-D1} \right) \left[1 - B\left(C_{T2} - y; \pi_{T0}, n_{B-D2} \right) \right], \tag{18.17}$$

and there are similar quantities for δ_{RNew} and δ_{TNew}. Values of the components of Q are then chosen to satisfy simultaneously

$$\delta_{R0} \times \delta_{TNew} \le \alpha_R, \ \delta_{RNew} \times \delta_{T0} \le \alpha_T \text{ and } \delta_{RNew} \times \delta_{TNew} \ge 1 - \beta. \tag{18.18}$$

There is a corresponding set of very complex equations if $\varphi \ne 1$ in equation (18.12). However, assuming independence between response and toxicity, that is $\varphi = 1$, gives designs which are close to optimal and so Bryant and Day (1995) recommend that this is adequate for general use. This assumption is implemented in the corresponding designs of $^S S_S$.

The number of subjects for Stage 1, the corresponding acceptable response and acceptable toxicity thresholds for entry into Stage 2, the total study size, and the corresponding final thresholds for acceptance of the test compound are given in **Table 18.3**.

18.3 Randomised Designs

Although many TE designs are single arm, there are situations in which it may be desirable to conduct a randomised trial, even though the intent of the trial is still TE in nature. Such trials allow for exploratory comparisons to be made between a new treatment and the current standard of care. The conclusions of the trial would not be confirmatory, but nonetheless the information generated from the trial would still be useful in understanding the potential efficacy of the new treatment. Thus such trials are likely to be designed in a manner close to the External-Pilot studies of **Chapter 16**. Nevertheless, in many cases, the sample size calculations for such trials have used the approaches discussed in **Chapters 4–7**. However, reflecting the non-confirmatory nature of these studies, typically a higher Type I error and/or a lower power would be used when computing the sample size required. Alternatively, a larger difference to be detected may be specified. Each of these would reduce the sample size chosen for the trial concerned.

Simon-Wittes-Ellenberg

There are situations whereby there are g (≥ 2) potential compounds available for use in the same type of patients and for eventual test in a Phase III trial against a current standard, but practicalities imply that only one of these can go forward for this subsequent evaluation. In such situations, the randomised Simon, Wittes and Ellenberg (1985) design selects the candidate drug from the g with the highest level of activity. Although details of the random allocation to the options process are not outlined here, this is a vital part of the design implementation. Details are provided by, for example, Machin and Fayers (2010).

The approach chooses the observed 'best' of the treatments for the eventual Phase III trial, however small the advantage is over the others. The trial size is determined in such a way that if a treatment exists for which the underlying efficacy is superior to the others by a specified amount, then it will be selected with a high probability.

When the difference in true response rates of the best and next best treatment is δ, then the probability of correct selection, P_{cs}, is smallest when there is a single best treatment and the other $g-1$ treatments are of equal but lower efficacy. The response rate of the worst treatment is denoted π_{Worst}.

For a specified response π, the probability that the best treatment produces the highest observed response rate is

$$Prob(Highest) = \sum_{i=0}^{m} f(i)\left[1 - B\left(i; \pi_{Worst} + \delta, m\right)\right], \tag{18.19}$$

and

$$f(i) = \left[B\left(i; \pi_{Worst}, m\right)\right]^{g-1} - \left[B\left(i-1; \pi_{Worst}, m\right)\right]^{g-1}, \tag{18.20}$$

where m is the number of subjects per treatment under test and $B(.)$ is the cumulative Binomial distribution of equation (1.12).

If there is a tie among the treatments for the largest observed response rate, then one of the tied treatments is randomly selected. Hence, in calculating the probability of correct selection, it is necessary to add to equation (18.19) the probability that the best treatment was selected after being tied with 1 or more of the other treatments for the greatest observed response rate. This is

$$Prob(Tie) = \sum_{i=0}^{m} \left[b(i; \pi_{Worst} + \delta, m) \sum_{j=1}^{g-1} \left(\frac{1}{j+1} \right) k(i, j) \right], \tag{18.21}$$

where $k(i, j) = \dfrac{(g-1)!}{j!(g-1-j)!} \left[b(i; \pi_{Worst}; m) \right]^{j} \left[B(i-1; \pi_{Worst}, m) \right]^{g-1-j}$.

The quantity $k(i, j)$ represents the probability that exactly j of the inferior treatments are tied for the largest number of observed responses among the $g-1$ inferior treatments, and this number of responses is i. The factor $\left(\dfrac{1}{j+1} \right)$ in equation (18.21) is the probability that the tie between the best and the j inferior treatments is randomly broken by selecting the best treatment.

The sum of expressions (18.19) and (18.21) gives the probability of correct selection, that is

$$P_{CS} = Prob(Highest) + Prob(Tie). \tag{18.22}$$

The corresponding tables for the number of patients per treatment group required is determined by searching for specified values of π_{Worst}, δ, and g, the value of m which provides a probability of correct selection equal to a set value for P_{CS}.

Except in extreme cases, when π_{Worst} is small or large, the sample size is relatively insensitive to these baseline response rates. Since precise knowledge of these may not be available, Liu (2001) proposes a conservative approach to trial design which involves using the largest sample size for each g and δ. Unfortunately, with $g \geq 4$ groups, these designs lead to relatively large randomised trials and this may limit their usefulness.

Table 18.4 gives the required sample size per treatment concerned, m, for a range of options of π_{Worst}, δ, and g for $P_{CS} = 0.9$.

18.4 Genomic Targets

The principles behind designs for trials involving genomic targets were discussed in **Chapter 15**, and these same principles also apply in the context of TEs.

Single Arm Design

In particular, the concept of 'enrichment' can be incorporated into many TEs. Thus, **Figure 18.1** is a single arm equivalent of **Figure 15.2**, and both involve pre-selecting only the diagnosis positive (D+) patients for inclusion into the study.

Similarly, the biomarker stratified design of **Figure 15.3** can be adapted and used by treating each of the D+ and diagnosis negative (D−) arms as two stand-alone single arm trials as in **Figure 18.2**. At the end of the study, if both the D+ and D− arms indicate an acceptable outcome, the drug under test

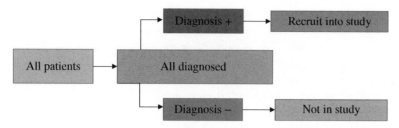

Figure 18.1 Enrichment Design for a TE Trial. (*See insert for color representation of the figure.*)

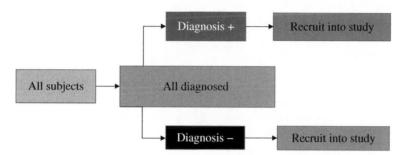

Figure 18.2 Biomarker stratified design for TE trials. (*See insert for color representation of the figure.*)

would be recommended for further development in an unselected (all patients) population. However if only the D+ arm appears active, the drug could be recommended for further testing only in the restricted group of patients who are all D+ patients. If only the D− arm is positive, that would suggest that further investigations of the diagnostic test are needed. Depending on the outcome of those investigations, further developments of the drug might be carried out on a further unselected population as the expectation would be that D+ patients should respond to the test better than D− ones.

Another option, when the TE design involves two stages, could be to make a decision at the end of Stage 1 to either stop the study or proceed with recruitment of unselected patients into Stage 2 or alternatively to proceed to just recruit D+ patients, depending on the results of Stage 1 in each arm.

Randomised Design

Freidlin, McShane, Polley, *et al* (2012) propose a randomised TE trial design that can be used to guide decision making for further development of an experimental therapy involving biomarkers. Depending on the TE trial results, a decision will then be made to either drop consideration of the new therapy or to perform a randomised Phase III trial (i) with an enrichment design, (ii) with a biomarker stratified design or (iii) without using the biomarker.

Randomised TE trials typically use an intermediate endpoint like progression-free survival (PFS) to obtain results earlier than those that would be obtained using overall survival (OS). This also allows the study to target larger treatment effects than might typically be expected for OS, resulting in smaller sample sizes needed. At the time the study is designed, there is some preliminary rationale suggesting that the D+ patients are likely to derive the most benefit from the new therapy, but benefit for the D− patients cannot be ruled out. Patients are randomly assigned to the experimental and control treatments, and the biomarker status of each patient is recorded. The idea is to use the observed treatment effects through the corresponding control over new treatment hazard ratio (*HR*) in each of the D+ and D– subgroups, as well as the overall value, to guide decision making.

With a specified sample size and after sufficient follow-up, a decision is made concerning further development of the new treatment and biomarker as described in **Figure 18.3**. In Step 1, the null hypothesis that PFS is the same for both treatment arms in the D+ subgroup is tested at the 1-sided $\alpha = 0.1$ significance level. If this test in Step 1 does not reject (that is, we have not demonstrated that the experimental treatment is better than the control in the D+ subgroup), then in Step 2A, the null hypothesis that PFS is the same for both treatment arms for all randomly assigned patients is tested at 1-sided $\alpha = 0.05$ significance. If this test in Step 2A does not reject, the design recommends no further testing of the new therapy. If this test in Step 2A does reject (that is, the new treatment is better than the control in the whole population), then the conclusion is that the new treatment is potentially active, but the biomarker is not useful. The design then recommends dropping the biomarker and performing a standard randomised Phase III trial.

If the test rejects the null hypothesis in Step 1 (that is, the new treatment is better than the control in the D+ subgroup), then the recommendation (Step 2B) is based on a 2-sided 80% confidence interval (*CI*) for the *HR* in the D– subgroup. If the whole *CI* is below a $HR = 1.3$, then there is strong evidence that the new treatment is, at best, only marginally helpful for the D– patients, and a biomarker enrichment Phase III trial is recommended. If the whole *CI* is above $HR = 1.5$, then there is evidence that the treatment works sufficiently well in the D– patients (and therefore the biomarker is not useful), and the recommendation is to drop the biomarker and perform a standard randomised Phase III trial. If neither of these conditions holds, then a Phase III biomarker-stratified design is recommended, because there is insufficient information on how well the treatment works in the D– subgroup.

With regard to sample size, because the underlying assumption is that the benefit of the new therapy is greatest among D+ patients, sample size considerations are driven by the D+ subgroup, and the techniques discussed in **Chapter 7** on sample sizes for the comparison of survival data can be used. We would also want to have approximately at least this many events in the D– subgroup to help with the decision making.

18.5   Bibliography

As we have indicated, TE designs with survival outcomes are discussed in detail by Case and Morgan (2003), those for a dual endpoint of response and toxicity by Bryant and Day (1995) and the selection design by Simon, Wittes and Ellenberg (1985). Alternative designs for survival endpoints have been proposed by Kwak and Jung (2014), Whitehead (2014), Mick, Crowley and Caroll (2000) as well as Cheung and Thall (2002). The Bayesian design of Johnson and Cook (2009) discussed in **Chapter 17** can also be adapted for survival data.

For TE trials involving genomic targets, further discussion of the approaches described, particularly in the context of using the Simon two-stage designs, can be found in Pusztai and Hess (2004) and Jones and Holmgren (2007). Other designs have also been used. Among these are the Randomized Discontinuation Design, described by Kopec, Abrahamowicz and Esdaile (1993) and implemented by Stadler (2007), which is particularly useful for the situation when the patient group most likely to benefit from a new agent is not clearly recognisable. The BATTLE trial of Kim, Herbst, Wistuba, *et al* (2011) uses an adaptive design approach to concurrently investigate four different treatment arms in lung cancer in a TE setting.

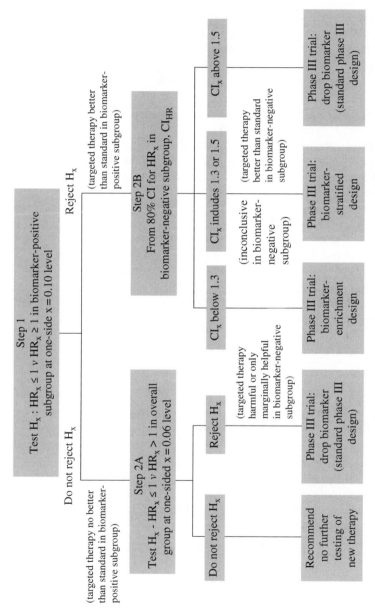

Figure 18.3 Decision algorithm for recommendation of, or not, a subsequent Phase III trial (from Freidlin, McShane, Polley and Korn, 2012).

18.6 Examples

Tables 18.1 and 18.2 and Equations 18.1, 18.4 and 18.5

Example 18.1   Case-Morgan Designs - Resectable pancreatic cancer

Case and Morgan (2003) consider the design of a Phase II trial of the effectiveness of adjuvant Gemcitabine and external beam radiotherapy in the treatment of patients with resectable pancreatic cancer and they planned to test the null hypothesis that 1-year survival is 35% or less. Suppose they plan an 80% power with an alternative 1-year survival of 50% for testing this hypothesis at a 1-sided 5% significance level.

In our notation, $T_{Sum} = 1$, $S_0(1) = 0.35$, $S_{New}(1) = 0.50$ and these imply from equation (18.1) death rates of $\lambda_0 = -log0.35 = 1.0498$ and $\lambda_{New} = -log0.5 = 0.6931$.

With $1 - \beta = 0.8$ and 1-sided $\alpha = 0.05$, $^S\!S_S$ begins by calculating the A'Hern (2001) single-stage sample size of **Chapter 17** with design parameters set as $\pi_0 = S_0(1)$ and $\pi_{New} = S_{New}(1)$. This gives $N_{A'H} = 68$, and the investigators anticipate that recruitment will take $D_{A-H} = 3$ years, which implies that $R = D_{A-H}/T_{Sum} = 3$ also.

EDA design

With $S_0(1) = 0.35$, $S_{New}(1) = 0$ and $R = 3$, Table 18.2 or $^S\!S_S$ suggests for the *EDA* design that Stage 1 recruits $n_{C-M1} = 40$, which will take $40/(68/3) = 1.76$ years at which time the interim analysis is to be conducted. For the study to continue into Stage 2, $z_{Interim}$ of equation (18.4) must exceed the critical value $C_1 = 0.328$. If Stage 2 is initiated, a further $n_{C-M2} = 39$ patients are required, taking an anticipated further $39/(68/3) = 1.72$ years to recruit. Hence, a total recruitment time of $D_{Accrual} = 1.76 + 1.72 = 3.4$ 8 years. Thus, the final analysis will occur, after a follow up period of $T_{Sum} = 1$ year post recruitment closure, at 4.48 years, at which time z_{Final} of equation (18.5) must exceed the critical value $C_2 = 1.544$ in order to conclude sufficient activity.

ETSL design

For this design, again with $N_{A'H} = 68$, $D_{A-H} = 3$ years and $R = 3$, **Table 18.2** or $^S\!S_S$ now gives $n_{C-M1} = 40$. This will take $45/(68/3) = 1.99$ years, at which time the interim analysis is to be conducted. For the study to continue into Stage 2, $z_{Interim}$ of equation (18.4) must exceed the critical value $C_1 = 0.609$. If Stage 2 is initiated, a further $n_{C-M2} = 39$ patients are required, taking an anticipated further $39/(68/3) = 1.72$ years to recruit. Hence, a total recruitment time of $D_{Accrual} = 1.99 + 1.72 = 3.71$ years. Thus, the final analysis will occur $T_{Sum} = 1$ year later at 4.71 years, at which time z_{Final} of equation (18.5) must exceed the critical value $C_2 = 1.497$.

In this example, the *ETSL* design (if completed to the end of Stage 2) requires 5 more patients to be recruited, a *higher* interim analysis threshold, but a *lower* final analysis threshold than the corresponding *EDA* design

Table 18.3

Example 18.2   Bryant-Day design - Ifosfamide and Vinorelbine in ovarian cancer

González-Martín, Crespo, García-López, *et al* (2002) used the Bryant-Day two-stage design with a cut-off point for the response rate of 10% and for severe toxicity of 25%. Severe toxicity was defined as grade 3-4 non-haematological toxicity, neutropenic fever or grade 4 thrombocytopenia. They do not provide full details of how the sample size was determined, but their choice of design specified a Stage

1 of 14 patients and a Stage 2 of a further 20 patients. In the event, in these advanced platinum–resistant ovarian cancer patients, the combination of Ifosfamide and Vinorelbine was evidently very toxic. Hence, the trial was closed after 12 patients with an observed toxicity level above the 25% contemplated.

In fact their study sample size is close to a design with $\alpha_R = \alpha_T = 0.1$, $\beta = 0.2$, $\pi_{R0} = 0.1$, $\pi_{RNew} = 0.3$; $\pi_{T0} = 0.75$ and $\pi_{TNew} = 0.90$. On this basis, the completed Stage 1 trial of 15 patients proceeds to Stage 2 if there are at least 2 responses *and* there are 10 or more patients with acceptable toxicity. The Stage 2 trial size involves a further 19 patients, to a total of 34 for the whole trial. Sufficient efficacy with acceptable toxicity would be concluded if there were 6 or more responses observed *and* 29 or more with acceptable toxicity.

Had they chosen instead the first design of **Table 18.3**, that is, $\alpha_R = \alpha_T = 0.1$, $\beta = 0.15$; $\pi_{R0} = 0.1$, $\pi_{RNew} = 0.3$; $\pi_{T0} = 0.6$ and $\pi_{TNew} = 0.8$, then Stage 1 consists of $n_{B-D1} = 19$ patients. The trial would proceed to Stage 2 if there are at least $C_{R1} = 2$ responses *and* there are also $C_{T1} = 12$ or more patients with acceptable toxicity. The Stage 2 trial size is a further 21 patients, to a total of $N_{B-D} = 40$ for the whole trial, and sufficient efficacy with acceptable toxicity would be concluded if there were $C_R = 7$ or more responses observed *and* $C_T = 28$ or more with acceptable toxicity.

Equation 5.4

Example 18.3 Randomised trial - Dengue fever
Low, Sung, Wijaya, *et al* (2014) conducted what they termed a 'proof-of-concept' trial in patients with dengue fever. The total sample size of 50 was determined using the approach discussed in **Chapter 5** for comparing two independent groups with continuous data. The design assumed a virological log reduction (VLR) between Placebo (*P*) and Celgosivir (*C*) of $\delta_{Plan} = \mu_C - \mu_P = 0.7$ VLR and $\sigma_{Plan} = 1.0$ VLR, hence $\Delta_{Plan} = 0.7$, and with a 5% 1-sided Type 1 error and power of 80%. The 1-sided test was chosen for the alternative hypothesis that the true difference in means δ is greater than 0.

In the event, the mean difference observed was $d = 0.22$ VLR, far less than anticipated while the SDs, $s_P = 0.75$ and $s_C = 1.07$, were close to the planned values.

Although termed a 'proof-of-concept' trial, formal statistical comparisons were made and the authors concluded 'Mean VLR was greater in patients given celgosivir than in those given placebo, but the difference was non-significant ... '. It would be important to note that even if a statistically significant difference had been observed, this would not be confirmatory given the exploratory nature of the trial as reflected in the relatively small sample size.

Planning that uses the considerations of **Chapter 16** is usually advised for trials of this type.

Table 18.4

Example 18.4 Simon-Wittes-Ellenburg design - Advanced non-small cell lung cancer
Leong, Toh, Lim, *et al* (2007) conducted a randomised Phase II trial of the $g = 3$ single-agents Gemcitabine, Vinorelbine and Docetaxel for the treatment of elderly and/or poor performance status patients with advanced non-small-cell lung cancer. The design was implemented with the probability of correctly selecting the best treatment assumed to be 90%. It was anticipated that the single-agent activity of each drug has a baseline response rate of approximately 20%. In order to detect a 15% superiority of the best treatment over the others, how many patients should be recruited per treatment for the trial?

For the difference in response rate $\delta = 0.15$, smallest response rate $\pi_{Worst} = 0.2$, probability of correct selection $P_{CS} = 0.90$ and treatment groups $g = 3$, Table 18.4 and $^S\!S_S$ give a sample size of $m = 44$ per treatment group. Thus, the total number of patients to be recruited is $N = gm = 3 \times 44 = 132$.

Example 18.5   Simon-Wittes-Ellenburg design- Non-Hodgkins' lymphoma

Itoh, Ohtsu, Fukuda, *et al* (2002) describe a randomised 2-group Phase II trial comparing dose-escalated CHOP (*DE*) with biweekly dose-intensified CHOP (*DI*) in newly diagnosed patients with advanced-stage aggressive non-Hodgkins' lymphoma. Their design anticipated at least a 65% complete response rate (*CR*) for both options. To achieve a 90% probability of selecting the better arm when the *CR* rate is 15% higher in one arm than the other, the authors state: ' … at least 30 patients would be required in each arm'. The detailed tabulations of **Table 18.4** and $^S\!S_S$ give 29 as opposed to 30.

In the event, they recruited 35 patients to each arm and observed response rates with *DE* and *DI* of 51% and 60% respectively. Both are lower than the 'at least 65%' that the investigators had anticipated. Their following randomised Phase III trial compares *DI* CHOP with the *Standard* CHOP regimen.

References

Technical

A'Hern RP (2001). Sample size tables for exact single stage phase II designs. *Statistics in Medicine*, **20**, 859–866.

Bryant J and Day R (1995). Incorporating toxicity considerations into the design of two-stage Phase II clinical trials. *Biometrics*, **51**, 1372–1383.

Case LD and Morgan TM (2003). Design of Phase II cancer trials evaluating survival probabilities. *BMC Medical Research Methodology*, **3**, 6.

Cheung YK and Thall PF (2002). Monitoring the rates of composite events with censored data in phase II clinical trials. *Biometrics*, **58**, 89–97.

Freidlin B, McShane LM, Polley MY and Korn EL (2012). Randomised Phase II trial designs with biomarkers. *Journal of Clinical Oncology*, **30**, 3304–3309.

Johnson VE and Cook JD (2009). Bayesian design of single-arm phase II clinical trials with continuous monitoring. *Clinical Trials*, **6**, 217–226.

Jones CL and Holmgren E (2007). An adaptive Simon two-stage design for Phase 2 studies of targeted therapies. *Contemporary Clinical Trials*, **28**, 654–661.

Kim ES, Herbst JJ, Wistuba II, Lee JJ, Blumenschein GR, Tsao A, Stewart DJ, Hicks ME, Erasmus J, Gupta S, Alden CM, Liu S, Tang X, Khuri FR, Tran HT, Johnson BE, Heymach JV, Mao L, Fossella F, Kies MS, Papadimitrakopoulou V, Davis SE, Lippman SM and Hong WK. (2011). The BATTLE trial: personalizing therapy for lung cancer. *Cancer Discovery*, **1**, 44–53.

Kopec JA, Abrahamowicz M and Esdaile JM (1993). Randomised discontinuation trials: utility and efficiency. *Journal of Clinical Epidemiology*, **46**, 959–971.

Kwak M and Jung S (2014). Phase II clinical trials with time-to-event endpoints: optimal two-stage designs with one sample log-rank test. *Statistics in Medicine*, **33**, 2004–2016.

Liu PY (2001). Phase II selection designs. In: Crowley J (ed) *Handbook of Statistics in Clinical Oncology*, Marcel Dekker Inc, New York, pp 119–127.

Machin D and Fayers PM (2010). *Randomized Clinical Trials*. Wiley-Blackwell, Chichester.

Mick R, Crowley JJ and Carroll RJ (2000). Phase II clinical trial design for noncytotoxic anticancer agents for which time to disease progression is the primary endpoint. *Controlled Clinical Trials*, **21**, 343–359.

Pusztai L and Hess KR (2004). Clinical trial design for microarray predictive marker discovery and assessment. *Annals of Oncology*, **15**, 1731–1737.

Simon R, Wittes RE and Ellenberg SS (1985). Randomized phase II clinical trials. *Cancer Treatment Reports*, **69**, 1375–1381.

Stadler WM (2007). The randomized discontinuation trial: a phase II design to assess growth-inhibitory agents. *Molecular Cancer Therapeutics*, **6**, 1180–1185.

Stadler WM, Rosner G, Small E, Hollis D, Rini B, Zaentz SD, Mahony J and Ratain MJ (2005). Successful implementation of the randomized discontinuation trial design: an application to the study of the putative antiangiogenic agent carboxyaminoimidazole in renal cell carcinoma-CALGB 69901. *Journal of Clinical Oncology*, **23**, 3726–3732.

Whitehead J (2014). One stage and two stage designs for phase II clinical trials with survival endpoints. *Statistics in Medicine*, **33**, 3830–3843.

Examples

González-Martín A, Crespo C, García-López JL, Pedraza M, Garrido P, Lastra E and Moyano A (2002). Ifosfamide and vinorelbine in advanced platinum-resistant ovarian cancer: excessive toxicity with a potentially active regimen. *Gynecologic Oncology*, **84**, 368–373.

Itoh K, Ohtsu T, Fukuda H, Sasaki Y, Ogura M, Morishima Y, Chou T, Aikawa K, Uike N, Mizorogi F, Ohno T, Ikeda S, Sai T, Taniwaki M, Kawano F, Niimi M, Hotta T, Shimoyama M and Tobinai K (2002). Randomized phase II study of biweekly CHOP and dose-escalated CHOP with prophylactic use of lenograstim (glycosylated G-CSF) in aggressive non-Hodgkin's lymphoma: Japan Clinical Oncology Group Study 9505. *Annals of Oncology*, **13**, 1347–1355.

Leong SS, Toh CK, Lim WT, Lin X, Tan SB, Poon D, Tay MH, Foo KF, Ho J and Tan EH (2007). A randomized phase II trial of single agent Gemcitabine, Vinorelbine or Docetaxel in patients with advanced non-small cell lung cancer who have poor performance status and/or are elderly. *Journal of Thoracic Oncology*, **2**, 230–236.

Low JG, Sung C, Wijaya L, Wei Y, Rathore APS, Watanabe S, Tan BH, Toh L, Chua LT, Hou Y, Chow A, Howe S, Chan WK, Tan KH, Chung JS, Cherng BP, Lye DC, Tambayah PA, Ng LC, Connolly J, Hibberd ML, Leo YS, Cheung YB, Ooi EE and Vasudevan SG (2014). Efficacy and safety of celgosivir in patients with dengue fever (CELADEN): a phase 1b, randomised, double-blind, placebo-controlled, proof-of-concept trial. *Lancet Infectious Diseases*, **14**, 706–715.

Table 18.1 Stage 1, n_{C-M1}, and Final, N, Sample Sizes and Thresholds C_1 and C_2 for the Case-Morgan Expected Duration of Accrual (*EDA*) design with 1-sided $\alpha = 0.05$.

$S_0(T)$	$S_{New}(T)$	R	Power $1-\beta=0.8$				Power $1-\beta=0.9$			
			C_1	C_2	n_{CM1}	N	C_1	C_2	n_{CM1}	N
0.30	0.45	2	0.166	1.567	46	75	0.082	1.590	65	102
		2.5	0.264	1.554	42	77	0.188	1.581	60	103
		3	0.322	1.544	39	78	0.252	1.574	57	105
	0.50	2	0.177	1.565	27	44	0.082	1.590	37	58
		2.5	0.270	1.552	24	45	0.193	1.579	34	59
		3	0.315	1.545	23	45	0.250	1.573	33	60
0.35	0.50	2	0.177	1.567	46	76	0.088	1.591	67	105
		2.5	0.270	1.553	42	78	0.192	1.580	62	107
		3	0.328	1.544	40	79	0.249	1.574	58	108
	0.55	2	0.188	1.564	28	46	0.097	1.590	37	58
		2.5	0.274	1.552	26	47	0.208	1.578	34	59
		3	0.330	1.543	24	48	0.252	1.574	33	60
0.40	0.55	2	0.180	1.567	48	80	0.094	1.591	66	103
		2.5	0.268	1.554	44	81	0.202	1.580	61	105
		3	0.318	1.547	41	82	0.249	1.574	57	106
	0.60	2	0.188	1.565	29	47	0.091	1.590	39	61
		2.5	0.286	1.550	26	48	0.217	1.577	36	63
		3	0.331	1.542	24	49	0.262	1.573	34	63
0.45	0.60	2	0.195	1.565	47	79	0.097	1.591	68	107
		2.5	0.280	1.553	43	80	0.211	1.579	63	110
		3	0.322	1.545	40	81	0.256	1.574	59	110
	0.65	2	0.185	1.567	29	47	0.108	1.590	38	59
		2.5	0.280	1.552	26	48	0.211	1.579	35	60
		3	0.331	1.544	24	49	0.262	1.573	33	61
0.50	0.65	2	0.192	1.567	47	77	0.105	1.590	65	102
		2.5	0.278	1.553	42	79	0.211	1.579	60	104
		3	0.322	1.546	40	80	0.256	1.574	56	105
	0.70	2	0.208	1.562	25	42	0.123	1.588	37	58
		2.5	0.289	1.550	23	43	0.209	1.579	34	59
		3	0.325	1.545	21	43	0.264	1.572	32	60
0.55	0.70	2	0.204	1.565	47	79	0.108	1.591	64	101
		2.5	0.292	1.552	43	80	0.224	1.578	59	103
		3	0.331	1.546	40	81	0.268	1.573	56	104
	0.75	2	0.205	1.564	25	42	0.117	1.589	35	55
		2.5	0.287	1.551	23	43	0.212	1.578	32	56
		3	0.346	1.541	22	43	0.256	1.574	30	57
0.60	0.75	2	0.201	1.567	42	70	0.126	1.589	59	94
		2.5	0.297	1.551	38	71	0.209	1.581	54	95
		3	0.331	1.546	36	72	0.265	1.574	51	96
	0.80	2	0.208	1.564	24	41	0.129	1.588	32	50
		2.5	0.293	1.552	22	42	0.220	1.579	29	50
		3	0.340	1.543	21	42	0.272	1.572	27	51
0.65	0.80	2	0.209	1.565	37	62	0.126	1.589	52	82
		2.5	0.296	1.552	34	63	0.218	1.579	48	84
		3	0.335	1.544	32	64	0.277	1.572	45	85
	0.85	2	0.211	1.565	21	35	0.126	1.589	29	46
		2.5	0.284	1.553	19	36	0.205	1.580	27	47
		3	0.346	1.542	18	36	0.271	1.573	26	48

Table 18.2 Stage 1, n_{C-M1}, and Final, N, Sample Sizes and Thresholds C_1 and C_2 for the Case-Morgan Expected Total Study Length (*ETSL*) design with 1-sided $\alpha = 0.05$.

$S_0(T)$	$S_{New}(T)$	R	C_1	C_2	n_{CM1}	N	C_1	C_2	n_{CM1}	N
			\multicolumn{4}{c}{Power $1-\beta = 0.8$}				
0.3	0.45	2	0.662	1.485	53	83	0.639	1.520	77	111
		2.5	0.634	1.490	48	83	0.611	1.525	70	111
		3	0.606	1.494	44	83	0.577	1.532	65	110
	0.50	2	0.667	1.482	31	48	0.634	1.521	44	63
		2.5	0.631	1.490	28	48	0.614	1.522	40	64
		3	0.617	1.492	26	48	0.583	1.528	37	63
0.35	0.5	2	0.664	1.486	54	84	0.637	1.522	79	115
		2.5	0.634	1.490	48	84	0.608	1.525	72	115
		3	0.609	1.497	45	84	0.591	1.529	67	114
	0.55	2	0.667	1.482	33	51	0.643	1.520	44	63
		2.5	0.634	1.490	29	51	0.605	1.526	40	63
		3	0.611	1.493	27	51	0.592	1.527	37	63
0.40	0.55	2	0.669	1.484	56	88	0.645	1.520	78	113
		2.5	0.639	1.491	50	88	0.604	1.528	70	112
		3	0.614	1.495	47	88	0.584	1.531	65	112
	0.60	2	0.671	1.484	33	52	0.646	1.520	46	67
		2.5	0.639	1.489	30	52	0.602	1.528	42	67
		3	0.621	1.492	28	52	0.584	1.531	39	67
0.45	0.60	2	0.669	1.484	55	87	0.649	1.522	81	117
		2.5	0.642	1.491	50	87	0.609	1.527	73	117
		3	0.615	1.494	46	87	0.589	1.530	68	117
	0.65	2	0.674	1.484	33	52	0.642	1.521	45	65
		2.5	0.644	1.487	30	52	0.611	1.526	40	65
		3	0.618	1.494	28	52	0.587	1.529	37	65
0.50	0.65	2	0.673	1.485	54	86	0.650	1.522	77	111
		2.5	0.639	1.491	49	85	0.618	1.525	69	111
		3	0.617	1.495	45	85	0.592	1.530	64	111
	0.70	2	0.675	1.483	29	46	0.653	1.520	44	63
		2.5	0.646	1.488	26	46	0.611	1.527	39	63
		3	0.628	1.491	24	46	0.589	1.530	37	63
0.55	0.70	2	0.672	1.487	55	87	0.650	1.522	75	110
		2.5	0.640	1.491	49	87	0.615	1.527	68	110
		3	0.616	1.495	46	86	0.596	1.529	64	110
	0.75	2	0.679	1.483	29	46	0.656	1.519	41	60
		2.5	0.639	1.491	26	46	0.620	1.524	37	60
		3	0.625	1.492	24	46	0.589	1.530	35	60
0.60	0.75	2	0.677	1.485	48	77	0.652	1.521	70	102
		2.5	0.645	1.490	44	77	0.618	1.528	63	101
		3	0.621	1.494	40	77	0.592	1.531	59	101
	0.80	2	0.683	1.482	28	45	0.650	1.522	37	54
		2.5	0.642	1.490	25	45	0.617	1.526	34	54
		3	0.623	1.494	24	45	0.593	1.530	31	54
0.65	0.80	2	0.680	1.484	43	68	0.656	1.521	61	90
		2.5	0.645	1.492	39	68	0.618	1.526	55	90
		3	0.625	1.493	36	68	0.592	1.530	52	90
	0.85	2	0.687	1.481	24	39	0.655	1.521	35	50
		2.5	0.644	1.490	22	39	0.620	1.526	31	50
		3	0.625	1.493	20	39	0.594	1.530	29	50

Table 18.3 Bryant and Day Response and Toxicity design.

Sample sizes and rejection criteria for π_{R0}, π_{RNew}, π_{T0} and π_{TNew} computed assuming $\phi = 1$ of equation (18.12). n_{B-D1} is the number of Stage 1 patients and N_{B-D} is the total to be accrued to both stages. At the end of Stage 1, Stage 2 will be activated if the number of responses is $\geq C_{R1}$ and when the number who experience acceptable toxicity is $\geq C_{T1}$. At the end of Stage 2, the treatment will be accepted for potential Phase III trial if both the number of responses is $\geq C_R$ and the number with acceptable toxicity is $\geq C_T$.

π_{R0}	π_{RNew}	π_{T0}	π_{TNew}	n_{B-D1}	C_{R1}	C_{T1}	N_{B-D}	C_R	C_T
				$\alpha_R = 0.10$; $\alpha_T = 0.10$; $\beta = 0.15$					
0.1	0.3	0.60	0.80	19	2	12	40	6	27
0.2	0.4	0.60	0.80	20	4	12	41	11	28
0.3	0.5	0.60	0.80	20	6	12	43	16	29
0.4	0.6	0.60	0.80	20	8	12	46	22	31
0.5	0.7	0.60	0.80	17	8	10	43	25	29
0.6	0.8	0.60	0.80	18	11	11	43	29	29
0.1	0.3	0.75	0.95	9	0	6	25	4	21
0.2	0.4	0.75	0.95	18	4	14	34	9	28
0.3	0.5	0.75	0.95	19	6	15	37	14	30
0.4	0.6	0.75	0.95	14	5	10	37	18	31
0.5	0.7	0.75	0.95	16	8	12	39	23	33
0.6	0.8	0.75	0.95	13	8	10	37	25	30
				$\alpha_R = 0.10$; $\alpha_T = 0.10$; $\beta = 0.10$					
0.1	0.3	0.60	0.80	21	2	13	46	7	31
0.2	0.4	0.60	0.80	24	5	15	54	14	36
0.3	0.5	0.60	0.80	23	7	14	57	21	38
0.4	0.6	0.60	0.80	25	10	15	53	25	36
0.5	0.7	0.60	0.80	22	11	13	52	30	35
0.6	0.8	0.60	0.80	20	12	12	49	33	33
0.1	0.3	0.75	0.95	14	1	11	34	5	28
0.2	0.4	0.75	0.95	18	3	13	37	10	31
0.3	0.5	0.75	0.95	22	7	17	46	17	38
0.4	0.6	0.75	0.95	22	9	17	46	22	38
0.5	0.7	0.75	0.95	20	10	15	43	25	36
0.6	0.8	0.75	0.95	19	12	15	43	29	35

Table 18.3 (Continued)

Sample sizes and rejection criteria for π_{R0}, π_{RNew}, π_{T0} and π_{TNew} computed assuming $\phi = 1$ of equation (18.12). n_{B-D1} is the number of Stage 1 patients and N_{B-D} is the total to be accrued to both stages. At the end of Stage 1, Stage 2 will be activated if the number of responses is $\geq C_{R1}$ and when the number who experience acceptable toxicity is $\geq C_{T1}$. At the end of Stage 2, the treatment will be accepted for potential Phase III trial if both the number of responses is $\geq C_R$ and the number with acceptable toxicity is $\geq C_T$.

π_{R0}	π_{RNew}	π_{T0}	π_{TNew}	n_{B-D1}	C_{R1}	C_{T1}	N_{B-D}	C_R	C_T
				$\alpha_R = 0.15$; $\alpha_T = 0.15$; $\beta = 0.15$					
0.1	0.3	0.60	0.80	15	1	9	30	4	20
0.2	0.4	0.60	0.80	17	3	10	36	9	24
0.3	0.5	0.60	0.80	19	5	11	33	12	22
0.4	0.6	0.60	0.80	20	8	12	37	17	25
0.5	0.7	0.60	0.80	17	8	10	37	21	25
0.6	0.8	0.60	0.80	14	8	8	33	22	22
0.1	0.3	0.75	0.95	12	1	9	22	3	18
0.2	0.4	0.75	0.95	12	2	9	28	7	23
0.3	0.5	0.75	0.95	13	3	9	27	10	22
0.4	0.6	0.75	0.95	17	7	13	30	14	24
0.5	0.7	0.75	0.95	17	9	13	30	17	24
0.6	0.8	0.75	0.95	14	8	11	25	17	20
				$\alpha_R = 0.15$; $\alpha_T = 0.15$; $\beta = 0.10$					
0.1	0.3	0.60	0.80	16	1	9	36	5	24
0.2	0.4	0.60	0.80	24	5	15	41	10	27
0.3	0.5	0.60	0.80	22	6	13	42	15	28
0.4	0.6	0.60	0.80	26	10	16	41	19	27
0.5	0.7	0.60	0.80	24	12	14	39	22	26
0.6	0.8	0.60	0.80	18	10	10	36	24	24
0.1	0.3	0.75	0.95	13	1	10	31	4	25
0.2	0.4	0.75	0.95	16	3	12	36	9	29
0.3	0.5	0.75	0.95	20	6	15	36	13	29
0.4	0.6	0.75	0.95	17	6	12	36	17	29
0.5	0.7	0.75	0.95	15	7	11	37	21	30
0.6	0.8	0.75	0.95	15	9	11	33	22	27

Table 18.4 Simon-Wittes-Ellenberg Design.

For a probability of correctly selecting the best treatment $P_{CS}=0.9$, the table gives the number of patients m in each group required to identify the best of g treatments under investigation for the worst response rate π_{Worst} anticipated and difference in response rate δ.

Smallest Response Rate,	Number of treatments, g				
π_{Worst}	2	3	4	5	6
	$\delta=0.1, P_{CS}=0.9$				
0.10	42	62	74	83	90
0.15	53	79	95	106	115
0.20	62	93	111	125	136
0.25	69	104	125	141	153
0.30	75	113	136	153	166
0.35	79	119	144	162	175
0.40	82	123	149	167	181
0.45	82	124	150	169	183
0.50	82	123	149	167	182
0.55	79	120	145	162	177
0.60	75	113	137	154	168
0.65	69	105	127	142	155
0.70	62	94	113	127	138
0.75	53	80	97	109	118
0.80	42	63	77	86	94
0.85	29	44	53	60	65
	$\delta=0.15, P_{CS}=0.9$				
0.10	21	31	37	41	45
0.15	26	38	45	51	55
0.20	29	44	52	59	64
0.25	32	48	58	65	71
0.30	35	52	62	70	76
0.35	36	54	65	73	79
0.40	37	55	67	75	81
0.45	37	55	67	75	81
0.50	36	54	65	73	80
0.55	35	52	63	71	77
0.60	32	49	59	66	72
0.65	29	44	53	60	65
0.70	26	39	47	53	57
0.75	21	32	38	43	47
0.80	16	24	29	32	35

Table 18.4 (Continued)

For a probability of correctly selecting the best treatment $P_{CS}=0.9$, the table gives the number of patients m in each group required to identify the best of g treatments under investigation for the worst response rate π_{Worst} anticipated and difference in response rate δ.

Smallest Response Rate,					

	$\delta=0.2, P_{CS}=0.9$				
	Number of treatments, g				
π_{Worst}	2	3	4	5	6
0.10	13	19	23	25	27
0.15	16	23	27	31	33
0.20	18	26	31	35	38
0.25	19	28	34	38	41
0.30	20	30	36	40	44
0.35	21	31	37	42	45
0.40	21	31	38	42	46
0.45	21	31	37	42	45
0.50	20	30	36	41	44
0.55	19	28	34	39	42
0.60	18	26	32	36	39
0.65	16	23	28	32	34
0.70	13	20	24	27	29
0.75	11	16	19	21	23

	$\delta=0.25, P_{CS}=0.9$				
0.10	9	13	16	18	19
0.15	11	16	19	21	22
0.20	12	17	21	23	25
0.25	13	19	22	25	27
0.30	13	19	23	26	28
0.35	13	20	24	27	29
0.40	13	20	24	27	29
0.45	13	20	24	26	29
0.50	13	19	23	25	28
0.55	12	18	21	24	26
0.60	11	16	19	22	23
0.65	9	14	17	19	20
0.70	8	11	13	15	16

19

The Correlation Coefficient

SUMMARY

The strength of the linear association between two continuous or ranked variables assessed in the same individuals is estimated by the Pearson or Spearmen correlation coefficients respectively. The formula for sample sizes to detect a correlation of a pre-specified magnitude is described. Recommendations as to what may be considered 'small', 'medium' and 'large' associations are indicated. The approach to identifying a lack of association, that is when there is truly no association between the two variables and so the correlation is zero, is included. Finally, sample sizes are described for situations when a study stipulates a pre-specified width of the confidence interval for the Pearson or Spearman correlation coefficient is required.

19.1   Introduction

An investigator may wish to show that two continuous measurements, such as the waist circumference and hip circumference in patients with a particular condition, are associated. Any association implies that as one measurement increases the other generally increases (or generally decreases) and this rate is approximately constant. In other circumstances, there may be a single variable to be assessed but its value is recorded by two different instruments designed to determine the same thing. In this case the two measurements may be anticipated to be in close agreement to each other.

The strength and direction (negative or positive) of an association is measured by either the Pearson or the Spearman correlation coefficient, ρ. In either case, a correlation of $\rho = 0$ indicates that there is no linear association between the two variables, while $\rho = +1$ or -1 indicates a perfect positive or negative linear correlation respectively. Strictly, the correlation coefficient measures the degree of *linear* relationship between two variables and so is inappropriate if the relationship appears to be non-linear.

Once the study is completed then, with the estimated correlation coefficient, r, a hypothesis test can be conducted. The corresponding null hypothesis is that the true or population correlation coefficient $\rho_{Pop} = 0$. A small p-value will then indicate evidence against that hypothesis. However, such an indication does not imply that ρ_{Pop} is necessarily distant from zero or close to the extremes of $+1$ or -1.

Sample Sizes for Clinical, Laboratory and Epidemiology Studies, Fourth Edition. David Machin, Michael J. Campbell, Say Beng Tan and Sze Huey Tan.
© 2018 John Wiley & Sons Ltd. Published 2018 by John Wiley & Sons Ltd.

19.2 Theory and Formulae

The correlation coefficient is a dimensionless quantity. As a consequence it can (itself) act as the index of the effect-size required for planning. Before the study, we need to specify the anticipated size of the correlation coefficient ρ that we think might represent the true correlation between the two variables. Clearly the smaller the true correlation coefficient, the larger the study has to be to detect it. To get a feel for the correlation coefficient between two continuous variables, we note that ρ^2 is the proportion of variance in either of the variables which may be accounted for by the other, using a linear relationship.

Usually the direction of the relationship will be specified in advance. For example, systolic and diastolic blood pressures are certain to be positively associated and so a 1-sided significance test is required for the analysis. In contrast, but perhaps less common, if one is estimating an association with no sign pre-specified, then a 2-sided test is warranted.

Suggested values of 0.1, 0.3 and 0.5 are regarded as 'small', 'medium' and 'large' effects for ρ in epidemiology, but for laboratory work, for example, much larger values may be anticipated.

Sample Size

To calculate appropriate sample sizes, we assume that we are investigating the association between two Normally distributed variables with correlation coefficient ρ. It can be shown that

$$u = \frac{1}{2} log\left[\frac{1+\rho}{1-\rho}\right] + \frac{\rho}{2(N-1)} \tag{19.1}$$

is approximately Normally distributed with standard deviation $1/\sqrt{N-3}$, where N is the sample size. This leads to the appropriate sample size to detect an anticipated correlation ρ_{Plan} for 1-sided significance level α and power of $1-\beta$ as

$$N = \frac{(z_{1-\alpha} + z_{1-\beta})^2}{u^2} + 3. \tag{19.2}$$

If a 2-sided test is appropriate then $z_{1-\alpha}$ is replaced by $z_{1-\alpha/2}$ in equation (19.2).

However, it should be emphasised that to calculate u for equation (19.2) we require some value for N (the number we are trying to estimate!) to substitute in (19.1). To circumvent this problem, an initial value for u is calculated as

$$u_0 = \frac{1}{2} log\left[\frac{1+\rho_{Plan}}{1-\rho_{Plan}}\right]. \tag{19.3}$$

This is the first term on the right hand side of (19.1). The value obtained is then used in (19.2) to give an initial value for N labelled N_0. This N_0 is then used in (19.1) to obtain a new value for u, say u_1, which is now used in (19.2) to obtain a revised sample size N_1. The whole iteration process is repeated until two consecutive values of N_i within unity of each other are found.

If Spearman's rank correlation is used, the same methods of sample size calculation apply. Sample sizes for the Pearson and Spearman correlation coefficients are given in **Table 19.1**.

Lack of Association

Cohen (1988) cites an example of a social psychologist planning an experiment in which college students would be subjected to two questionnaires, one on personality, y_{Person}, and one on social desirability, y_{Social}. He wishes to show that $y_{Personality}$ and y_{Social} are *not* associated. In this the object is to 'prove the null hypothesis' which in any study with a finite sample size is not possible. To circumvent this difficulty we presume an investigator may be willing to effectively assume that $\rho = 0$ when it is observed to be small. Thus the situation is restructured as an attempt to demonstrate that ρ is indeed small. Thus, the design team will specify a small absolute value of ρ_{Plan}. Further, a Type I error, α, corresponds to the probability the null hypothesis is rejected when it is actually true while the Type II error, β, is the probability that the null hypothesis is not rejected when it is actually false. For lack of association studies, α is set larger than the usual 0.05 while β is relatively smaller and less than 0.1. The corresponding sample size is then obtained from equation (19.2).

Confidence Intervals

Pearson

For an estimated correlation coefficient r_P based on N subjects, an approximate $100(1-\alpha)\%$ confidence interval (CI) for the Pearson correlation coefficient, ρ_P, is estimated by

$$r - z_{1-\alpha/2} \frac{\left(1-r^2\right)}{\sqrt{N-3}} \text{ to } r + z_{1-\alpha/2} \frac{\left(1-r^2\right)}{\sqrt{N-3}}. \tag{19.4}$$

The sample size required to estimate a planned correlation coefficient, ρ_{Plan}, with a pre-specified width, w, of the CI is given by

$$N_P^0 = \frac{4z_{1-\alpha/2}^2 \left(1-\rho_{Plan}^2\right)^2}{w^2} + 3. \tag{19.5}$$

However, this equation is only accurate if the sample size turns out to be relatively large (>55) and $|\rho_{Plan}| < 0.7$. A more accurate estimate is given by the following

$$N_P^{Final} = \left(N_P^0 - 3\right)\left(\frac{w_0}{W}\right)^2 + 3, \tag{19.6}$$

where

$$w_0 = \left[\frac{\exp(2U)-1}{\exp(2U)+1}\right] - \left[\frac{\exp(2L)-1}{\exp(2L)+1}\right], \tag{19.7}$$

$$U = \frac{1}{2}\log\left(\frac{1+\rho_{Plan}}{1-\rho_{Plan}}\right) + \theta \times \frac{z_{1-\alpha/2}}{\sqrt{N_P^0-3}} \text{ and } L = \frac{1}{2}\log\left(\frac{1+\rho_{Plan}}{1-\rho_{Plan}}\right) - \theta \times \frac{z_{1-\alpha/2}}{\sqrt{N_P^0-3}} \tag{19.8}$$

and $\theta = \theta_P = 1$.

Spearman

The corresponding CI expression for the Spearman rank correlation is

$$r - z_{1-\alpha/2} \frac{(1-r^2)}{\sqrt{N-3}} \sqrt{1 + \frac{r^2}{2}} \text{ to } r + z_{1-\alpha/2} \frac{(1-r^2)}{\sqrt{N-3}} \sqrt{1 + \frac{r^2}{2}}, \tag{19.9}$$

while the sample size required to estimate a planned correlation coefficient, ρ_{Plan}, with a pre-specified width, w, of the CI is now given by

$$N_S^0 = \frac{4 z_{1-\alpha/2}^2 \left(1 - \rho_{Plan}^2\right)^2 \left(1 + \frac{\rho_{Plan}^2}{2}\right)}{w^2} + 3. \tag{19.10}$$

Since the multiplier $\left(1 + \frac{\rho_{Plan}^2}{2}\right)$ will range from 1 when $\rho_{Plan} = 0$ to 1.5 when $\rho_{Plan} = 1$, sample sizes will be larger than those studies involving the Pearson correlation coefficient of the same magnitude.

A more accurate sample size estimate is provided by replacing in equation (19.6) N_P^0 by N_S^0 and in equation (19.8) θ by

$$\theta_S = \sqrt{1 + \frac{\rho_{Plan}^2}{2}}. \tag{19.11}$$

Tables 19.2 and 19.3 respectively give sample sizes for a range of pre-specified widths for the confidence intervals for the Pearson and Spearman correlation coefficients. Both tables use the more accurate approach, as does SS_S, when computing sample sizes.

19.3 Practical Considerations

Apart from α and β, all that is necessary to determine a sample size is to specify ρ_{Plan}. However, consideration should also be given to the anticipated data to be collected. These should cover as broad a range as possible for both variables concerned as the wider their ranges, the more sensitive the study will be. Thus a repeat study of that summarized in **Figure 19.1** should cover a similar (and wide) range of waist and hip circumference values. The study should not be confined to individuals close to the mean waist and hip circumference values of 72.7 and 97.3 cm respectively. Also investigators should be aware of the possible undue influence of outlier observations such as those indicated in **Figure 19.1** which are distant from the main cloud of data points. In this case, excluding these from the calculations reduces the estimated correlation to $r = 0.74$ although this has little impact on the study conclusions.

For situations in which the Spearman correlation is appropriate, it is important to have sufficient categories in both variables concerned, certainly five or more, and also to avoid tied values in each variable, which can be difficult if there are only a few categories.

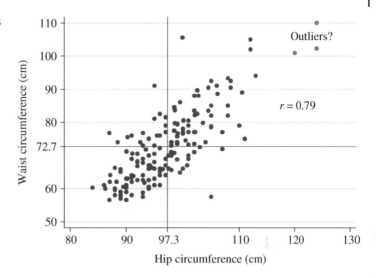

Figure 19.1 Scatter plot of waist versus hip circumference in 166 individuals. (*See insert for color representation of the figure.*)

19.4 Bibliography

Cohen (1988) described sample sizes for tests of the significance of the correlation coefficient and suggests values, in the context of epidemiological studies, indicative of small, medium and large planning values. Bonett and Wright (2000) describe the large sample approximations of equations (19.5) and (19.10) for determining sample size for a given width of the CI for the Pearson and Spearman correlation coefficients respectively. They also give the more accurate expressions for these through the appropriate use of equation (19.6) which are of particular use as $|\rho_{Plan}|$ approaches unity. These latter expressions form the basis for the sample sizes given in **Table 19.2, Table 19.3** and S_S. The differences in various methods for computing a sample size for a CI of a correlation coefficient are discussed by Moinester and Gottfried (2014).

19.5 Examples and Use of the Tables

> For one-sided test size, $\alpha = 0.05$, $z_{0.95} = 1.6449$.
> For two-sided, $\alpha = 0.05$ and 0.20, $z_{0.975} = 1.9600$ and $z_{0.90} = 1.2816$.
> For a one-sided, $1 - \beta = 0.8$, 0.9, and 0.95, $z_{0.80} = 0.8416$, $z_{0.90} = 1.2816$, and $z_{0.95} = 1.6449$ respectively.

Table 19.1 and Equations 19.1, 19.2 and 19.3

Example 19.1 Pearson correlation - Sample size - Forced expiratory volume and forced vital capacity Suppose that patients with a certain lung disease are available at a clinic and one wishes to test if there is a significant correlation between forced expiratory volume in 1 second (FEV_1) and the forced vital capacity (FVC) in these patients. A positive correlation is assumed, and so the eventual test of significance will be 1-sided. Studies in similar types of patients had suggested that the correlation might be close to 0.6.

Here setting $\rho_{Plan} = 0.6$, in the first part of equation (19.1), provides an initial value for the iteration to calculate the sample size required as $u_0 = \frac{1}{2}\log\left[\frac{1+0.6}{1-0.6}\right] = 0.6931$. Substituting this in equation (19.2), assuming a 1-sided $\alpha = 0.05$ and $1-\beta = 0.8$ and hence $z_{0.95} = 1.6449$ and $z_{0.80} = 0.8416$, gives

$$N_0 = \frac{(1.6449+0.8416)^2}{0.6931^2} + 3 = 15.9 \approx 16. \text{ Following this, } u_1 = \frac{1}{2}\log\left[\frac{1+0.6}{1-0.6}\right] + \frac{0.6}{2(16-1)} = 0.7131 \text{ with}$$

$$N_1 = \frac{(1.6449+0.8416)^2}{0.7131^2} + 3 = 15.2 \text{ or } 16 \text{ once more. Thus the iteration process needs to go no further.}$$

The same value is obtained from **Table 19.1** or directly from $^{S}S_{S}$. The study requires at least $N = 16$ subjects on which both FEV_1 and FVC are measured.

In this example the initial estimate of sample size, N_0, provides the appropriate value. Hence the iteration was unnecessary although this can only be verified to be the case by conducting this next iteration. In practice, the process usually converges after 2 iterations.

Table 19.1 and Equations 19.2 and 19.3

Example 19.2 Pearson correlation - Medium sized study – Nursing home residents
As one component of a study to validate the Harmful Behaviors Scale (HBS) as a measure of direct and indirect self-destructive behaviours in 610 nursing home residents aged 65 and older, Draper, Bridaty, Low, *et al* (2002) reported a Pearson correlation of 0.679 with the Behavioral Pathology in Alzheimer's Disease Rating Scale (BEHAVE-AD). No details of how the sample size for the study was determined are provided.

A repeat study is planned but in a smaller nursing home with residents of less challenging conditions. What sample size is required?

On the basis of the earlier study, a positive correlation is anticipated so a 1-sided test appears appropriate. The plan is to set $\alpha = 0.05$, $\beta = 0.1$, but as the patients are less challenging, a smaller correlation is anticipated so that $\rho_{Plan} = 0.3$, and the sample size is anticipated to be relatively large. Use of equation (19.3) gives $u_0 = \frac{1}{2}\log\left[\frac{1+0.3}{1-0.3}\right] = 0.3095$ and equation (19.2) gives

$$N = \frac{(1.6449+1.2816)^2}{0.3095^2} + 3 = 89.41 + 3 = 92.41 \text{ or } 93. \text{ The more accurate Table 19.1, or directly from}$$

$^{S}S_{S}$, give $N = 92$. On this basis a study of 100 patients might be conducted.

Table 19.1 and Equations 19.2 and 19.3

Example 19.3 Spearman correlation - Temporomandibular joint osteoarthritis
Cömert Kiliç, Kiliç and Sümbüllü (2015, Table 5) reported estimates of the Spearman rank correlation coefficients, ρ_S, between several clinical signs and measures assessed using cone beam computed tomography findings including the severity of osteophyte formation (*OF*) and severity of sclerosis (*S*) in the condylar head in patients with temporomandibular joint osteoarthritis. The clinical signs were assessed by the patients themselves using a Visual Analogue Scale (VAS). *OF* was determined by the length of bony outgrowth on the condyle and was then divided into 4 categories

Clinical sign	r_S	Test size, α 1-sided	Test size, α 2-sided	Power $1 - \beta$	Sample size N
Osteophyte formation (*OF*)					
Masticatory efficiency	0.073	-	0.05	0.8	1,471
Painless MIO*	0.157	-	0.05	0.8	317
Lateral motion	−0.003	-	0.05	0.8	872,096
Sclerosis (*S*)					
Masticatory efficiency	−0.264	0.05	-	0.8	88
Painless MIO*	−0.192	0.05	-	0.8	167
Lateral motion	−0.242	0.05	-	0.8	105

*MIO: Maximum inter-incisal opening.

Figure 19.2 Spearman rank correlation coefficients between clinical signs and cone beam computed tomography findings with minimal sample sizes suggested by equation (19.2) (part data from Cömert Kiliç, Kiliç and Sümbüllü, 2015, Table 5).

(Absent, <1 mm, 1-2 mm, and >2 mm). Similarly there were four categories for *S* (0: Absence, 1: Slight, with a minimal increase in Thickness of the Condylar Cortical Bone (TCCB), 2: Moderate, with a moderate increase in TCCB, 3: Extensive, with a profound increase in TCCB). The study included information from 76 patients and a selection of their findings are given in **Figure 19.2**.

The estimated Spearman correlations in **Figure 19.2** with respect to *OF* are all small and differ in sign so that it is not surprising that the use of equations (19.2) and (19.3) or S_S, with 2-sided $\alpha = 0.05$ and $1 - \beta = 0.8$ and the values given in **Figure 19.2** used as planning values, would result in the very large sample sizes indicated if a repeat study to confirm these results were to be anticipated. On the other hand, the Spearman correlations for *S* are all negative and so a 1-sided α would be appropriate. They are also larger. Both of these features result in the corresponding sample sizes being smaller than for *OF*. Nevertheless, even for the largest correlation in magnitude, $\rho_S = -0.264$ between *S* and masticatory efficiency suggests $N = 88$ patients, which is larger than the initial study involving 76 patients.

Table 19.1 and Equation 19.2

Example 19.4 Lack of association - Personality and social desirability
A psychologist wishes to plan an experiment in which medical students are asked questions from which measures of personality and social desirability can be obtained. The investigator wishes to show that these two variables are not associated. How many students must he recruit to his study?

In such a situation, the psychologist may be willing to accept that a small value of the observed correlation, say $\rho = 0.1$, indicates a lack of association. In addition a large 2-sided $\alpha = 0.2$ is chosen and small $\beta = 0.05$. From these equation (19.1) gives $u_0 = \frac{1}{2} log \left[\frac{1 + 0.1}{1 - 0.1} \right] = 0.1003$. Substituting this in equation (19.2), with $z_{0.80} = 1.2816$ and $z_{0.95} = 1.6449$, we have $N_0 = \frac{(1.2816 + 1.6449)^2}{0.1003^2} + 3 = 854.3 \approx 855$. As

N_0 is so large, no further iteration is required. **Table 19.1** gives $N = 853$. Using ${}^S S_S$ with 2-sided $\alpha = 0.2$, $1 - \beta = 0.95$ but with $\rho_{Plan} = 0.095$ (which is very close to 0.1) gives $N = 946$, while if we set $\rho_{Plan} = 0.105$ (also very close to 0.1), $N = 774$. These large disparities in sample size illustrate how crucial the planning value of the correlation coefficient is when designing a study to conclude a lack of association.

Table 19.2 and Equations 19.5, 19.6, 19.7 and 19.8

Example 19.5   Pearson - Width of confidence interval - Forced expiratory volume and forced vital capacity

Suppose the investigators in *Example 19.1* postulated $\rho_{Plan} = 0.6$ and were concerned to estimate the correlation coefficient to have a required 95% CI of width 0.2. This would imply a CI from 0.5 to 0.7. The corresponding sample size, with 2-sided $\alpha = 0.05$ and $w = 0.2$, is given from equation (19.5) as

$$N_P^0 = \frac{4 \times 1.96^2 \left(1 - 0.6^2\right)^2}{0.2^2} + 3 = 160.35 \text{ or } 161.$$ Alternatively, the more precise calculations associated

with equation (19.6) give a very similar figure of 160.53 or $N_P^{Final} = 161$ once more.

However, had the investigators postulated $\rho_{Plan} = 0.9$ then equation (19.5) indicates $N_P^0 = 17$, whereas the more accurate (19.6) gives a larger value of $N_P^{Final} = 21$.

The corresponding entries for $\rho_{Plan} = 0.6$ and 0.9 from **Table 19.2** or ${}^S S_S$ are $N_P^{Final} = 162$ and 21 respectively.

Table 19.3 and Equations 19.7, 19.8, 19.10 and 19.11

Example 19.6   Spearman – Width of confidence interval - Temporomandibular joint osteoarthritis **Figure 19.2** gives the estimated Spearman correlation coefficient between the severity of sclerosis (S) and masticatory efficiency (ME) as $r_S = -0.264$ as quoted by Cömert Kiliç, Kiliç and Sümbüllü (2015). This is based on information from $N = 76$ patients. The corresponding 95% CI calculated using equation (19.9) is from $-0.264 - 1.96 \times \dfrac{\left[1 - \left(-0.264\right)^2\right]}{\sqrt{76 - 3}} \times \sqrt{1 + \dfrac{\left(-0.264\right)^2}{2}}$ to

$-0.264 + 1.96 \times \dfrac{\left[1 - \left(-0.264\right)^2\right]}{\sqrt{76 - 3}} \times \sqrt{1 + \dfrac{\left(-0.264\right)^2}{2}}$ or -0.477 to -0.051.

This has a large width, $w = 0.477 - 0.051 \approx 0.4$. If a confirmatory study is planned with $\rho_{Plan} = -0.264$ but with a smaller $w = 0.3$, then equation (19.10) gives

$$N_S^0 = \frac{4 \times 1.96^2 \times \left[1 - \left(-0.264\right)^2\right]^2 \times \left[1 + \dfrac{\left(-0.264\right)^2}{2}\right]}{0.3^2} + 3 = 154.$$

This increases to $N_S^0 = 345$ if $w = 0.2$. For $\rho_{Plan} = -0.3$, $w = 0.2$, the sample size for a 95% CI from the more accurate **Table 19.3** and ${}^S S_S$ gives $N_S^{Final} = 335$, which is a little smaller. However, for correlations of larger magnitudes, a difference between the two approaches becomes apparent. Thus, for a 95% CI of $w = 0.2$ and $\rho_{Plan} = -0.9$, $N_S^0 = 23$, while $N_S^{Final} = 28$ or 20% larger.

References

Technical

Bonett DG and Wright TA (2000). Sample size requirements for estimating Pearson, Kendall and Spearman correlations. *Psychometrika*, **65**, 23–28.

Cohen J (1988). *Statistical Power Analysis for Behavioral Sciences*, (2nd edn) Lawrence Earlbaum, New Jersey.

Moinester M and Gottfried R (2014). Sample size estimation for correlations with pre-specified confidence interval. *The Quantitative Methods for Psychology*, **10**, 124–130.

Examples

Cömert Kiliç S, Kiliç N and Sümbüllü MA (2015). Temporomandibular joint osteoarthritis: cone beam computed tomography findings, clinical features, and correlations. *International Journal of Oral & Maxillofacial Surgery*, **44**, 1268–1274.

Draper B, Brodaty H, Low L-F, Richards V, Paton H and Lie D (2002). Self-destructive behaviors in nursing home residents. *Journal of the American Geriatrics Society*, **50**, 354–358.

Table 19.1 Sample sizes for detecting a statistically significant Pearson or Spearman correlation coefficient [Equations 19.1, 19.2 and 19.3].

	α		Power, $1-\beta$		
ρ_{Plan}	1-sided	2-sided	0.8	0.9	0.95
0.1	0.025	0.05	782	1046	1293
	0.05	0.10	617	853	1078
	0.10	0.20	450	655	853
0.2	0.025	0.05	193	258	319
	0.05	0.10	153	211	266
	0.10	0.20	112	162	211
0.3	0.025	0.05	84	112	138
	0.05	0.10	67	92	116
	0.10	0.20	50	71	92
0.4	0.025	0.05	46	61	75
	0.05	0.10	37	50	63
	0.10	0.20	28	39	50
0.5	0.025	0.05	29	37	46
	0.05	0.10	23	31	39
	0.10	0.20	18	24	31
0.6	0.025	0.05	19	25	30
	0.05	0.10	16	21	25
	0.10	0.20	12	16	21
0.7	0.025	0.05	13	17	20
	0.05	0.10	11	14	17
	0.10	0.20	9	12	14
0.8	0.025	0.05	10	12	14
	0.05	0.10	8	10	12
	0.10	0.20	7	8	10
0.9	0.025	0.05	7	8	9
	0.05	0.10	6	7	8
	0.10	0.20	5	6	7

Table 19.2 Sample sizes for a pre-specified width of the 2-sided confidence interval for a Pearson correlation coefficient [Equations 19.5, 19.6, 19.7 and 19.8].

CI Width (*w*)	0.10		0.15		0.20	
100(1 − *α*)% CI	95	99	95	99	95	99
ρ_{Plan}						
0.1	1508	2601	671	1156	378	650
0.2	1418	2446	631	1088	356	612
0.3	1275	2198	568	977	321	550
0.4	1087	1874	484	834	274	470
0.5	868	1495	388	666	220	376
0.6	634	1092	284	488	162	276
0.7	405	697	183	313	105	179
0.8	206	352	95	161	56	94
0.9	63	106	32	53	21	34

Table 19.3 Sample sizes for a pre-specified width of the 2-sided confidence interval for a Spearman correlation coefficient [Equations 19.7, 19.8, 19.10 and 19.11].

CI Width (*w*)	0.10		0.15		0.20	
100(1 − *α*)% CI	95	99	95	99	95	99
ρ_{Plan}						
0.1	1515	2614	6741	1161	380	653
0.2	1446	2495	643	1109	363	624
0.3	1332	2297	593	1021	335	575
0.4	1173	2024	523	900	295	507
0.5	976	1682	436	749	247	422
0.6	747	1287	335	575	190	325
0.7	503	866	227	388	130	221
0.8	270	464	124	211	73	123
0.9	87	148	44	73	29	47

20

Observer Agreement Studies

SUMMARY
In this chapter we describe sample size calculations for observer agreement studies, with respect to the degree of either self-agreement of a single observer assessing the same material twice or agreement between two observers both independently assessing the same specimens, for example, to make a decision with respect to a definitive diagnosis. In these situations, when binary decisions are to be made, sample sizes are then based on the pre-specified width of the confidence interval (CI) of either the estimated probability of lack of reproducibility (disagreement) or alternatively Cohen's κ statistic.
For a study design comprising two observers in which both individually assess and make a diagnosis for all of the specimens on one occasion and then make a second assessment on a random sub-sample of these, then the lack of reproducibility and disagreement are both estimated within the same study. In which case, the final sample size depends on pre-specified CI widths of each of these components.
When the measures taken by the reviewer(s) are continuous in nature, then sample size for agreement is determined by the required width of the CI for the intra-class correlation coefficient.

20.1   Introduction

Assessing the results of diagnostic procedures and the effects of therapies often involves some degree of subjective judgment. Observer agreement studies are conducted to investigate the reproducibility and level of consensus on such assessments. Typically, several observers (in general we term them readers to avoid confusion between observers and observations) make assessments on each of a series of specimens (assumed as one per subject or patient depending on the context) and their assessments are compared. For example, to examine the thickness measurement in cutaneous malignant melanoma, the two readers would evaluate histo-pathology slides from a series of patients and record their estimates of the thickness. In other circumstances, the assessments made are binary, such as a decision on the presence or absence of metastases on liver scintigraphy charts.

Initially, we consider observer agreement studies in which the specimens concerned are either re-reviewed by the same reader to check his or her own reproducibility or where two readers assess all specimens once and the agreement (often reported as disagreement) between them is determined.

However, an important concern relevant to study design is the presence of both within-reader and between-reader variation. The apparent disagreement between readers may be due to either one of these components or both. It is important to distinguish between them, as any action taken to reduce

Sample Sizes for Clinical, Laboratory and Epidemiology Studies, Fourth Edition. David Machin, Michael J. Campbell, Say Beng Tan and Sze Huey Tan.
© 2018 John Wiley & Sons Ltd. Published 2018 by John Wiley & Sons Ltd.

disagreement will depend on which type of variation dominates. To do this requires at least two readers each making at least two repeated observations of the same specimens.

Consequently, we consider observer agreement studies where (i) each reader assesses all specimens twice and (ii) where each reader assesses a proportion of the specimens twice and the remainder only once.

Observer-agreement studies are designed to estimate the level of reader agreement and so sample sizes are usually based on the achievement of sufficient precision of the estimate as expressed by the desired width of the relevant CI rather than by a test of a hypothesis.

Moreover, there are often no obvious hypotheses to test. The hypothesis of perfect agreement between readers is unrealistic as it can be refuted by a single case of disagreement and the hypothesis of agreement purely by chance is also unrealistic. Nevertheless, we describe a hypothesis testing approach to sample size for a continuous outcome in which a minimally acceptable inter-observer agreement (or reliability) is pre-specified.

20.2   Binary Outcomes

Agreement or Reproducibility

The basic structure of the study design can be either of two forms:

i) *Agreement*: two readers and a between-reader comparison of the same specimens are made.
ii) *Reproducibility*: a single reader makes two assessments of each specimen and then a within-reader comparison is made.

Suppose two readers make a diagnostic decision after examining a specimen taken from a patient; then how likely is it that the two readers draw the same diagnostic conclusion? If we assume the question is whether or not a particular disease is present or absent, then this review process generates, for each of the specimens reviewed, one of the four possible binary pairs (0, 0), (1, 0), (0, 1) and (1, 1) as indicated in **Figure 20.1**.

From **Figure 20.1**, the estimates of the proportion of times the reader(s) agree(s), π_{Agree}, or disagree, π_{DisAg}, are respectively

$$p_{Agree} = \frac{d_{00} + d_{11}}{m_{Repeat}} \quad \text{and} \quad p_{DisAg} = \frac{d_{10} + d_{01}}{m_{Repeat}}. \tag{20.1}$$

Second Review(er)	First review(er)		
	Absent (0)	Present (1)	Total
Absent (0)	d_{00}	d_{01}	
Present (1)	d_{10}	d_{11}	
Total			m_{Repeat}

Figure 20.1 Possible outcomes for (i) two readers each reviewing the same specimens only once to determine the level of between-reader disagreement or (ii) a single reader reviewing the same material on two occasions to determine their own lack of reproducibility.

Sample size

If the corresponding anticipated value for the probability of disagreement, π_{DisAg}, is not too close to zero and the sample size is anticipated to be reasonably large, then the CI for the estimate p_{DisAg} of π_{DisAg} takes the following symmetric (limits equally above and below p_{DisAg}) form

$$L = p_{DisAg} - z_{1-\alpha/2}\sqrt{\frac{p_{DisAg}\left(1-p_{DisAg}\right)}{m_{Repeat}}} \text{ to } U = p_{DisAg} + z_{1-\alpha/2}\sqrt{\frac{p_{DisAg}\left(1-p_{DisAg}\right)}{m_{Repeat}}}. \tag{20.2}$$

At the planning stage of a study, the true π_{DisAg} will be anticipated by the investigating team as π_{Plan}. In which case, the planning value of the CI width can be set as:

$$W_{Plan} = 2z_{1-\alpha/2}\sqrt{\frac{\pi_{Plan}\left(1-\pi_{Plan}\right)}{m_{Repeat}}}. \tag{20.3}$$

Thus, if the width of the anticipated $100(1-\alpha)\%$ CI of W_{DisAg} is pre-specified as W_{Plan}, then equation (20.3) can be rearranged to give the sample size required as

$$m_{Repeat} = 4\frac{\pi_{Plan}\left(1-\pi_{Plan}\right)}{W_{Plan}^2}z_{1-\alpha/2}^2 = 4\Omega_{Plan}z_{1-\alpha/2}^2. \tag{20.4}$$

This expression will not be reliable if π_{Plan} is set close to either 0 or 1. In general, as described in equation (1.19), it is better to use the *recommended* method to calculate the CIs as the corresponding L and U become increasingly more asymmetric as values of π_{DisAg} decline from 0.4 to 0.05, which is the typical range of disagreement values found in such studies. The sample size required is therefore better given by:

$$m_{Specimens} = \left[\left(2\Omega_{DisAg}-1\right) + \sqrt{\left(2\Omega_{DisAg}-1\right)^2 + \frac{1}{W_{DisAg}^2} - 1}\right]z_{1-\alpha/2}^2. \tag{20.5}$$

In **Table 20.1**, it is this latter expression which gives the sample sizes for 2-sided 90% and 95% CIs for a range of planning values for π_{DisAg} and W_{DisAg}.

Agreement and Reproducibility

If replicate observations on *some* (not necessarily all) specimens are included within the study conducted by the same two readers, then the between- and within-reader variation allows the disagreement as well as the reproducibility to be quantified.

Two readers with each reader making two assessments of each specimen

In this situation, each specimen examined by a reader, say A, has an unknown 'true' assessment, but owing to difficulties of assessment or other reasons, the reader sometimes makes an 'error' and records a result opposite to his own 'true' assessment with this probability denoted ξ_A.

Further, suppose that the true assessment of A for a particular specimen drawn at random would be to diagnose the condition as present (denoted 1) and this has the probability Θ_{A1}. The corresponding probability of diagnosing the condition as absent (denoted 0) is Θ_{A0}. Similarly for the second reader, B, we have ξ_B, Θ_{B1} and Θ_{B0}.

These probabilities can be combined into four binary-pair outcomes, to give $\Theta_{00} = \Theta_{A0} \times \Theta_{B0}$ and similarly Θ_{01}, Θ_{10} and Θ_{11} from which $\Theta_{DisAg} = \Theta_{01} + \Theta_{10}$ is the probability that the readers truly disagree. The proportion Θ_{DisAg} represents the true between-reader variation, having extracted the contribution to the disagreement made by the within-reader variation. If $\Theta_{01} = \Theta_{10} = 0$ then there is no between-reader disagreement.

Thus, a possible two stage design is that in Stage I, independently of the other, each reader assesses the same set of N specimens once. For Stage II, a random sample of a given size, m_{Repeat}, of these same specimens is selected and each reader then conducts a further review. Each reader will make $T = N + m_{Repeat}$ assessments and so $2T$ observations are recorded in all.

Within-reader variation - Reproducibility

For a reader in Stage II, the degree of reproducibility between their Stage I and Stage II reviews is quantified by the probability of making a chance error in diagnosis, ξ. This is the probability of ascribing a 0 to a diagnosis when it should be 1, or a 1 to a diagnosis that should be 0. The estimate of this probability is

$$\xi = \left(1 - \sqrt{1 - 2\pi_{DisAg}}\right) / 2, \tag{20.6}$$

where π_{DisAg} is the true proportion of specimens in which the reader differs from his or herself. This has an approximate $100(1 - \alpha)\%$ CI,

$$L = \xi - z_{1-\alpha/2} \times SE(\xi) \text{ to } U = \xi + z_{1-\alpha/2} \times SE(\xi), \tag{20.7}$$

where $SE(\xi) = \sqrt{\dfrac{\xi(1-\xi)[1-2\xi(1-\xi)]}{2(1-2\xi)^2 m_{Repeat}}}$. Thus the width of the CI is given by

$$w_\xi = 2\sqrt{\dfrac{\xi(1-\xi)[1-2\xi(1-\xi)]}{2(1-2\xi)^2 m_{Repeat}}} z_{1-\alpha/2}. \tag{20.8}$$

It follows from equation (20.8) that for a specified w_ξ set equal to w_{Plan} the requisite number of specimens to review by each reader is

$$m_{Repeat} = \dfrac{2\xi(1-\xi)[1-2\xi(1-\xi)]}{(1-2\xi)^2 w_{Plan}^2} z_{1-\alpha/2}^2. \tag{20.9}$$

Table 20.2 gives the number of specimens, m_{Repeat}, each to be assessed twice, for a range of values of ξ, w_ξ, and 2-sided CIs of 90% and 95%. In this situation, the combined number of assessments actually made by both readers is $T = 2m_{Repeat}$.

Between-reader Variation - Agreement

As each reader, A and B, makes m_{Repeat} diagnoses, estimates of the associated measures of reproducibly for each, that is ξ_A and ξ_B respectively, are obtained as well as estimates of θ_{01}, which is the probability that on the first assessment reader A says 0 and reader B says 1, and θ_{10}, which is the probability with the positions of A and B reversed. From these, the estimated probability of their disagreement is

$$\Theta_{DisAg} = \frac{\theta_{10} + \theta_{01} - \left[\left(1 - \xi_A\right)\xi_B + \xi_A\left(1 - \xi_B\right)\right]}{\left(1 - 2\xi_A\right)\left(1 - 2\xi_B\right)}. \tag{20.10}$$

At the design stage of a study, there will usually be no reason to expect one reader to have a greater error rate than the other, so we assume from now on that $\xi_A = \xi_B = \xi$. Consequently, equation (20.10) now becomes

$$\Theta_{DisAg} = \frac{\theta_{10} + \theta_{01} - 2\xi\left(1 - \xi\right)}{\left(1 - 2\xi\right)^2}. \tag{20.11}$$

It follows that the associated CI takes the form

$$L = \Theta_{DisAg} - z_{1-\alpha/2} \times SE\left(\Theta_{DisAg}\right) \text{ to } U = \Theta_{DisAg} + z_{1-\alpha/2} \times SE\left(\Theta_{DisAg}\right) \tag{20.12}$$

The corresponding expression for the $SE(\Theta_{DisAg})$ is complicated and is detailed below equation (20.13). Nevertheless, the width of the CI can be expressed algebraically and so, for the given ξ and m_{Repeat}, from equation (20.9), together with planning values of Θ and W_Θ, a sample size can be obtained. However, equation (20.11) implies that the choice of planning values of ξ and Θ should be consistent with the constraint that $(\theta_{10} + \theta_{01})$ is a probability and must therefore be < 1. So it is important to check that the particular design characteristics chosen by the investigators are consistent with this.

Sample size

As the design of the study is to estimate both *reproducibility* and *agreement*, the final sample size chosen must be sufficient to meet both these objectives. In order to achieve this, the number of specimens and the final number of repeats required for the study is established based on the following considerations. The first step is to calculate m_{Repeat} from equation (20.9). Once this is established a planning value for Θ_{DisAg} is required together with the corresponding precision, w_Θ, for the $100(1 - \gamma)\%$ CI. The required study size is then based on the following considerations.

(i) Minimise the number of specimens assessed twice by each reader

If it is desired to minimise the number of specimens assessed twice by each reader then, for the width of the $100(1 - \gamma)\%$ CI set as w_Θ, the required number is

$$N = \frac{m_{Repeat}\left(E - Bm_{Repeat}\right)}{Cm_{Repeat} - D}, \tag{20.13}$$

where $\quad B = \dfrac{G(1-2F)^2 w_\Theta^2}{4z_{1-\gamma/2}^2}$, $\quad C = \dfrac{(H-G)(1-2F)^2 w_\Theta^2}{4z_{1-\gamma/2}^2}$, $\quad D = (H-G)F(1-F)(1-2\Theta_{DisAg})^2/2, E =$

$H(H-G) + F(1-2\Theta_{DisAg})^2 \left[\dfrac{G(1-F)}{2} - H(1-2F) \right]$, with $F = 2\xi(1-\xi)$, $G = (2F - F^2)/4$ and $H =$

$\Theta_{DisAg}(1-\Theta_{DisAg}) + F(1-F)(1-2\Theta_{DisAg})^2$.

(ii) Minimise the total number of specimens

If it is desired, when all subjects are assessed twice, to minimise the total number of specimens required to achieve the desired precision in Θ_{Dis}, then the sample size is

$$N_{Eq} = \frac{4\left[\Theta_{DisAg}(1-\Theta_{DisAg})(1-2F-2F^2) + 3F^2/4 \right] z_{1-\gamma/2}^2}{w_\Theta^2 (1-2F)^2}. \tag{20.14}$$

Since $F = 2\xi(1-\xi)$, this equation depends only on specified values for ξ, Θ_{DisAg}, w_Θ and γ. **Table 20.3** gives the number of specimens, each assessed twice by each reader, required to yield a given CI width of Θ_{DisAg}.

(iii) Minimise the total number of assessments

If it is desired to minimise the total number of assessments, $T = N + m_{Repeat}$, then the optimal number of repeat assessments that achieves this is given by

$$m_{Opt} = \frac{D}{C}\left[1 + \sqrt{\frac{CE-BD}{CD-BD}} \right], \tag{20.15}$$

where B, C, D and E are defined as above. N_{Opt} is then determined from (20.13) by replacing m_{Repeat} by m_{Opt}. In some situations, equation (20.15) may give a value of m_{Opt} greater than N_{Eq}. In this case, the design with all N_{Eq} specimens assessed twice by each reader is also the design that minimises the total number of assessments, T.

Practical Issues

To assist in the planning of reader agreement studies, **Figure 20.2** lists the planning values that have to be specified in order to calculate the appropriate number of specimens required for the two readers to review. In circumstances when both reproducibility and agreement are to be assessed in one study, the numbers necessary for reproducibility may or may not be sufficient for agreement. This can only be determined by completing the calculations indicated in the 'Yes' column of **Figure 20.2** after which the different quantities m_{Repeat}, N, N_{Eq}, m_{Opt} and N_{Opt} can be compared with the planning needs of objectives (i), (ii) or (iii).

Cohen's Kappa, κ

Inter-observer agreement can also be assessed using Cohen's κ, which takes the form

$$\kappa = \frac{\pi_{Agree} - \pi_{Chance}}{1 - \pi_{Chance}} \qquad\qquad (20.16)$$

where π_{Agree} is the proportion of reader pairs exhibiting perfect agreement and π_{Chance} the proportion expected to show agreement by chance alone. From **Figure 20.1**, $p_{Agree} = (d_{00} + d_{11})/m_{Repeat}$ and so to obtain the expected agreement we use the row and column totals to estimate the expected numbers agreeing for each category.

Need to separate observer variation into between-and within-reader components	
No	Yes
Planning rate of observer disagreement: π_{DisA}, Precision required: W_{Plan} Required 2-sided CI: $(1-\alpha)\%$ Equation (20.5), **Table 20.1** Number of specimens: $m_{Specimens}$	Planning error rate for each observer: ξ Precision required: w_ξ Required 2-sided CI: $(1-\alpha)\%$ Equation (20.9), **Table 20.2** Number of duplicate observations: m_{Repeat}
Cohen's kappa	Planning rate of observer disagreement: Θ_{DisAg} Precision required: w_Θ Required 2-sided CI: $(1-\gamma)\%$
Planning value: κ Planning rate of observer disagreement: π_{DisAg}, Precision required: W_κ Required 2-sided CI: $(1-\alpha)\%$ Equation (20.18), **Table 20.4** Number of specimens: m_κ	**(i) Minimise the number of specimens assessed twice by each reader**
	Equation (20.13) Number of specimens required: N
	(ii) Minimise the total number of specimens
	Equation (20.14), **Table 20.3** m_{Repeat} and N constrained to be equal: N_{Eq}
	(iii) Minimise the total number of assessments
	Equation (20.15)
	Number of duplicate observations: m_{Opt}
	Equation (20.13)
	Number of specimens required: N_{Opt}

Figure 20.2 Steps for sample size determination for reader-agreement studies based on binary endpoints.

For a negative agreement (Absent, Absent), the expected proportion is the product of $\dfrac{d_{01}+d_{00}}{m_{Repeat}}$ and $\dfrac{d_{10}+d_{00}}{m_{Repeat}}$, giving $\dfrac{(d_{01}+d_{00})(d_{10}+d_{00})}{m_{Repeat}^2}$. Likewise, for a positive agreement, the expected propor-

tion is $\dfrac{(d_{10}+d_{11})(d_{01}+d_{11})}{m_{Repeat}^2}$. Therefore, the expected proportion of agreements for the whole table is

the sum of these two terms, that is

$$p_{Agree} = \frac{(d_{01}+d_{00})(d_{10}+d_{00})}{m_{Repeat}^2} + \frac{(d_{10}+d_{11})(d_{01}+d_{11})}{m_{Repeat}^2}. \tag{20.17}$$

Study size
Suppose the same two readers each assess every specimen independently; then, if κ is not too close to 0 or 1, for a specified width W_κ of the $100(1-\alpha)\%$ CI, the number of specimens to review is given by

$$m_\kappa = \frac{4(1-\kappa)}{W_\kappa^2}\left[(1-\kappa)(1-2\kappa)+\frac{\kappa(2-\kappa)}{2\pi_{DisAg}\left(1-\pi_{DisAg}\right)}\right]z_{1-\alpha/2}^2. \tag{20.18}$$

The planning values that have to be specified by the study design team are listed in the 'No' column of **Figure 20.2**, while **Table 20.4** gives the number of specimens required, m_κ, for a range of values of κ, π_{DisAg}, W_κ, and 2-sided CIs of 90% and 95%.

20.3 Continuous Outcomes

Intra-Class Correlation Coefficient

The intra-class correlation (ICC), ρ, is the equivalent to Cohen's κ when the readers are asked to record on a continuous rather than on a binary scale. Further, it allows more than two readers to be compared. It is defined by

$$\rho = \frac{\sigma_{Between}^2}{\sigma_{Within}^2+\sigma_{Between}^2}, \tag{20.19}$$

where σ_{Within}^2 and $\sigma_{Between}^2$ are the within- and between-reader components of the variance.

Study Size – confidence interval approach
Suppose that k readers each assess the specimens independently; then, for a pre-specified ρ_{Plan} and width of the $100(1-\alpha)\%$ CI, W_ρ, the number of specimens required is

$$m_{Specimens} = \frac{8z_{1-\alpha/2}^2\left(1-\rho_{Plan}\right)^2\left[1+(k-1)\rho_{Plan}\right]^2}{k(k-1)W_\rho^2}+1. \tag{20.20}$$

However, if $k = 2$ and $\rho_{Plan} \geq 0.7$, the number of specimens required is increased to

$$m_{Corrected} = m_{Specimens} + 5\rho_{Plan}.$$ (20.21)

The design choice implies the number of observations, $T_{Obs} = km_{Specimens}$, are to be recorded.

The number of specimens required is given in **Table 20.5** for different values of k, ρ_{Plan} and W_ρ for 90% and 95% CIs.

Study size – Hypothesis testing approach

To estimate the study size, a minimally acceptable level of inter-observer reliability, say ρ_0, has to be specified. Further, ρ_{Plan} is then set as the value that is anticipated from the study. For this purpose the effect size is

$$C_0 = \frac{1 + k\left[\dfrac{\rho_0}{1 - \rho_0}\right]}{1 + k\left[\dfrac{\rho_{Plan}}{1 - \rho_{Plan}}\right]}.$$ (20.22)

For a given number of observations, $N_{Obs} = km_{Specimens}$, the design choice corresponds to choosing a balance between the number of readers, k, and the number of specimens, $m_{Specimens}$.

The number of specimens then required for a 1-sided alternative hypothesis, and hence with 1-sided significance α and power $1 - \beta$, is given by

$$m_{Specimens} = 1 + \frac{2k\left(z_{1-\alpha} + z_{1-\beta}\right)^2}{(k-1)\left[logC_0\right]^2}.$$ (20.23)

The corresponding sample sizes are given in **Table 20.6** for a range of values of ρ_0, ρ_1 and k for 1-sided $\alpha = 0.05$ and $\beta = 0.8$ and 0.9. Although many of the entries suggest the number of specimens required may be less than (say) 10, we suggest that all planned studies should have that number as the minimum requirement.

Cautionary notes

Equation (20.23) is more sensitive to different values of ρ than (20.20) of the CI approach. For example, under a null hypothesis of $\rho_0 = 0.7$, 1-sided $\alpha = 0.05$, 1-sided $\beta = 0.2$ and $k = 3$, from equation (20.23) with $\rho_{Plan} = 0.725$, 0.75 and 0.80, we require 1,603, 374 and 80 specimens respectively. This large reduction is caused by relatively small changes to ρ_{Plan} that result in large changes of the effect size C_0 of equation (20.22), and this ultimately affects the corresponding sample size. In comparison, sample sizes required to estimate ρ with a 95% CI of $W_\rho = 0.2$ from (20.20) are 60, 52 and 36, which are relatively modest and do not differ by such a degree.

20.4   Bibliography

Newcombe and Altman (2000, pp 46-47) provide the basic requirements which lead to equation (20.5). Freedman, Parmar and Baker (1993) derive of the sample-size formulae (20.9) to (20.15). Cantor (1996) describes the situation in which π_{DisAg} is different for each of the two raters. For Cohen's

κ, Donner and Eliasziw (1992) give the $SE(\kappa)$ from which (20.18) is then derived. Cicchetti (2001) gives a general discussion of the problem of estimating a valid sample size in this area. He points out that clinically useful results can be obtained with relatively modest values of κ, and there is diminishing gain from increasing the sample size much above 100. Bonett (2002) proposed the CI approach to sample size calculation of equations (20.20) and (20.21) for the intraclass correlation coefficient, while Walter, Eliasziw and Donner (1998) suggest a hypothesis testing approach and define the effect size, C_0, of equation (20.22) for this purpose with the sample size given by equation (20.23).

20.5 Examples and Use of the Tables

Table 2.2
For two-sided test size, $\alpha = 0.05$, $z_{0.975} = 1.96$.
For one-sided test size, $\alpha = 0.05$, $z_{0.95} = 1.6449$.
For one-sided $1 - \beta = 0.8$, $z_{0.8} = 0.8416$.

Table 20.1 and Equations 20.4 and 20.5

Example 20.1   Two readers - No replicate observations - Disagreement
It is anticipated that two readers will have a probability of disagreement of approximately 25%, but it is desired to estimate this with a 95% CI of width 10%. How many observations should be made?

Here, $\pi_{DisAg} = 0.25$, $W_{Dis} = 0.1$ and hence, $\Omega_{DisAg} = \dfrac{0.25 \times (1 - 0.25)}{0.1^2} = 18.75$. Then with 2-sided $\alpha = 0.05$, equation (20.4) gives $m_{Two} = 4 \times 18.75 \times 1.96^2 = 288.12$ or 289. This agrees closely with the more precise calculations of equation (20.5), which gives $m_{Rec} = \left[[(2 \times 18.75) - 1] + \sqrt{[(2 \times 18.75) - 1]^2 + \dfrac{1}{0.1^1}} - 1 \right] \times 1.96^2 = 285.55$ or 286 as does **Table 20.1**. So for such a study, this implies that the two readers examine the same 300 specimens independently.

However, as the anticipated value of π_{DisAg} reduces in value, **Figure 20.3** shows an increasing disparity between the sample sizes obtained by (20.4) and (20.5). Further, the symmetric nature of equation (20.4) provides an impossible CI when $\pi_{DisAg} = 0.025$.

Table 20.2 and Equation 20.9

Example 20.2   Single observer error - Second assessment of specimens
A reader wishes to establish their own probability of error, ξ, for making a particular diagnosis from patient specimens and plans a study involving two assessments per specimen and judges his own probability of error as 5%. If a 95% CI of width 0.1 is specified, how many repeat observations should be made?

Here, $\xi = 0.05$, $w_\xi = 0.1$ and for 2-sided $\alpha = 0.05$, equation (20.9) gives $m_{Repeat} = \dfrac{2 \times 0.05 \times (1 - 0.05) \left[1 - (2 \times 0.05) + 2 \times 0.05^2 \right] 1.96^2}{0.1^2 (1 - (2 \times 0.05))^2} = 40.78$. This implies that the reader should repeat

π_{Dis}	m_{Two}	Anticipated 2-sided 95%CI		m_{Re}	Anticipated 2-sided 95%CI	
		L	U		L	U
0.25	289	0.200	0.300	286	0.203	0.303
0.20	246	0.150	0.250	245	0.155	0.255
0.15	196	0.100	0.200	196	0.107	0.207
0.10	139	0.050	0.150	141	0.061	0.161
0.05	73	0.000	0.100	83	0.020	0.120
0.025	38	−0.025	0.075	56	0.006	0.105
		Impossible range				

Figure 20.3 Diverging sample sizes between the Large sample, m_{Two}, and Recommended, m_{Rec}, methods for varying proportions of disagreement, π_{DisAg}, for a given width of the 95% CI $W_{DisAg} = 0.1$.

the assessments on approximately 40 specimens. Alternatively, direct entry into **Table 20.2** gives $m_{Repeat} = 41$. However if, in this example, the width of the interval was set with $w_\xi > 0.1$, then no sample size is returned in **Table 20.2** as this requirement implies the lower limit of the CI for ξ would take impossible negative values.

Tables 20.2 and 20.3 and Equations 20.9, 20.13, 20.14 and 20.15

Example 20.3 Reader reproducibility and disagreement - Urothelial dysplasia
In illustrating their methodology, Freedman, Parmar and Baker (1993) use the results of the study conducted by Richards, Parmar, Anderson, *et al* (1991) to determine agreement with respect to the presence of urothelial dysplasia as determined from biopsies. These suggest design values for individual reader error as 0.15 and for true disagreement as 0.2. Further, the width of the 95% CI for the observer error is set as 0.15, that for the true disagreement is set at 0.2, and a repeat study is planned to have two readers.

Reproducibility and disagreement
Thus, the planning values are $\xi = 0.15$, $w\xi = 0.15$ and 2-sided $\alpha = 0.05$. Then from equation (20.9), the appropriate number of specimens required to each be assessed twice by two readers is

$$m_{Repeat} = \frac{2 \times 0.15 \times (1 - 0.15) \times [1 - 2 \times 0.15 \times (1 - 0.15)]}{[1 - (2 \times 0.15)]^2 \times 0.15^2} \times 1.96^2 = 66.19 \text{ or } 67. \text{ This can also be obtained}$$

from **Table 20.2**.

Then use of equation (20.13) with $\xi = 0.15$ and $m_{Repeat} = 67$, together with $\Theta_{DisAg} = 0.2$ and $w_\Theta = 0.2$, leads to the number of specimens to be reviewed as $N = 1,164$.

Disagreement only

Alternatively, from **Table 20.3**, which tabulates equation (20.14), for a 95% CI with $\Theta_{DisAg} = 0.2$ and $w_\Theta = 0.2$, but now with reproducibility $\xi = 0.15$ given rather than to be estimated in the study, the same desired precision for Θ_{DisAg} can be obtained from $N_{Eq} = 171$ specimens each assessed twice, hence $T_{Obs} = 342$.

Using (20.15), which is anticipated to minimise T_{Obs}, gives $m_{Opt} = 550$. However, this is now greater than $N_{Eq} = 171$. As a consequence using N_{Eq}, rather than m_{Opt}, actually minimises the total number of assessments for this situation.

Table 20.4 and Equation 20.18

Example 20.4   Cohen's Kappa - Use of 5-L triage for emergency medicine

As part of a study to evaluate the 5-Level (5-L) triage conducted by nurses for suitable action with patients admitted to Accident & Emergency (A&E) hospital departments, Travers, Waller, Bowling, *et al* (2002) reported a weighted kappa statistic, κ_{Weight}, between triage nurse ratings compared to an expert consensus rating of 0.68.

Suppose this level of consensus is anticipated in a confirmatory study conducted in a different A&E setting; how large a study should be conducted?

As several authors, including Fayers and Machin (2016, p109), have expressed reservations about the use of κ_{Weight}, it is planned only to report the unweighted κ.

The investigators choose $\pi_{DisAg} = 0.35$, anticipate $\kappa_{Plan} = 0.7$ and wish to determine this with $W\kappa = 0.1$ for a 2-sided 95% CI. Then, from equation (20.18), $m_\kappa = \dfrac{4(1-0.7)}{0.1^2}\left[(1-0.7)\left[1-(2\times0.7)\right]+\dfrac{0.7(2-0.7)}{2\times0.35(1-0.35)}\right]1.96^2 = 866.66$ or 867. **Table 20.4** shows how sensitive m_κ is to the size of W_κ.

Thus, in this situation, as W_κ increases from 0.125 to 0.2, the corresponding sample size decreases quite dramatically from 555 to 217. Further, sample sizes decrease as π_{DisAg} approaches 0.5 and also decrease with an increasing anticipated κ.

The planning requirements specified in this example suggest about 900 A&E admissions are required for whom 5-L triage ratings by the nurses are to be completed, all of which are subsequently *blind* assessed by the expert panel. However, the study of Travers, Waller, Bowling, *et al* (2002) involved only 300 or so samples. In many situations large sample sizes are often difficult to obtain.

Table 20.5 and Equations 20.20 and 20.21

Example 20.5   Intraclass correlation - Confidence Interval approach - Information needs in cardiac rehabilitation

De Melo Ghisi, dos Santos, Bonin, *et al* (2014) describe a psychometric evaluation of the English language Information Needs in Cardiac Rehabilitation (INCR) scale for suitability in the Portuguese language in a random sample of 30 from 3,000 cardiac rehabilitation (CR) patients from Brazil. The test-retest reliability of the scale was evaluated by the intraclass correlation coefficient, ρ_{INCR}. A total of 55 values were reported, one for each question of the INCR scale, with a median value of 0.74 (range 0.37 to 0.93), and a minimum standard of $\rho_{INCR} = 0.7$ was set for inclusion in the (revised) final scale. In fact, 15 (27.3%) of the ICCs failed to meet this criterion but only 4 were dropped from the (revised) Portuguese version.

This is a test-retest by the same $m_{INCR} = 30$ patients. Inspection of the final column with $k = 2$ of **Table 20.5**, which tabulates equations (20.20) and (20.21), suggests that for the majority of the 55 intraclass correlations reported, the width of the corresponding 95% CIs, were they to be calculated, would exceed $W_\rho = 0.2$. This implies that the lower limit (L) of these intervals would fall below the desired threshold of $\rho_{INCR} = 0.7$, suggesting that a larger sample of patients would have been more appropriate for this study. For example, if $\rho_{INCR} = 0.7$, $k = 2$, then for a 95% CI of width $W_\rho = 0.2$, **Table 20.5** indicates that $m_{INCR} = 105$ patients would be required.

Table 20.5 and Equations 20.20 and 20.21

Example 20.6 Intra-class correlation - Confidence interval approach - Active colonic Crohn's disease

As part of a study described by D'Haens, Löwenberg, Samaan, *et al* (2015) investigating the safety and feasibility of a second generation pillcam colon capsule endoscope (PCCE-2) for assessing active colonic Crohn's disease, inter-observer agreement was undertaken of PCCE-2 recordings by independent readers. The corresponding ICC values obtained are summarised in **Figure 20.4**. Each of these ICCs has an associated width of the corresponding 95% CI in excess of $W\rho = 0.5$.

Suppose we wished to repeat the study using the ICCs originally determined for planning purposes but require to estimate ρ to within ± 0.1, that is, have a 95% CI width of $W_\rho = 0.2$. The original study includes $k = 2$ assessors and 20 recordings. How is the number of specimens required influenced by adding a further assessor?

If we take 2-sided $\alpha = 0.05$, $k = 2$, $\rho_{Plan} = 0.67$, then equation (20.20) suggests $m_{Spec} =$

$$1 + \frac{8 \times 1.96^2 (1 - 0.67)^2 \left[1 + (2 - 1) \times 0.67\right]^2}{2 \times (2 - 1) \times 0.2^2} = 117.67 \text{ or } 118 \text{ recordings are required. This is confirmed}$$

approximately by the use of **Table 20.5** with $\rho_{Plan} = 0.65$, which gives $m_{Spec} = 130$.

If an extra assessor is involved, hence $k = 3$, then the number of recordings to assess is reduced to 78. The corresponding reductions for $k = 2$ and 3 assessors for $\rho_{Plan} = 0.66$ of **Figure 20.4** are 124 to 81, and for $\rho_{Plan} = 0.61$ are 153 to 97.

Table 20.6 and Equations 20.22 and 20.23

Example 20.7 Intra-class correlation - Hypothesis testing approach - Gross motor function

Walter, Eliasziw and Donner (1998) describe a study in which therapists are assessing children with Down's syndrome using the Gross Motor Functional Measure (GMFM). This has been validated for use in children with cerebral palsy, and it was felt necessary to check its validity in children with a

Index		ICC (ρ)	95% CI
Crohn's Disease Endoscopic Index of Severity	CDEIS	0.67	0.35 to 0.86
Simple Endoscopic Score for Crohn's Disease	SES-CD	0.66	0.32 to 0.85
Global Evaluation of Lesion	GELS	0.61	0.25 to 0.83

Figure 20.4 Intraclass correlations (ICC) established when evaluating a second generation pillcam colon capsule endoscope (from D'Haens, Löwenberg, Samaan, *et al*, 2015).

different condition. Suppose the investigators were hoping for an inter-rater reliability of at least 0.85 in the study of the GMFM assessments and had determined that a reliability of 0.7 or higher would be acceptable. Hence, the null hypothesis H_0: $\rho_0 = 0.7$ and the alternative H_1: $\rho_1 = 0.85$. For practical reasons no child could be seen more than $k = 4$ times and approximately 30 children were available. Thus the design options were restricted to a choice of $k = 2$, 3 or 4.

For $\rho_0 = 0.7$, $\rho_{Plan} = 0.85$ and $k = 2$, 3 and 4, equation (20.22) gives the respective effect sizes $C_0 = 0.4594$, 0.4444 and 0.4366. For 1-sided significance of 5% and 80% power, equation (20.23)

gives when $k = 2$, $m_{Children} = 1 + \dfrac{2 \times 2 \times (1.6449 + 0.8416)^2}{(2-1)[log 0.4594]^2} = 1 + 40.9 = 41.9$ or 42. The corresponding

number of observations is $N_{Obs} = k \, m_{Children} = 84$, while for $k = 3$, $m_{Children} = 30$ and $N_{Obs} = 90$ and when $k = 4$, $m_{Children} = 26$ and $N_{Obs} = 104$ are required.

In the design with the minimum number of observations, $N_{Obs} = 84$, and so 42 children would each be seen twice. However, the restriction in numbers of children to no more than 30 eliminates the possibility of this design. In which case, the investigators might opt for $k = 3$ observations per child involving all 30 children.

Table 20.6 shows that one design that would involve 30 children concerns $\rho_0 = 0.5$, $\rho_{Plan} = 0.8$, $k = 2$ observations per child and would have 1-sided $\alpha = 0.05$ and $1 - \beta = 0.8$.

Table 20.6 and Equations 20.22 and 20.23

Example 20.8   Inter-rater reliability - Hypothesis testing approach - Spinal cord injury
Basso, Velozo, Lorenz, *et al* (2015) investigate the interrater reliability of the Neuromuscular Recovery Scale (NRS) for the spinal cord using the hypothesis testing approach. They hoped for an inter-rater reliability of at least 0.8 and specified a reliability of 0.5 or higher would be acceptable. Hence, the null hypothesis H_0: $\rho_0 = 0.5$ and the alternative H_{Alt}: $\rho_{Plan} = 0.8$. In addition, they specified that $k = 15$ raters would be involved, but in the methods section of their paper, they do not explicitly specify the values of 1-sided α and β.

For $\rho_0 = 0.5$, $\rho_{Plan} = 0.8$ and $k = 15$, equation (20.22) gives the respective effect size

$C_0 = \dfrac{1 + 15 \times [0.5 / (1 - 0.5)]}{1 + 15 \times [0.8 / (1 - 0.8)]} = 0.2623$. Assuming a 1-sided $\alpha = 0.05$ and 1-sided $\beta = 0.2$, equation

(20.23) gives $m_{Subjects} = 1 + \dfrac{2 \times 15 (1.6449 + 0.8416)^2}{(15 - 1) \times [log 0.2623]^2} = 8.40$ or 9.

Thus the number of observations to record in this study would be $N_{Obs} = k \times m_{Subjects} = 15 \times 9 = 135$. If the design had planned for $k = 10$ or even 5 raters, then C_0 increases to 0.2683 and 0.2857 respectively with corresponding values for $m_{Subjects}$ of 8.94 or 9 (as for $k = 15$) and 10.85 or 11.

Increasing the null hypothesis value to $\rho_0 = 0.6$ but retaining the other planning values gives, for the number of raters $k = 5$, 10, 15 and 20, the number of subjects required as 19.89, 16.52, 15.56 and 15.56 respectively. These are much larger than those obtained earlier but nevertheless also suggest that, as the number of raters increases, there may be little gain beyond having $k = 10$.

References

Technical

Bonett DG (2002). Sample size requirements for estimating intraclass correlations with desired precision. *Statistics in Medicine*, **21**, 1331–1335.

Cantor AB (1996). Sample size calculations for Cohen's kappa. *Psychological Methods*, **2**, 150–153.

Cicchetti DV (2001). The precision of reliability and validity estimates re-visited: distinguishing between clinical and statistical significance of sample size requirements. *Journal of Clinical and Experimental Neuropsychology*, **23**, 695–700.

Donner A and Eliasziw M (1992). A goodness-of-fit approach to inference procedures for the kappa statistic: confidence interval construction, significance-testing and sample size estimation. *Statistics in Medicine*, **11**, 1511–1519.

Fayers PM and Machin D (2016). *Quality of Life; The Assessment, Analysis and Reporting of Patient-reported Outcomes.* (3rd edn) Wiley-Blackwell, Chichester.

Freedman LS, Parmar MKB and Baker SG (1993). The design of observer agreement studies with binary assessments. *Statistics in Medicine*, **12**, 165–179.

Newcombe RG and Altman DG (2000). Proportions and their differences. In Altman DG, Machin D, Bryant TN and Gardner MJ (eds), *Statistics with Confidence*, (2nd edn) BMJ Books, London.

Walter SD, Eliasziw M and Donner A (1998) Sample size and optimal designs for reliability studies. *Statistics in Medicine*, **17**, 101–110.

Examples

Basso DM, Velozo C, Lorenz D, Suter S and Behrman AL (2015). Interrater reliability of the neuromuscular recovery scale for spinal cord injury. *Archives of Physical Medicine and Rehabilitation*, **96**, 1397–1403.

D'Haens G, Löwenberg M, Samaan MA, Franchimont D, Ponsioen C, van den Brink GR, Fockens P, Bossuyt P, Amininejad L, Rafamannar G, Lensink EM and Van Gossum AM (2015). Safety and feasibility of using the second-generation pillcam colon capsule to assess active colonic Crohn's disease. *Clinical Gastoenterology and Hepatology*, **13**, 1480–1486.

Ghisi GL, dos Santos RZ, Bonin CBD, Roussenq S, Grace SL, Oh P and Benetti M (2014). Validation of a Portuguese version of the Information Needs in Cardiac Rehabilitation (INCR) scale in Brazil. *Heart & Lung*, **43**, 192–197.

Richards B, Parmar MKB, Anderson CK, Ansell ID, Grigor K, Hall RR, Morley AR, Mostofi FK, Risdon RA and Uscinska BM (1991). Interpretation of biopsies of "normal" urothelium in patients with superficial bladder cancer. *British Journal of Urology*, **67**, 369–375.

Travers DA, Waller AE, Bowling JM, Flowers D and Tintinalli J (2002). Five-level triage system more effective than Three-level in tertiary emergency department. *Journal of Emergency Nursing*, **28**, 395–400.

Walter SD, Eliasziw M and Donner A (1998). Sample size and optimal designs for reliability studies. *Statistics in Medicine*, **17**, 101–110.

Table 20.1 Sample size, m_{Repeat}, required to observe a pre-specified confidence interval width, W_{DisAg}, for an anticipated proportion of disagreements, π_{DisAg}, between two readers [Equation 20.5].

	Confidence Interval (CI)							
	90%				95%			
	Planned width of 2-sided CI, W_{DisAg}				Planned width of 2-sided CI, W_{DisAg}			
π_{DisAg}	0.05	0.1	0.15	0.2	0.05	0.1	0.15	0.2
0.01	76	30	18	12	108	43	25	17
0.02	107	36	20	14	152	52	29	19
0.03	142	43	23	15	201	61	33	21
0.04	178	51	26	16	252	72	37	23
0.05	214	59	29	18	304	83	41	25
0.06	251	67	32	20	356	95	46	28
0.07	287	75	35	21	407	107	50	30
0.08	323	83	39	23	458	118	55	32
0.09	358	92	42	25	508	130	60	35
0.10	392	100	45	26	554	139	62	35
0.11	426	108	49	28	604	153	69	40
0.12	459	116	52	30	651	164	74	42
0.13	491	123	55	31	696	175	78	44
0.14	522	131	58	33	741	186	83	47
0.15	552	138	62	35	784	196	87	49
0.16	582	146	65	36	826	206	92	51
0.17	611	153	68	38	867	216	96	54
0.18	639	159	71	40	907	226	100	56
0.19	666	166	73	41	945	236	104	58
0.20	692	172	76	43	982	245	108	60
0.25	810	202	89	49	1,150	286	126	70
0.30	907	226	99	55	1,288	320	141	78
0.35	983	244	107	60	1,395	347	152	84
0.40	1,037	258	113	63	1,472	366	161	89
0.45	1,069	266	117	65	1,518	377	166	92
0.50	1,080	268	118	65	1,533	381	167	93

Table 20.2 Required number of specimens each assessed twice, $m_{Specimens}$, by two readers to yield a confidence interval of a given width, w_ξ, for the probability of making a chance error in diagnosis, ξ. [Equation 20.9].

| | Planned width of 2-sided 90% CI, w_ξ | | | | | Planned width of 2-sided 95% CI, w_ξ | | | | |
ξ	0.1	0.125	0.15	0.175	0.2	0.1	0.125	0.15	0.175	0.2
0.05	29	–	–	–	–	41	–	–	–	–
0.06	35	–	–	–	–	50	–	–	–	–
0.07	42	27	–	–	–	59	38	–	–	–
0.08	49	31	22	–	–	69	44	32	–	–
0.09	56	36	25	18	–	79	51	35	18	–
0.10	63	40	28	21	16	89	57	40	29	23
0.11	71	45	32	23	18	100	64	45	33	25
0.12	79	50	35	26	20	111	71	50	37	28
0.13	87	56	39	29	22	123	79	55	41	31
0.14	96	62	43	32	24	136	87	61	45	34

Table 20.2 (Continued)

ξ	Planned width of 2-sided 90% CI, w_ξ					Planned width of 2-sided 95% CI, w_ξ				
	0.1	0.125	0.15	0.175	0.2	0.1	0.125	0.15	0.175	0.2
0.15	105	68	47	35	27	149	96	67	49	38
0.16	116	74	52	38	29	164	105	73	54	41
0.17	126	81	56	42	32	179	115	80	59	45
0.18	138	88	62	45	35	196	125	87	64	49
0.19	150	96	67	49	38	213	137	95	70	54
0.20	164	105	73	54	41	233	149	104	76	59
0.21	179	115	80	59	45	254	163	113	83	64
0.22	195	125	87	64	49	277	177	123	91	70
0.23	213	136	95	70	54	302	193	134	99	76
0.24	232	149	104	76	58	330	211	147	108	83
0.25	254	163	113	83	64	361	231	161	118	91

Table 20.3 Total number of specimens, N, required, each assessed twice by each reader, to yield a given confidence interval width of the probability of their disagreement, Θ_{DisAg}. [Equation 20.14].

Θ_{DisAg}	ξ	Planned width of 2-sided 90% CI, w_Θ				Planned width of 2-sided 95% CI, w_Θ			
		0.05	0.1	0.15	0.2	0.05	0.1	0.15	0.2
0.10	0.05	515	129	58	33	732	183	82	46
	0.10	804	201	90	51	1,142	286	127	72
	0.15	1,464	366	163	92	2,078	520	231	130
0.15	0.05	711	178	79	45	1,010	253	113	64
	0.10	1,032	258	115	65	1,466	367	163	92
	0.15	1,707	427	190	107	2,424	606	270	152
0.20	0.05	881	221	98	56	1,251	313	139	79
	0.10	1,230	308	137	77	1,746	437	194	110
	0.15	1,918	480	214	120	2,723	681	303	171
0.25	0.05	1,025	257	114	65	1,455	364	162	91
	0.10	1,397	350	156	88	1,984	496	221	124
	0.15	2,097	525	233	132	2,977	745	331	187
0.30	0.05	1,142	286	127	72	1,622	406	181	102
	0.10	1,534	384	171	96	2,178	545	242	137
	0.15	2,243	561	250	141	3,184	796	354	199
0.35	0.05	1,234	309	138	78	1,752	438	195	110
	0.10	1,640	410	183	103	2,329	583	259	146
	0.15	2,356	589	262	148	3,345	837	372	210
0.40	0.05	1,299	325	145	82	1,844	461	205	116
	0.10	1,716	429	191	108	2,437	610	271	153
	0.15	2,437	610	271	153	3,460	865	385	217
0.45	0.05	1,338	335	149	84	1,900	475	212	119
	0.10	1,762	441	196	111	2,501	626	278	157
	0.15	2,486	622	277	156	3,529	883	393	221
0.50	0.05	1,351	338	151	85	1,919	480	214	120
	0.10	1,777	445	198	112	2,523	631	281	158
	0.15	2,502	626	278	157	3,553	889	395	223

Table 20.4 Number of specimens required, m_κ, to observe a given confidence interval width for inter-observer agreement using Cohen's Kappa, κ [Equation 20.18].

If $\pi_{DiAgs} > 0.5$ enter the table with $1 - \pi_{DisAg}$.

		Planned width of 2-sided 90% CI, W_κ					Planned width of 2-sided 95% CI, W_κ				
π_{DisAg}	κ	0.1	0.125	0.15	0.175	0.2	0.1	0.125	0.15	0.175	0.2
0.05	0.4	4,453	2,850	1,979	1,454	1,114	6,322	4,046	2,810	2,065	1,581
	0.5	4,272	2,735	1,899	1,395	1,068	6,066	3,882	2,696	1,981	1,517
	0.6	3,794	2,428	1,686	1,239	949	5,386	3,447	2,394	1,759	1,347
	0.7	3,071	1,966	1,365	1,003	768	4,361	2,791	1,938	1,424	1,091
	0.8	2,162	1,384	961	706	541	3,069	1,964	1,364	1,003	768
	0.9	1,120	717	498	366	280	1,589	1,017	707	519	398
0.10	0.4	2,387	1,528	1,061	1,061	597	3,389	2,169	1,507	1,107	848
	0.5	2,255	1,443	1,003	737	564	3,202	2,049	1,423	1,046	801
	0.6	1,986	1,271	883	649	497	2,820	1,805	1,253	921	705
	0.7	1,603	1,026	713	524	401	2,276	1,457	1,012	743	569
	0.8	1,129	723	502	369	283	1,603	1,026	713	524	401
	0.9	587	376	261	192	147	833	534	371	272	209
0.15	0.4	1,708	1,093	759	558	427	2,425	1,552	1,078	792	607
	0.5	1,592	1,019	708	520	398	2,260	1,447	1,004	738	565
	0.6	1,392	891	619	455	348	1,976	1,265	879	646	494
	0.7	1,120	717	498	366	280	1,590	1,018	707	520	398
	0.8	789	505	351	258	198	1,121	717	498	366	281
	0.9	412	264	183	135	103	585	374	260	191	147
0.20	0.4	1,377	882	612	450	345	1,955	1,251	869	639	489
	0.5	1,269	812	564	415	318	1,801	1,153	801	588	451
	0.6	1,102	706	490	360	276	1,565	1,002	696	511	392
	0.7	885	566	394	289	222	1,256	804	559	410	314
	0.8	624	399	278	204	156	886	567	394	290	222
	0.9	327	209	145	107	82	464	297	206	152	116
0.25	0.4	1,187	760	528	388	297	1,685	1,078	749	550	422
	0.5	1,083	693	481	354	271	1,537	984	683	502	385
	0.6	936	599	416	306	234	1,328	850	591	434	332
	0.7	749	480	333	245	188	1,064	681	473	348	266
	0.8	529	338	235	173	133	750	480	334	245	188
	0.9	278	178	124	91	70	394	252	175	129	99

Table 20.4 (Continued)

If $\pi_{DisAg} > 0.5$ enter the Table with $1 - \pi_{DisAg}$. Each cell gives the number of specimens, m_κ.

π_{DisAg}	κ	Planned width of 2-sided 90% CI, W_κ					Planned width of 2-sided 95% CI, W_κ				
		0.1	0.125	0.15	0.175	0.2	0.1	0.125	0.15	0.175	0.2
0.30	0.4	1,068	684	475	349	267	1,516	970	674	495	379
	0.5	967	619	430	316	242	1,372	879	610	448	343
	0.6	832	532	370	208	208	1,181	756	525	386	296
	0.7	665	426	296	217	167	944	604	420	309	236
	0.8	469	301	209	154	118	666	426	296	218	167
	0.9	247	158	110	81	62	350	224	156	115	88
0.35	0.4	992	635	441	324	248	1,408	901	626	460	352
	0.5	892	571	397	292	223	1,267	811	563	414	317
	0.6	765	490	340	250	192	1,086	695	483	355	272
	0.7	611	391	272	200	153	867	555	386	283	217
	0.8	431	276	192	141	108	612	392	272	200	153
	0.9	227	146	101	75	57	323	207	144	106	81
0.40	0.4	944	604	420	309	236	1,340	858	596	438	335
	0.5	846	542	376	277	212	1,201	769	534	392	301
	0.6	723	463	322	237	181	1,027	657	457	336	257
	0.7	577	369	257	189	145	819	524	364	268	205
	0.8	407	261	181	133	102	578	370	257	189	145
	0.9	215	138	96	71	54	305	195	136	100	77
0.45	0.4	918	588	408	300	230	1,303	834	579	426	326
	0.5	820	525	365	268	205	1,165	746	518	381	292
	0.6	700	448	312	229	175	994	637	442	325	249
	0.7	558	358	248	183	140	793	507	353	259	199
	0.8	394	253	176	129	99	560	358	249	183	140
	0.9	208	133	93	68	52	296	189	132	97	74
0.50	0.4	910	582	405	297	228	1,291	827	574	422	323
	0.5	812	520	361	266	203	1,153	738	513	377	289
	0.6	693	444	308	227	174	984	630	438	322	246
	0.7	552	354	246	181	138	784	502	349	256	196
	0.8	390	250	174	128	98	554	355	246	181	139
	0.9	206	132	92	68	52	292	187	130	96	73

Table 20.5 Sample sizes required to estimate an intra-class correlation for a pre-specified confidence interval width [Equations 20.20 and 20.21].

Each cell gives the number of specimens, $m_{Specimens}$. Hence, the total number of observations for the study is $T_{Obs} = k \times m_{Specimens}$.

CI	k	ρ_{Plan}	0.05	0.075	0.1	0.125	0.15	0.175	0.2
						Planned width of 2-sided CI, W_ρ			
90%	2	0.60	1,775	790	445	285	199	146	112
		0.65	1,445	643	362	232	162	119	92
		0.70	1,131	505	286	185	130	97	75
		0.75	834	374	212	138	97	73	57
		0.80	567	255	146	95	68	51	41
		0.85	339	154	85	59	43	33	27
	3	0.60	1,119	498	281	180	126	93	71
		0.65	937	417	235	151	105	78	60
		0.70	750	334	189	121	85	63	48
		0.75	565	252	142	92	64	48	37
		0.80	392	175	99	64	45	33	26
		0.85	238	107	61	39	28	21	16
	4	0.60	907	404	228	146	102	75	58
		0.65	771	343	194	125	87	64	50
		0.70	626	279	158	101	71	52	41
		0.75	478	213	121	78	54	40	31
		0.80	335	150	85	55	39	29	22
		0.85	206	92	53	34	24	18	14
95%	2	0.60	2,519	1,120	631	404	281	207	159
		0.65	2,051	913	514	329	229	169	130
		0.70	1,604	716	405	261	183	136	105
		0.75	1,182	528	299	193	136	101	79
		0.80	802	360	205	133	94	71	55
		0.85	479	216	120	81	58	44	35
	3	0.60	1,588	707	398	255	178	131	101
		0.65	1,329	592	333	214	149	110	84
		0.70	1,064	474	267	171	120	88	68
		0.75	802	357	202	130	90	67	52
		0.80	555	248	140	90	63	47	36
		0.85	338	151	86	55	39	29	23
	4	0.60	1,286	573	323	207	144	106	82
		0.65	1,094	487	275	176	123	91	70
		0.70	887	395	223	143	100	74	57
		0.75	678	302	171	110	77	57	44
		0.80	475	212	120	77	54	40	31
		0.85	292	131	74	48	34	25	20

Table 20.6 Sample sizes required to observe a given intra-class correlation using the hypothesis testing approach with 1-sided $\alpha = 0.05$ for different numbers of readers, k [Equations 20.22 and 20.23].

Each cell gives the number of specimens required, $m_{Specimens}$. Hence, the total number of observations for the study is $T = k \times m_{Specimens}$.

		Power $1-\beta=0.8$					Power $1-\beta=0.9$				
		Number of readers, k					Number of readers, k				
ρ_0	ρ_1	2	3	4	5	10	2	3	4	5	10
0.1	0.2	591	252	157	115	55	818	349	217	159	76
	0.3	143	65	43	33	18	197	90	59	45	24
	0.4	61	30	20	16	10	83	41	28	22	13
	0.5	32	17	12	10	7	44	23	16	13	8
	0.6	19	11	8	7	5	26	14	11	9	6
	0.7	12	7	6	5	4	16	10	7	6	5
	0.8	8	5	4	4	3	10	6	5	5	4
	0.9	5	4	3	3	2	6	4	4	3	3
0.2	0.3	544	262	178	140	82	752	362	246	193	113
	0.4	128	65	46	37	24	177	90	64	51	32
	0.5	53	29	21	18	12	73	39	29	24	16
	0.6	27	16	12	10	7	37	21	16	14	10
	0.7	15	10	8	7	5	21	13	10	9	7
	0.8	9	6	5	5	4	12	8	6	6	5
	0.9	5	4	3	3	3	7	5	4	4	3
0.3	0.4	476	252	184	151	101	659	349	254	209	139
	0.5	109	61	46	38	27	150	84	63	53	37
	0.6	44	26	20	17	13	60	35	27	23	17
	0.7	21	10	11	9	7	29	18	14	13	10
	0.8	11	6	6	6	5	15	10	8	7	6
	0.9	6	4	4	4	3	8	6	5	4	4
0.4	0.5	393	226	173	147	107	544	312	239	204	148
	0.6	87	52	41	36	27	119	71	56	49	37
	0.7	33	21	17	15	12	45	28	23	20	16
	0.8	15	10	9	8	6	20	13	11	10	8
	0.9	7	5	5	4	4	9	7	6	5	5
0.5	0.6	300	184	147	129	99	415	255	203	178	137
	0.7	63	40	33	29	23	86	55	45	40	32
	0.8	22	15	13	11	9	30	20	17	15	12
	0.9	9	6	6	5	5	12	8	7	7	6
0.6	0.7	205	134	110	99	80	284	184	152	136	110
	0.8	39	27	22	20	17	54	36	31	28	23
	0.9	12	9	7	7	6	16	11	10	9	8
0.7	0.8	117	80	68	62	52	162	110	94	85	71
	0.9	18	13	12	11	9	25	18	16	14	12
0.8	0.9	46	33	29	27	23	63	45	39	36	31

21

Reference Intervals and Receiver Operating Curves

SUMMARY

An important part of the process of examining a patient is to check clinical measures taken from the patient against a 'normal' or 'reference' range of values. Evidence of the measure lying outside these values may be taken as indicative of the need for further investigation. In this chapter we describe sample sizes for establishing such reference intervals. The value of disease screening tests are often summarised by their sensitivity and specificity, and so sample sizes for comparing a diagnostic test's sensitivity to that of a standard as well as for the comparison between two tests are given. We also describe sample size calculations for determining receiver operating curves which are utilised for distinguishing diseased from non-diseased subjects.

21.1   Introduction

When a physician is in the process of establishing a diagnosis in a patient who presents with particular symptoms, the patient may be subjected to a series of tests, the results from which may then suggest an appropriate course of action. For example, a patient complaining of not feeling well may be tested for the presence of a bacterium in their urine. On the basis of the reading obtained, the patient may then be compared with the normal range of values expected from healthy individuals, and if the patient's values are outside the range, then infection is suspected. It is this infection that is then presumed to be the cause of 'not feeling well'.

The objective of a study to establish a normal range or reference interval (RI) is to define the interval for a particular clinical measurement within which the majority of values, often 95%, of a defined population will lie.

Such an interval is then used as a screen in a clinical context to identify patients presenting with particular symptoms that are 'outside' this interval—the purpose being to give an indication of a possible pathology causing their symptoms. However, for truly diagnostic purposes, merely being outside the RI is not sufficient as it is necessary to know the range of values of patients with the disease in question rather than the range for the general population at large. For example, in patients suspected of liver cancer, it is routine to take blood samples from which their α-feta protein (AFP) levels are determined. A high level is indicative of liver cancer although further and more detailed examination may be required to confirm the presumed diagnosis. The judgement as to whether or not a particular patient has a high AFP is made by comparison with AFP measured in individuals who are known to be free of the disease in question. In most circumstances, the range of values of

Sample Sizes for Clinical, Laboratory and Epidemiology Studies, Fourth Edition. David Machin, Michael J. Campbell, Say Beng Tan and Sze Huey Tan.
© 2018 John Wiley & Sons Ltd. Published 2018 by John Wiley & Sons Ltd.

AFP in patients who do indeed have liver cancer will overlap with those from healthy subjects who are presumed free of the disease. In view of this overlap, and to help distinguish the diseased from the non-diseased, receiver operating curves (ROC) are constructed to help determine the best cut-point value of the measure of concern for definitive diagnosis.

In clinical practice, diagnostic tests are never used in healthy persons but only in groups for which the need for the diagnostic test is indicated. These will include some patients without the disease in question and others with the disease present at various levels of severity. Consequently, the best approach to evaluate the diagnostic accuracy of a new diagnostic test is to use a sample of patients for whom the test is indicated. A careful description of the eligibility characteristics of this group needs to be provided. The patients in this group will undergo the new diagnostic test and also the reference test by which they will be categorised as non-diseased or diseased. The reference test is usually the currently accepted best available and feasible diagnostic tool to determine the presence or absence of the disease in question. Thus, for every patient, there are their test results and the ultimate clinical decision on their diagnosis.

21.2   Reference Intervals

Choosing the Subjects

Samples are taken from populations of individuals to provide estimates of the parameters of which we are interested—in our situation the cut-off-point(s) of the Reference Interval (RI) indicating boundaries of high (and/or low) values. The purpose of summarising the behaviour of a particular group is usually to draw some inference about a wider population of which the group is a sample. Thus although a group of volunteers may comprise the sample and are duly investigated, the usual object is to represent the RI of the general population as a whole. The wider population will include the healthy as well as those who are not. As a consequence, it is clearly important that the 'volunteers' are chosen carefully so that they do indeed reflect the population as a whole and not a particular subset of that population. If the 'volunteers' are selected at random from the population of interest then the calculated RI will be an estimate of the true RI of that population. If they are not, then it is no longer clear what the interval obtained represents and at worst it may not even be appropriate for clinical use.

Normal Distribution

If the continuous variable that has been measured has a Normal distribution, then the data $x_1, x_2, ..., x_N$ from the N subjects can be summarised by the sample mean, $\bar{x}$, and sample SD, s. These provide estimates of the associated population mean, μ and σ, respectively.

In this situation, the $100 (1 - \alpha)$% RI is estimated by

$$\bar{x} - z_{1-\alpha/2}s \text{ to } \bar{x} + z_{1-\alpha/2}s. \tag{21.1}$$

Often a 95% RI is required in which case $\alpha = 0.05$ and, from **Table 1.1**, $z_{1-\alpha/2} = z_{0.975} = 1.96$.

If we denote the cut-points defining the lower and upper limits of this RI by R_{Lower} and R_{Upper}, then its width is

$$W_{RI} = R_{Upper} - R_{Lower} = 2z_{1-\alpha/2}s. \tag{21.2}$$

Study size

A key property of any RI is the precision with which the cut-points are estimated. Thus of particular relevance to design are the width of the CIs for the estimated cut-points R_{Lower} and R_{Upper}. If the sample is large ($N > 100$), then the standard error (SE) of these cut points is

$$SE\left(R_{Lower}\right) = SE\left(R_{Upper}\right) = \sigma\sqrt{\frac{3}{N}} = 1.7321\frac{\sigma}{\sqrt{N}} \tag{21.3}$$

Thus the approximate $100(1 - \gamma)\%$ CI for the true cut at R_{Lower} is

$$R_{Lower} - z_{1-\gamma/2} \times 1.7321\frac{s}{\sqrt{N}} \text{ to } R_{Lower} + z_{1-\gamma/2} \times 1.7321\frac{s}{\sqrt{N}}, \tag{21.4}$$

and there is a similar expression for R_{Upper}. The width of each of these CIs is

$$W_{Cut} = 2 \times z_{1-\gamma/2} \times 1.7321\frac{s}{\sqrt{N}}. \tag{21.5}$$

One design criteria for determining an appropriate study size to establish a RI is to fix a value for the ratio of W_{Cut} to W_{RI}. The design therefore sets $\rho_{Plan} = \dfrac{W_{Cut}}{W_{RI}}$ to some pre-specified value. In this case it follows, from dividing equation (21.5) by (21.2) and rearranging, that the sample size is estimated by

$$N = 3\left[\frac{z_{1-\gamma/2}}{\rho_{Plan} z_{1-\alpha/2}}\right]^2. \tag{21.6}$$

For the particular case when $\alpha = \gamma$, equation (21.6) simplifies to

$$N = \frac{3}{\rho_{Plan}^2}. \tag{21.7}$$

Values of N for differing ratios, ρ, for combinations of CIs of 80%, 90% and 95% for the cut-point and 90%, 95% and 99% RIs are given in **Table 21.1**.

Non-normal Situation

Logarithmic transformation

If the continuous data do not have a Normal distribution then, in some circumstances, a logarithmic transformation of the data may have to be made. In which case, the RI for $y = log\, x$ will take the form of equation (21.1) but with y replacing x in the calculation of the mean and SD. However, the corresponding RI on the x-scale is then obtained from the antilogarithms of the lower and upper limits of this range. That is, the RI for x is

$$exp\left(\bar{y} - z_{1-a/2}s_y\right) \text{ to } exp\left(\bar{y} + z_{1-a/2}s_y\right). \tag{21.8}$$

Nevertheless, the sample size can still be estimated by equations (21.6) and (21.7) if the width of the RI is provided.

Ranked data

If the continuous data cannot be transformed to the Normal distribution form, then a RI can still be calculated. In this case, the data $x_1, x_2, \ldots x_N$ are first ranked from largest to smallest. These are then labelled $x_{(1)}, x_{(2)}, \ldots x_{(j)}, \ldots, x_{(N)}$. The lower limit of the $100(1 - \alpha)$% RI is then $x_{(j)}$, where $j = N\alpha/2$ (interpolating between adjacent observations if $N\alpha/2$ is not an integer). Similarly, the upper limit is the observation corresponding to $j = N(1 - \alpha/2)$. These limits provide an *empirical* RI.

The ranks of the lower and upper limits of a $100(1 - \gamma)$% CI for any quantile q are:

$$r_q = Nq - \left[z_{1-\gamma/2} \times \sqrt{Nq(1-q)} \right] \qquad (21.9)$$
$$s_q = 1 + Nq + \left[z_{1-\gamma/2} \times \sqrt{Nq(1-q)} \right].$$

Once these values are rounded to the nearest integer, they provide the r_qth and s_qth observations in this ranking and hence the relevant lower and upper confidence limits. To determine those for R_{Lower}, one sets $q = \alpha/2$ in equation (21.9), and for R_{Upper}, $q = 1 - \alpha/2$ is used.

However, these are the *ranks* of the observed values corresponding to R_{Lower} and R_{Upper}, not the values themselves, and so there is no equivalent algebraic form to W_{Cut} of equation (21.5) in this case. However, an approximate *SE* is provided that is appropriate for quantiles estimated using ranks *but* assuming these ranks had arisen from data having a Normal distribution form. This gives, in place of equation (21.3),

$$SE\left(R_{Lower}\right) = SE\left(R_{Upper}\right) = \eta \frac{\sigma}{\sqrt{N}}, \qquad (21.10)$$

where

$$\eta = \frac{\sqrt{(\gamma/2)\left[1 - (\gamma/2)\right]}}{\phi_{1-\gamma/2}}, \qquad (21.11)$$

and $\phi_{1-\gamma/2} = \frac{1}{\sqrt{2\pi}} exp\left(-\frac{1}{2} z_{1-\gamma/2}^2\right)$ is the height of the Normal distribution of **Figure 1.1** at $z_{1-\gamma/2}$.

Thus, an approximation to the $100(1 - \gamma)$% CI for the true R_{Lower} of the $100(1 - \alpha)$% RI is

$$R_{Lower} - z_{1-\gamma/2} \times \eta \frac{\sigma}{\sqrt{N}} \text{ to } R_{Lower} + z_{1-\gamma/2} \times \eta \frac{\sigma}{\sqrt{N}}. \qquad (21.12)$$

This CI has width

$$W = 2z_{1-\gamma/2} \times \eta \frac{\sigma}{\sqrt{N}}. \qquad (21.13)$$

Study size

Sample size is determined by first using equation (21.6) to give $N_{Initial}$ and then this is inflated to give

$$N_{Rank} = \frac{\eta}{\sqrt{3}} N_{Initial} = \sqrt{3}\eta \left[\frac{z_{1-\gamma/2}}{\rho_{Plan} z_{1-\alpha/2}} \right]^2. \tag{21.14}$$

This will lead to a larger study size to establish a RI than is given by (21.6). This is why, if at all possible, transforming the scale of measurement to one that is approximately Normal in distribution is very desirable.

Values of N_{Rank} for differing ratios, ρ, for combinations of CIs of 80%, 90% and 95% for the cut-point and 90%, 95% and 99% RIs are given in **Table 21.2**.

21.3 Sensitivity and Specificity

Diagnostic test results are often given in the form of a continuous variable, such as diastolic blood pressure or haemoglobin level. However, for the purposes of diagnosis of a particular disease or condition, a cut-point along this scale is required. Thus, for every laboratory test or diagnostic procedure with the corresponding cut-point chosen, if the disease is present the probability that the test will be positive is required. The sensitivity of the test, Se, is the proportion of those with the disease who also have a positive test result. Conversely, if the disease is absent, the probability that the test result will be negative is required. Thus the specificity of the test, Sp, is the proportion of those without the disease who also have a negative test result.

One Sample Design

Sample size

In this situation, if the proportion anticipated to have the disease is $\pi_{Disease}$, then the number of subjects, $N_{Subjects}$, necessary to show that a given Se_{Plan} differs from a target value, Se_{Known}, for a given 1-sided significance level α and a power $(1 - \beta)$ is given by

$$N_{Subjects} = \frac{\left\{ z_{1-\alpha/2} \sqrt{Se_{Known}(1 - Se_{Known})} + z_{1-\beta} \sqrt{Se_{Plan}(1 - Se_{Plan})} \right\}^2}{\pi_{Disease}(Se_{Plan} - Se_{Known})^2}. \tag{21.15}$$

Table 21.3 gives $N_{Subjects}$ for differing values of Se_{Known}, Se_{Plan} and $\pi_{Disease}$ for 1-sided $\alpha = 0.05$ and $1 - \beta = 0.8$ and 0.9.

This is a large sample approximation and Li and Fine (2004) have indicated how the exact method using the binomial probabilities may be calculated. Their methodology is implemented in $^{SS}_{SS}$.

Two Sample Design

Independent groups

If two diagnostic tests, say A and B, are to be compared then the total number of individuals required, randomised on a 1: φ basis, is given by

$$N_{Subjects} = \left(\frac{1+\varphi}{\varphi}\right) \frac{\left\{z_{1-\alpha/2}\sqrt{\left[(1+\varphi)\overline{Se}(1-\overline{Se})\right]} + z_{1-\beta}\sqrt{\left[\varphi Se_A(1-Se_A) + Se_B(1-Se_B)\right]}\right\}^2}{\pi_{Disease}(Se_B - Se_A)^2}. \tag{21.16}$$

where $\overline{Se} = (Se_A + \varphi Se_B)/(1+\varphi)$. Hence the number of tests required in the two groups are $n_A = N_{Subjects}/(1+\varphi)$ and $n_B = \varphi N_{Subjects}/(1+\varphi)$ respectively.

Table 21.4 gives $N_{Subjects}$ for differing values of Se_A, Se_B and $\pi_{Disease}$ for 1-sided $\alpha = 0.05$ and $1 - \beta = 0.8$ and 0.9.

Paired design

If two diagnostic tests are to be compared but both tests are conducted within the same subjects, then this is a paired design. In this case each subject has two diagnostic outcomes determined, one from A the other from B. These may or may not agree with each other. Given a significance level α and a power $(1 - \beta)$, the number of subjects required is

$$N_{Subjects} = \frac{\left\{z_{1-\alpha/2}\Lambda + z_{1-\beta}\sqrt{\Lambda^2 - \zeta^2(3+\Lambda)/4}\right\}^2}{\pi_{Disease}\Lambda\zeta^2}, \tag{21.17}$$

where $\Lambda = (1 - Se_A)Se_B + (1 - Se_B)Se_A$ and $\zeta = (1 - Se_A)Se_B - (1 - Se_B)Se_A$.

Table 21.5 gives $N_{Subjects}$ for differing values of Se_A, Se_B and $\pi_{Disease}$ for 1-sided $\alpha = 0.05$ and $1 - \beta = 0.8$ and 0.9.

It is important to stress that once the sample size to receive both tests has been established then the order in which they are determined from the patient should be randomised half to have Test A followed by Test B and half in the reverse order.

21.4 Receiver Operating Curvess

When a diagnostic test produces a continuous measurement, then a diagnostic cut-point is selected. This is then used ultimately to divide future subjects into those who are suspected of having the disease and those who are not. This diagnostic cut-point is determined by first calculating Se and Sp at each potential cut-point along the measurement scale.

The Se of a diagnostic test is the proportion of those *with* the disease who also have a positive diagnostic result. It is also termed the True Positive Rate (TPR). On the other hand, the Sp is the proportion of those *without* the disease who also have a *negative* result, that is, they do not have the disease and their test is beneath the cut-point. Those who do not have the disease but have a test value above the cut-point are termed False Positive (FP). The corresponding rate $FPR = (1 - Sp)$.

Once a study is completed, Se on the (vertical) y-axis is plotted against $(1 - Sp)$ on the (horizontal) x-axis for each possible cut-point to produce the Receiver Operating Curve (ROC).

In order to divide the diseased from the non-diseased, the final (diagnostic) cut-point, *Cut*, chosen is usually made at a point that provides a sensible balance between Se and Sp. For a particular test this requires an assessment of the relative medical consequences, and costs, of making a FP diagnosis of the presence of a disease or a false negative (FN) diagnosis and thereby not diagnosing a disease that is indeed present.

A perfect diagnostic test would be one with no FP or no FN outcomes and the corresponding ROC would be represented by a line that starts at the origin and follows the y-axis to a $Se = 1$, while keeping a FPT of $(1 - Sp) = 0$, and then moves horizontally parallel to the x-axis until it reaches $(1 - Sp) = 1$.

A test that produces FP results at the same rate as FN results would produce a ROC on the diagonal line $y = x$.

Study size

Because evaluation of a diagnostic test is determined through the ROC, this requires two subject groups, the diseased and the non-diseased. If the objective of a study is to determine the area, AUC, under a ROC, then the corresponding estimated $100(1 - \alpha)\%$ CI is given by

$$AUC - z_{1-\alpha/2} \frac{\sigma}{\sqrt{m_{Disease}}} \text{ to } AUC + z_{1-\alpha/2} \frac{\sigma}{\sqrt{m_{Disease}}}. \tag{21.18}$$

Here, σ is the SD and it is a rather complex function of the anticipated ratio of non-diseased subjects to diseased patients, $R = m_{Non-disease}/m_{Disease}$, and the required Se (the TPR) and Sp (FPR). It is given by

$$\sigma = \frac{1}{2\sqrt{\pi}} exp\left[-\frac{1}{4}Z^2\right] \sqrt{\left(1 + \frac{1}{R} + \frac{5Z^2}{8} + \frac{Z^2}{8R}\right)}, \tag{21.19}$$

where $Z = z_{1-FPR} - z_{1-TPR}$ can be evaluated using **Table 1.1**.

If the width of the CI is set as ω, then the number of cases with the disease in question for inclusion in the study is

$$m_{Disease} = 4\left[\frac{\sigma_{Plan}}{\omega}\right]^2 z_{1-\alpha/2}^2. \tag{21.20}$$

The corresponding number of non-diseased subjects required is then $m_{Non-disease} = R \times m_{Disease}$. Thus, the final estimated total study size is

$$N = m_{Disease} + R \times m_{Disease} = m_{Disease} + m_{Non-disease}. \tag{21.21}$$

Values of $m_{Disease}$ for CI of 90% and 95% of differing width for combinations of FPR and TPR, $R = 1$, 1.5, 2 and 2.5, are given in **Table 21.6**.

21.5 Bibliography

Harris and Boyd (1995) give the large sample estimate of the standard error of cut points of equation (21.3) which lead to the sample size of equation (21.6). Practical values for $\rho = W_{Cut}/W_{RI}$ suggested by Linnet (1987) range from 0.1 to 0.3. The ranks of the lower and upper limits of a $100(1 - \gamma)\%$ CI for any quantile of equation (21.9) are given by Campbell and Gardner (2000). Li and Fine (2004) provide sample size formulae for determining sensitivity and specificity in a variety of situations including equations (21.15), (21.16) and (21.17). Obuchowski and McClish (1997), who refer to the AUC as the accuracy of the test, derive equation (21.19) for input into equation (21.20).

21.6 Examples and Use of the Tables

Table 2.2
For a RI a 5% two-sided CI, $\alpha = 0.05$, $z_{0.975} = 1.96$. For a Cut a 10% two-sided CI, $\gamma = 0.1$, $z_{0.8} = 1.6449$. For a 5% one-sided test, $\alpha = 0.05$, $z_{0.95} = 1.6449$. For a 5% two-sided test, $\alpha = 0.05$, $z_{0.975} = 1.96$. For one-sided $1 - \beta = 0.8$, $z_{0.8} = 0.8416$. A 10% FPR is equivalent to setting a one-sided, $\alpha = 0.1$, $z_{0.9} = 1.2816$. A 45% TPR is equivalent to setting a one-sided, $\alpha = 0.45$, $z_{0.55} = 0.1257$.

Table 21.1 and Equation 21.6

Example 21.1   RI - Normal distribution - Myocardial iron deposition
Anderson, Holden, Davis, *et al* (2001) established normal ranges for T2-star (T2*) values in the heart. T2* is measured using a magnetic resonance technique which can quantify myocardial iron deposition, the levels of which indicate the need for ventricular dysfunction treatment. They quote a 95% normal range for T2* as 36 to 68 ms obtained from 15 healthy volunteers (9 males, 6 females, aged 26 – 39).

We presume that we are planning to estimate the 95% RI for myocardial T2* and we have the above study available. From their study, $W_{Reference} = 68 - 36 = 32$ ms and we intend to quote a 90% *CI* for the cut-point(s) so determined.

Use of equation (21.6) with 2-sided $\alpha = 0.05$, 2-sided $\gamma = 0.1$ and $\rho_{Plan} = 0.1$ gives $N = 3 \times [1.6449/(0.1 \times 1.96)]^2 = 211.29 \approx 212$. Direct entry into **Table 21.1** or use of ^SS_S with a 95% RI ($\alpha = 0.05$), a 90% CI ($\gamma = 0.10$) for the cut-point and $\rho_{Plan} = 0.1$ gives $N = 212$ subjects. Had $\rho_{Plan} = 0.2$ been specified, then $N = 53$ subjects are required.

These estimates of study size contrast markedly with the 15 volunteers used by Anderson, Holden, Davis, *et al* (2001). In terms of the design criteria we have introduced here, their study corresponds to the use of $\rho_{Plan} = 0.38$, which is outside the upper limit of the range of values recommended by Linnet (1987).

Table 21.2 and Equations 21.11 and 21.14

Example 21.2   RI - Non-Normal distribution - Cerebrospinal fluid opening pressure
Whiteley, Al-Shahi, Warlow, *et al* (2006) conducted a study involving the prospective recording of the cerebrospinal fluid (CSF) opening pressure in 242 adults who had had a lumbar puncture. Their objective was to obtain the 95% RI for lumbar CSF opening pressure and relate this to the body mass index.

In their report, the authors plotted the distribution of CSF opening pressures in the 242 subjects and used a Kolmogorov-Smirnov test to conclude that the data were not Normally distributed. They then used a non-parametric approach to calculate the 95% RI. No mention was made of how they arrived at a sample size of 242.

Assuming that the authors wish a 95% RI (2-sided $\alpha = 0.05$) and 90% CI for the cut (2-sided $\gamma = 0.10$) and $\rho_{Plan} = 0.1$, then, from equation (21.11), $\phi_{0.95} = \frac{1}{\sqrt{2\pi}} exp\left(-\frac{1.6449^2}{2}\right) = 0.1031$, and

$$\eta = \frac{\sqrt{(0.1/2)\left[1-(0.1/2)\right]}}{0.1031} = 2.1139.$$ Use of equation (21.14) then gives $N_{Final} = \sqrt{3} \times 2.1139 \times$

$$\left[\frac{1.6449}{0.1 \times 1.96}\right]^2 = 258.88$$ or approximately 260 individuals. Direct entry into **Table 21.2** or use of $\boxed{^SS_S}$

give $N = 258$ subjects.

The sample size of 242 utilised by Whiteley, Al-Shahi, Warlow, *et al* (2006) would correspond to setting $\alpha = 0.05$, $\gamma = 0.10$ and $\rho_{Plan} \approx 0.103$ in $\boxed{^SS_S}$.

Table 21.3 and Equation 21.15

Example 21.3   Sensitivity - Single sample - Excessive daytime somnolence (EDS)
Hosselet, Ayappa, Norman, *et al* (2001) conducted a study to evaluate the utility of various measures of sleep-disordered breathing (SDB) to find that which best identifies excessive daytime somnolence (EDS). They concluded that a total respiratory disturbance index (RDI_{Total} – sum of apnoea, hypopnoea, and flow limitation events) of 18 events per hour or more had the best discriminant ability. This was then tested prospectively in 103 subjects, of whom 68 had EDS and 35 did not, giving a disease prevalence of $p_{Disease} = 68/103 = 0.66$. The sensitivity of the test was reported to be 86%.

In a confirmatory study of the value of RDI_{Total} as a screen for EDS, how many subjects need to be recruited?

Suppose the new investigators feel that the subject population in the confirmatory study may differ in several respects from the earlier study and so anticipate that the sensitivity of the test may be somewhat higher at $Se_{Plan} = 0.95$, with the disease prevalence lower at $\pi_{Disease} = 0.55$. Then assuming a 1-sided test of 2.5% and a power of 80%, with $Se_{Known} = 0.86$, equation (21.15) gives

$$N_{Subjects} = \frac{\left\{1.96 \times \sqrt{0.86(1-0.86)} + 0.8416 \times \sqrt{0.95(1-0.95)}\right\}^2}{0.55 \times (0.95-0.86)^2} = 167.38 \text{ or approximately 168 patients.}$$

Using the more accurate exact binomial approach implemented in $\boxed{^SS_S}$ gives $N = 164$. This latter approach is also used to generate the values given in **Table 21.3**, where, for example, if $Se_{Known} = 0.8$, $Se_{Plan} = 0.9$ and $\pi_{Disease} = 0.5$, the required sample size would be $N = 164$.

Tables 21.4 and 21.5 and Equations 21.16 and 21.17

Example 21.4   Sensitivity - Two group - Periodontal disease
Nomura, Tamaki, Tanaka, *et al* (2006) conducted a study to evaluate the utility of various salivary enzyme tests for screening of periodontitis. Amongst the biochemical markers, salivary lactate dehydrogenase (LDH), with a cut at 371 IU/L, appeared the best and free haemoglobin (f-HB), with a cut at 0.5 IU/L, the worst, with sensitivities 0.66 and 0.27 respectively.

Parallel group

If a repeat study is planned, how many subjects are needed if only one test can be given to each individual? The anticipated proportion with periodontal disease is anticipated to be 1 in 4.

If the difference anticipated is the same as that observed by Nomura, Tamaki, Tanaka, *et al* (2006), then the planning difference is $Se_B - Se_A = 0.66 - 0.27 = 0.39$ and $\pi_{Disease} = 0.25$. Thus, for a 2-sided test of 5% and power 80%, the total number with the disease required using equation (21.16) is, for $\varphi = 1$

and $\overline{Se} = \dfrac{0.27 + 0.66}{2} = 0.465,$

$$N_{Subjects} = \left(\dfrac{1+1}{1}\right)\dfrac{\left\{1.96 \times \sqrt{\left[(1+1) \times 0.465 \times (1-0.465)\right]} + 0.8416 \times \sqrt{\left[1 \times 0.27 \times (1-0.27) + 0.66 \times (1-0.66)\right]}\right\}^2}{0.25 \times (0.66 - 0.39)^2}$$

= 195.70 or 196.

Using the more precise approach implemented in $^{S}S_{S}$ also gives $N = 196$. Alternatively, **Table 21.4** could be used with a 2-sided test of 5% and power 80%. Since the table does not have the particular input values tabulated, the nearest values of $Se_A = 0.3$, $Se_B = 0.7$ and $\pi_{Disease} = 0.3$ would need to be used to give $N = 156$.

Paired groups

If it were possible to make both diagnostic tests in each individual, then a paired design using equation (21.17) could be used for determining sample size. Thus in this situation $\Lambda = (1 - Se_A)Se_B + (1 - Se_B)Se_A = 0.58$, $\zeta = (1 - Se_A)Se_B - (1 - Se_B)Se_A = 0.40$ and $\pi_{Dieases} = 0.3$, hence

$$N_{Subjects} = \dfrac{\left\{1.96 \times 0.58 + 0.8416\sqrt{0.58^2 - 0.40^2 (3 + 0.58)/4}\right\}^2}{0.3 \times 0.58 \times 0.40^2} = 81.54 \text{ or } 82.$$ This implies that 41

subjects are assigned to each of the diagnostic sequences AB and BA.

In this situation, the choice of a paired design rather than parallel groups reduces the size of the proposed study considerably.

Using $^{S}S_{S}$ or **Table 21.5** with 2-sided $\alpha = 0.05$, power 80%, $Se_A = 0.3$, $Se_B = 0.7$ and $\pi_{Disease} = 0.3$ gives $N = 82$.

Table 21.6 and Equations 21.19 and 21.20

Example 21.5 AUC of ROC - Cartilage abnormalities

Obuchowski and McClish (1997) consider the planning of a study to estimate the accuracy of magnetic resonance imaging (MRI) for detecting cartilage abnormalities in patients with symptomatic knees. Patients in the study were to undergo MRI for arthroscopy, which is considered the gold standard for determining the presence/absence of abnormalities. Following a 5-point scoring, it was anticipated that 40% of patients will have a cartilage abnormality, so $R = 60/40 = 1.5$. They stipulated an anticipated specificity of 90%, a sensitivity of 45% and the width of the corresponding 95% CI as $\omega = 0.1$.

The anticipated Sp and Se imply $FPR = 0.1$ and $TPR = 0.45$ and the corresponding 1-sided values $z_{0.9} = 1.2816$ and $z_{0.55} = 0.1257$. Hence equation (21.19) with $Z = 1.2816 - 0.1257 = 1.1559$ then gives

$$\sigma_{Plan} = \dfrac{1}{2\sqrt{\pi}} exp\left(-\dfrac{1.1599^2}{4}\right)\sqrt{\left(1 + \dfrac{1}{1.5} + \dfrac{5 \times 1.1559^2}{8} + \dfrac{1.1559^2}{8 \times 1.5}\right)} = 0.3265.$$ Using this in equation

(21.20), for a 95% *CI*, $m_{Disease} = 4\left[\dfrac{0.3265^2}{0.1^2} \times 1.96^2\right] = 163.82$ or approximately 164 subjects is obtained.

This differs marginally from $m_{Disease} = 161$ given by Obuchowski and McClish (1997, p1538), no doubt due to rounding errors.

Finally, $m_{Non-Disease} = R \times m_{Disease} = 1.5 \times 164 = 246$ so that the final estimated study size is $N = m_{Disease} + m_{Non-Disease} = 410$. Using $^{S}S_{S}$ directly leads to $N = 410$. However, **Table 21.6** does not have TPR = 0.45 tabulated, but using TPR = 0.40 with FPR = 0.1, $R = 1.5$, $\omega = 0.1$, $m_{Disease} = 176$ with the corresponding total sample size required would be $N = 2.5 \times 176 = 440$ subjects.

References

Technical

Campbell MJ and Gardner MJ (2000). Medians and their differences. In: Altman DG, Machin D, Bryant TN and Gardner MJ (eds) *Statistics with Confidence*. (2nd edn) British Medical Journal, London, 171–190.

Harris EK and Boyd JC (1995). *Statistical Bases of Reference Values in Laboratory Medicine*. Marcel Dekker, New York.

Li J and Fine J (2004). On sample size for sensitivity and specificity in prospective diagnostic accuracy studies. *Statistics in Medicine*, **23**, 2537–2550.

Linnet K (1987). Two-stage transformation systems for normalization of reference distributions evaluated. *Clinical Chemistry*, **33**, 381–386.

Obuchowski NA and McClish DN (1997). Sample size determination for diagnostic accuracy studies involving binormal ROC curve indices. *Statistics in Medicine*, **16**, 1529–1542.

Examples

Anderson LJ, Holden S, Davis B, Prescott E, Charrier CC, Bunce NH, Firmin DN, Wonke B, Porter J, Walker JM and Pennell DJ (2001). Cardiovascular T2-star (T2*) magnetic resonance for the early diagnosis of myocardial iron overload. *European Heart Journal*, **22**, 2171–2179.

Hosselet J-J, Ayappa I, Norman RG, Krieger AC and Rapoport DM (2001). Classification of sleep-disordered breathing. *American Journal of Respiratory Critical Care Medicine*, **163**, 398–405.

Nomura Y, Tamaki Y, Tanaka T, Arakawa H, Tsurumoto A, Kirimura K, Sato T, Hanada N and Kamoi K (2006). Screening of periodontitis with salivary enzyme tests. *Journal of Oral Science*, **48**, 177–183.

Whiteley W, Al-Shahi R, Warlow CP, Zeideler M and Lueck CJ (2006). CSF opening pressure: Reference interval and the effect of body mass index. *Neurology*, **67**, 1690–1691.

Table 21.1 Sample Sizes in order to obtain a pre-specified width of the confidence interval for the Cut-off value defining a limit of a Reference Interval for a continuous outcome measure having an assumed Normal distribution [Equation 21.6].

Each cell gives the total number of subjects, *N*, that should be entered into study.

Reference Interval		2-sided Confidence Interval for the estimated cut-off		
		100(1 − γ)%		
100(1 − α)%	ρ	80%	90%	95%
90%	0.025	2,914	4,800	6,816
	0.05	729	1,200	1,704
	0.075	324	534	758
	0.1	183	300	426
	0.125	117	192	273
	0.15	81	134	190
	0.175	60	98	140
	0.2	46	75	107
	0.3	21	34	48
	0.4	12	19	27
95%	0.025	2,053	3,381	4,800
	0.05	514	846	1,200
	0.075	229	376	534
	0.1	129	212	300
	0.125	83	136	192
	0.15	58	94	134
	0.175	42	69	98
	0.2	33	53	75
	0.3	15	24	34
	0.4	9	14	19
99%	0.025	1,189	1,958	2,780
	0.05	298	490	695
	0.075	133	218	309
	0.1	75	123	174
	0.125	48	79	112
	0.15	34	55	78
	0.175	25	40	57
	0.2	19	31	44
	0.3	9	14	20
	0.4	5	8	11

Table 21.2 Sample sizes in order to obtain a pre-specified width of the confidence interval for the Cut-off value defining a limit of a Reference Interval for a continuous outcome measure having an Non-Normal distribution [Equations 21.11 and 21.14].

Each cell gives the total number of patients, N, that should be entered into study.

Reference Interval		2-sided Confidence Interval of the estimated Cut-off		
		$100(1-\gamma)\%$		
$100(1-\alpha)\%$		80%	90%	95%
90%	0.025	2,876	5,857	10,512
	0.05	719	1,465	2,628
	0.075	320	651	1,168
	0.1	180	367	657
	0.125	116	235	421
	0.15	80	163	292
	0.175	59	120	215
	0.2	45	92	165
	0.3	20	41	73
	0.4	12	23	42
95%	0.025	2,026	4,125	7,403
	0.05	507	1,032	1,851
	0.075	226	459	823
	0.1	127	258	463
	0.125	82	165	297
	0.15	57	115	206
	0.175	42	85	152
	0.2	32	65	116
	0.3	15	29	52
	0.4	8	17	29
99%	0.025	1,173	2,389	4,287
	0.05	294	598	1,072
	0.075	131	266	477
	0.1	74	150	268
	0.125	47	96	172
	0.15	33	67	120
	0.175	24	49	88
	0.2	19	38	67
	0.3	9	19	30
	0.4	6	10	17

Table 21.3 Single group sample sizes required to observe a given sensitivity and specificity in diagnostic accuracy studies [Approximated by Equation 21.15].

Each cell gives the number of subjects for the study, *N*.

		1-sided $\alpha = 0.05$; Power $1-\beta = 0.8$				
		Disease Prevalence, $\pi_{Disease}$				
Se_{Known}	Se_{Plan}	0.05	0.1	0.3	0.5	0.7
0.1	0.2	1,560	780	260	156	112
	0.3	500	250	84	50	36
	0.4	260	130	44	26	19
	0.5	160	80	27	16	12
	0.6	120	60	20	12	9
	0.7	100	50	17	10	8
	0.8	60	30	10	6	5
	0.9	40	20	7	4	3
0.2	0.3	2,320	1,160	387	232	166
	0.4	700	350	117	70	50
	0.5	340	170	57	34	25
	0.6	200	100	34	20	15
	0.7	140	70	24	14	10
	0.8	80	40	14	8	6
	0.9	40	20	7	4	3
0.3	0.4	2,880	1,440	480	288	206
	0.5	780	390	130	78	56
	0.6	340	170	57	34	25
	0.7	200	100	34	20	15
	0.8	140	70	24	14	10
	0.9	100	50	17	10	8
0.4	0.5	3,160	1,580	527	316	226
	0.6	840	420	140	84	61
	0.7	380	190	64	38	28
	0.8	220	110	37	22	16
	0.9	120	60	20	12	9
0.5	0.6	3,160	1,580	527	316	226
	0.7	740	370	124	74	53
	0.8	360	180	60	36	26
	0.9	140	80	27	16	12
0.6	0.7	2,860	1,430	477	286	205
	0.8	720	360	120	72	52
	0.9	280	140	47	28	20
0.7	0.8	2,380	1,190	397	238	170
	0.9	560	280	94	56	40
0.8	0.9	1640	820	274	164	118

Table 21.3 (Continued)

Each cell gives the number of subjects for the study, *N*.

		1-sided $\alpha=0.05$; Power $1-\beta=0.9$				
		Disease Prevalence, $\pi_{Disease}$				
Se_{Known}	Se_{Plan}	0.05	0.1	0.3	0.5	0.7
0.1	0.2	2,180	1,090	364	218	156
	0.3	660	330	110	66	48
	0.4	360	180	60	36	26
	0.5	240	120	40	24	18
	0.6	140	70	24	14	10
	0.7	120	60	20	12	9
	0.8	100	50	17	10	8
	0.9	60	30	10	6	5
0.2	0.3	3,200	1,600	534	320	229
	0.4	940	470	157	94	68
	0.5	420	210	70	42	31
	0.6	260	130	44	26	19
	0.7	180	90	30	18	13
	0.8	120	60	20	12	9
	0.9	80	40	14	8	6
0.3	0.4	3,860	1,930	644	386	276
	0.5	1,060	530	177	106	76
	0.6	500	250	84	50	36
	0.7	280	140	47	28	20
	0.8	180	90	30	18	13
	0.9	100	50	17	10	8
0.4	0.5	4,280	2,140	714	428	306
	0.6	1,120	560	187	112	80
	0.7	500	250	84	50	36
	0.8	260	130	44	26	19
	0.9	160	80	27	16	12
0.5	0.6	4,260	2,130	710	426	305
	0.7	1060	530	177	106	76
	0.8	460	230	77	46	33
	0.9	220	110	37	22	16
0.6	0.7	3,940	1,970	657	394	282
	0.8	900	450	150	90	65
	0.9	340	170	57	34	25
0.7	0.8	3,280	1,640	547	328	235
	0.9	740	370	124	74	53
0.8	0.9	2240	1120	374	224	160

Table 21.4 Sample sizes required for a two group unpaired design for given sensitivity and specificity in diagnostic accuracy studies [Equation 21.16].

Each cell gives the total number of subjects for the study, *N*.

		2-sided $\alpha = 0.05$; Power $1 - \beta = 0.8$				
		Disease Prevalence, $\pi_{Disease}$				
Se_A	Se_B	0.05	0.1	0.3	0.5	0.7
0.1	0.2	7,959	3,980	1,327	796	569
	0.3	2,464	1,232	411	247	176
	0.4	1,260	630	210	126	90
	0.5	776	388	130	78	56
	0.6	522	261	87	53	38
	0.7	368	184	62	37	27
	0.8	265	133	45	27	19
	0.9	190	95	32	19	14
0.2	0.3	11,727	5,864	1,955	1,173	838
	0.4	3,249	1,625	542	325	233
	0.5	1,540	770	257	154	110
	0.6	894	447	149	90	64
	0.7	573	287	96	58	41
	0.8	386	193	65	39	28
	0.9	265	133	45	27	19
0.3	0.4	14,238	7,119	2,373	1,424	1,017
	0.5	3,720	1,860	620	372	266
	0.6	1,679	840	280	168	120
	0.7	933	467	156	94	67
	0.8	573	287	96	58	41
	0.9	368	184	62	37	27
0.4	0.5	15,494	7,747	2,583	1,550	1,107
	0.6	3,877	1,939	647	388	277
	0.7	1,679	840	280	168	120
	0.8	894	447	149	90	64
	0.9	522	261	87	53	38
0.5	0.6	15,494	7,747	2,583	1,550	1,107
	0.7	3,720	1,860	620	372	266
	0.8	1,540	770	257	154	110
	0.9	776	388	130	78	56
0.6	0.7	14,238	7,119	2,373	1,424	1,017
	0.8	3,249	1,625	542	325	233
	0.9	1,260	630	210	126	90
0.7	0.8	11,727	5,864	1,955	1,173	838
	0.9	2,464	1,232	411	247	176
0.8	0.9	7,959	3,980	1,327	796	569

Table 21.4 (Continued)

Each cell gives the total number of subjects for the study, *N*

		2-sided $\alpha = 0.05$; Power $1 - \beta = 0.9$				
		Disease Prevalence, $\pi_{Disease}$				
Se_A	Se_B	0.05	0.1	0.3	0.5	0.7
0.1	0.2	10,635	5,318	1,7734	1064	760
	0.3	3,279	1,640	547	328	235
	0.4	1,667	834	278	167	120
	0.5	1,018	509	170	102	73
	0.6	678	339	113	68	49
	0.7	472	236	79	48	34
	0.8	334	167	56	34	24
	0.9	233	117	39	24	17
0.2	0.3	15,678	7,839	2,613	1,568	1,120
	0.4	4,330	2,165	722	433	310
	0.5	2,041	1,021	341	205	146
	0.6	1,176	588	196	118	84
	0.7	746	373	125	75	54
	0.8	496	248	83	50	36
	0.9	334	167	56	34	24
0.3	0.4	19,041	9,521	3,174	1,905	1,361
	0.5	4,960	2,480	827	496	355
	0.6	2,228	1,114	372	223	160
	0.7	1,229	615	205	123	88
	0.8	746	373	125	75	54
	0.9	472	236	79	48	34
0.4	0.5	20,722	10,361	3454	2,073	1,481
	0.6	5,171	2,586	862	518	370
	0.7	2,228	1,114	372	223	160
	0.8	1,176	588	196	118	84
	0.9	678	339	113	68	49
0.5	0.6	20,722	10,361	3,454	2,073	1,481
	0.7	4,960	2,480	827	496	355
	0.8	2,041	1,021	341	205	146
	0.9	1,018	509	170	102	73
0.6	0.7	19,041	9,521	3,174	1,905	,361
	0.8	4,330	2,165	722	433	310
	0.9	1,667	834	278	167	120
0.7	0.8	15,678	7,839	2,613	1,568	1,120
	0.9	3,279	1,640	547	328	235
0.8	0.9	10,635	5,318	1,773	1,064	760

Table 21.5 Sample sizes required for a two group matched pair design for given sensitivity and specificity in diagnostic accuracy studies. [Equation 21.17].

Each cell gives the total number of subjects for the study, *N*.

		2-sided $\alpha=0.05$; Power $1-\beta=0.8$				
		Disease Prevalence, $\pi_{Disease}$				
Se_A	Se_B	0.05	0.1	0.3	0.5	0.7
0.1	0.2	3,931	1,966	656	394	281
	0.3	1,212	606	202	122	87
	0.4	628	314	105	63	45
	0.5	397	199	67	40	29
	0.6	278	139	47	28	20
	0.7	207	104	35	21	15
	0.8	160	80	27	16	12
	0.9	126	63	21	13	9
0.2	0.3	5,860	2,930	977	586	419
	0.4	1,632	816	272	164	117
	0.5	785	393	131	79	57
	0.6	467	234	78	47	34
	0.7	310	155	52	31	23
	0.8	220	110	37	22	16
	0.9	160	80	27	16	12
0.3	0.4	7,132	3,566	1,189	714	510
	0.5	1,878	939	313	188	135
	0.6	861	431	144	87	62
	0.7	490	245	82	49	35
	0.8	310	155	52	31	23
	0.9	207	104	35	21	15
0.4	0.5	7,766	3,883	1,295	777	555
	0.6	1,959	980	327	196	140
	0.7	861	431	144	87	62
	0.8	467	234	78	47	34
	0.9	278	139	47	28	20
0.5	0.6	7,766	3,883	1,295	777	555
	0.7	1,878	939	313	188	135
	0.8	785	393	131	79	57
	0.9	397	199	67	40	29
0.6	0.7	7,132	3,566	1,189	714	510
	0.8	1632	816	272	164	117
	0.9	628	314	105	63	45
0.7	0.8	5,860	2,930	977	586	419
	0.9	1,212	606	202	122	87
0.8	0.9	3,931	1,966	656	394	281

Table 21.5 (Continued)

Each cell gives the total number of subjects for the study, N.

		2-sided $\alpha = 0.05$; Power $1 - \beta = 0.9$				
		Disease Prevalence, $\pi_{Disease}$				
Se_A	Se_B	0.05	0.1	0.3	0.5	0.7
0.1	0.2	5,199	2,600	867	520	372
	0.3	1,572	786	262	158	113
	0.4	798	399	133	80	57
	0.5	494	247	83	50	36
	0.6	339	170	57	34	25
	0.7	247	124	42	25	18
	0.8	186	93	31	19	14
	0.9	142	71	24	15	11
0.2	0.3	7,800	3,900	1,300	780	558
	0.4	2,145	1,073	358	215	154
	0.5	1,014	507	169	102	73
	0.6	592	296	99	60	43
	0.7	384	192	64	39	28
	0.8	264	132	44	27	19
	0.9	186	93	31	19	14
0.3	0.4	9,510	4,755	1,585	951	680
	0.5	2,479	1,240	414	248	178
	0.6	1,119	560	187	112	80
	0.7	623	312	104	63	45
	0.8	384	192	64	39	28
	0.9	247	124	42	25	18
0.4	0.5	10,262	5,181	1,727	1,037	741
	0.6	2,589	1,295	432	259	185
	0.7	1,119	560	187	112	80
	0.8	592	296	99	60	43
	0.9	339	170	57	34	25
0.5	0.6	10,362	5,181	1,727	1,037	741
	0.7	2,479	1,240	414	248	178
	0.8	1,014	507	169	102	73
	0.9	494	247	83	50	36
0.6	0.7	9,510	4,755	1,585	951	680
	0.8	2,145	1,073	358	215	154
	0.9	798	399	133	80	57
0.7	0.8	7,800	3,900	1,300	780	558
	0.9	1,572	786	262	158	113
0.8	0.9	5,199	2,600	867	520	372

Table 21.6 Sample sizes required to observe a given 2-sided confidence interval width for the AUC of a ROC [Equations 21.18 and 21.19].

R is the ratio of diseased to non-diseased individuals in the target group. Each cell gives the number of subjects for each group, m. Hence, the total sample size for the study is $N = (1 + R)m$.

R	FPR	TPR	Width of 2-sided 90% CI, ω				Width of 2-sided 95% CI, ω			
			0.05	0.1	0.15	0.2	0.05	0.1	0.15	0.2
1	0.1	0.4	568	142	64	36	806	202	90	51
		0.5	490	123	55	31	696	174	78	44
		0.6	400	100	45	25	568	142	64	36
		0.7	300	75	34	19	426	107	48	27
		0.8	195	49	22	13	277	70	31	18
		0.9	90	23	10	6	127	32	15	8
	0.2	0.4	655	164	73	41	930	233	104	59
		0.5	612	153	68	39	869	218	97	55
		0.6	549	138	61	35	779	195	87	49
		0.7	461	116	52	29	655	164	73	41
		0.8	345	87	39	22	490	123	55	31
		0.9	195	49	22	13	277	70	31	18
	0.3	0.4	683	171	76	43	969	243	108	61
		0.5	663	166	74	42	941	236	105	59
		0.6	625	157	70	40	887	222	99	56
		0.7	562	141	63	36	798	200	89	50
		0.8	461	116	52	29	655	164	73	41
		0.9	300	75	34	19	426	107	48	27
1.5	0.1	0.4	492	124	56	32	698	176	78	44
		0.5	430	108	48	28	610	154	68	40
		0.6	354	90	40	24	504	126	56	32
		0.7	270	68	30	18	382	96	44	24
		0.8	176	44	20	12	250	64	28	16
		0.9	82	22	10	6	116	30	14	8
	0.2	0.4	554	140	62	36	788	198	88	50
		0.5	526	132	60	34	746	188	84	48
		0.6	476	120	54	30	676	170	76	44
		0.7	406	102	46	26	576	144	64	36
		0.8	308	78	36	20	436	110	50	28
		0.9	176	44	20	12	250	64	28	16
	0.3	0.4	572	144	64	36	812	204	92	52
		0.5	560	140	64	36	794	200	90	50
		0.6	534	134	60	34	758	190	86	48
		0.7	488	122	56	32	692	174	78	44
		0.8	406	102	46	26	576	144	64	36
		0.9	270	68	30	18	382	96	44	24

Table 21.6 (Continued)

R is the ratio of diseased to non-diseased individuals in the target group. Each cell gives the number of subjects for each group, *m*. Hence, the total sample size for the study is $N = (1 + R)m$.

R	FPR	TPR	Width of 2-sided 90% CI, ω				Width of 2-sided 95% CI, ω			
			0.05	0.1	0.15	0.2	0.05	0.1	0.15	0.2
2	0.1	0.4	453	114	51	29	642	161	72	41
		0.5	399	100	45	25	566	142	63	36
		0.6	331	83	37	21	470	118	53	30
		0.7	253	64	29	16	359	90	40	23
		0.8	167	42	19	11	237	60	27	15
		0.9	78	20	9	5	111	28	13	7
	0.2	0.4	504	126	56	32	715	179	80	45
		0.5	481	121	54	31	683	171	76	43
		0.6	440	110	49	28	625	157	70	40
		0.7	378	95	42	24	536	134	60	34
		0.8	289	73	33	19	409	103	46	26
		0.9	167	42	19	11	237	60	27	15
	0.3	0.4	515	129	58	33	732	183	82	46
		0.5	508	127	57	32	721	181	81	46
		0.6	488	122	55	31	693	174	77	44
		0.7	449	113	50	29	637	160	71	40
		0.8	378	95	42	24	536	134	60	34
		0.9	253	64	29	16	359	90	40	23
2.5	0.1	0.4	430	108	48	27	610	153	68	39
		0.5	381	96	43	24	540	135	60	34
		0.6	318	80	36	20	451	113	51	29
		0.7	243	61	27	16	345	87	39	22
		0.8	161	41	18	11	229	58	26	15
		0.9	76	19	9	5	107	27	12	7
	0.2	0.4	474	119	53	30	673	169	75	43
		0.5	455	114	51	29	645	162	72	41
		0.6	418	105	47	27	594	149	66	38
		0.7	361	91	41	23	512	128	57	32
		0.8	277	70	31	18	393	99	44	25
		0.9	161	41	18	11	229	58	26	15
	0.3	0.4	482	121	54	31	684	171	76	43
		0.5	477	120	53	30	676	169	76	43
		0.6	461	116	52	29	654	164	73	41
		0.7	426	107	48	27	605	152	68	38
		0.8	361	91	41	23	512	128	57	32
		0.9	243	61	27	16	345	87	39	22

22

Sample Size Software $^{S}S_{S}$

SUMMARY

The Sample Size Software, $^{S}S_{S}$, implements many of the sample size computation methods discussed in this book.

22.1 Introduction

The primary function of $^{S}S_{S}$ is as a sample size calculator, which can be accessed under **Sample Size Calculator** in the main menu, to compute sample sizes corresponding to various choices of input values. The calculator takes the format of a spreadsheet to facilitate the calculation of sample sizes for up to eight sets of design options, with the additional functionality to print out the associated sample sizes computed. This range of options is intended to facilitate discussion amongst the investigating team during the planning stages of a study as to the appropriate eventual sample size to be used. The use of $^{S}S_{S}$ is available for many methods discussed in the book except those of **Chapter 15** Genomics Targets and Dose-finding Studies and **Chapter 16** Feasibility and Pilot Studies.

22.2 System Requirements

It is essential to make sure that your PC meets the minimum system requirements of the program in order for it to run smoothly. If you are experiencing poor performance, kindly check to make sure that your system hardware supports the requirements. The minimum system requirements are:

- Operating System: Windows 10, 8.1, 8, 7 (SP1)
- CPU: 1.6 GHz or faster processor
- RAM: 1GB;
- Hard Drive: 200 MB of free space

Sample Sizes for Clinical, Laboratory and Epidemiology Studies, Fourth Edition. David Machin, Michael J. Campbell, Say Beng Tan and Sze Huey Tan.
© 2018 John Wiley & Sons Ltd. Published 2018 by John Wiley & Sons Ltd.

22.3   Installation Instructions

To download and install the software, go to www.wiley.com/go/machin/samplesizes4e and click on the "Click to Download" button. This will download a zipped folder onto your computer. Open the zipped folder and click on the SSSInstaller.msi file. Then follow the instructions that appear on the screen to install the software.

There may be situations during the installation of the software whereby the system will prompt the user that his/her system files are older than the version required by the software. Should this happen, the user should run Windows Update, which comes with the operating system, so as to update the system files from the Microsoft website, prior to re-installing ^SS_S.

22.4   Help Guide

For more details on using ^SS_S, users can refer to the Help file available under **Help** in the main menu of the software.

Cumulative References

Abdullah K, Thorpe KE, Mamak E, Maguire JL, Birken CS, Fehlings D, Hanley AJ, Macarthur C, Zlotkin SH and Parkin PC (2015). An internal pilot study for a randomized trial aimed at evaluating the effectiveness of iron interventions in children with non-anemic iron deficiency: the OptEC trial. *Trials*, **16**, 303. [16]

Abernethy AP, Currow DC, Frith P, Fazekas BS, McHugh A and Bui C (2003). Randomised, double blind, placebo controlled crossover trial of sustained release morphine for the management of refractory dyspnoea. *British Medical Journal*, **327**, 523–528. [8]

Adams G, Gulliford MC, Ukoumunne OC, Eldridge S, Chinn S and MJ (2004). Patterns of intra-cluster correlation from primary care research to inform study design and analysis. *Journal of Clinical Epidemiology*, **57**, 785–794. [12]

A'Hern RP (2001). Sample size tables for exact single stage phase II designs. *Statistics in Medicine*, **20**, 859–866. [2, 17, 18]

Altman DG (1991). *Practical Statistics for Medical Research*. Chapman & Hall/CRC, Boca Raton. [20]

Altman DG and Gardner MJ (2000). Means and their differences. In Altman DG, Machin D, Bryant TN and Gardner MJ (eds). *Statistics with Confidence*, 2nd edn. British Medical Journal Books, London, 31–32. [9]

Anderson LJ, Holden S, Davis B, Prescott E, Charrier CC, Bunce NH, Firmin DN, Wonke B, Porter J, Walker JM and Pennell DJ (2001). Cardiovascular T2-star (T2*) magnetic resonance for the early diagnosis of myocardial iron overload. *European Heart Journal*, **22**, 2171–2179. [21]

Ang ES-W, Lee S-T, Gan CS-G, See PG-J, Chan Y-H, Ng L-H and Machin D (2001). Evaluating the role of alternative therapy in burn wound management: randomized trial comparing Moist Exposed Burn Ointment with conventional methods in the management of patients with second-degree burns. *Medscape General Medicine*. **3**, 3. [3]

Arain M, Campbell MJ, Cooper CL and Lancaster GA (2010). What is a pilot or feasibility study? A review of current practice and editorial policy. *BMC Medical Research Methodology*, **10**, 67. [16]

Atiwannapat P, Thaipisuttikul P, Poopityastaporn P and Katekaew W (2016). Active versus receptive group music therapy for major depressive disorder – A pilot study. *Complementary Therapies in Medicine*, **26**, 141–145. [16]

Avery KNL, Williamson P, Gamble C, O'Connell E, Metcalfe C, Davidson P and Williams H (2015). Informing efficient randomised controlled trials: exploration of challenges in developing progression criteria for internal pilot studies. *Trials*, **16**(Suppl 2), P10. [16]

Sample Sizes for Clinical, Laboratory and Epidemiology Studies, Fourth Edition. David Machin, Michael J. Campbell, Say Beng Tan and Sze Huey Tan.
© 2018 John Wiley & Sons Ltd. Published 2018 by John Wiley & Sons Ltd.

Bacchetti P, McCulloch CE and Segal MR (2008). Simple, defensible sample sizes based on cost efficiency. *Biometrics*, **64**, 577–585. [2]

Bacchetti P, Wolf LE, Segal MR and McCulloch CE (2005). Ethics and sample size. *American Journal of Epidemiology*, **161**, 105–110. [2]

Baron-Cohen S, Scott FJ, Allison C, Williams J, Bolton P, Matthews FE and Brayne C (2009). Prevalence of autism-spectrum conditions: UK school-based population study. *British Journal of Psychiatry*, **194**, 500–509. [9]

Basso DM, Velozo C, Lorenz D, Suter S and Behrman AL (2015). Interrater reliability of the neuromuscular recovery scale for spinal cord injury. *Archives of Physical Medicine and Rehabilitation*, **96**, 1397–1403. [20]

Batistatou E, Roberts C and Roberts S (2014). Sample size and power calculations for trials and quasi-experimental studies with clustering. *The Stata Journal*, **14**, 159–175. [12]

Beitz A, Riphaus A, Meining A, Kronshage T, Geist C, Wagenpfeil S, Weber A, Jung A, Bajbouj M, Pox C, Schneider G, Schmid RM, Wehrmann T and von Delius S (2012). Capnographic monitoring reduces the incidence of arterial oxygen desaturation and hypoxemia during propofol sedation for colonoscopy: A randomized, controlled study (ColoCap Study). *The American Journal of Gastroenterology*, **107**, 1205–1220. [3]

Bidwell G, Sahu A, Edwards R, Harrison RA, Thornton J and Kelly SP (2005). Perceptions of blindness related to smoking: a hospital-based cross-sectional study. *Eye*, **19**, 945–948. [9]

Birkett MA and Day SJ (1994). Internal pilot studies for estimating sample size. *Statistics in Medicine*, **13**, 2455–2463. [16]

Biswas S, Liu DD, Lee JJ and Berry DA (2009). Bayesian clinical trials at the University of Texas M. D. Anderson Cancer Centre. *Clinical Trials*, **6**, 205–216. [17]

Bonett DG (2002). Sample size requirements for estimating the intraclass correlations with desired precision. *Statistics in Medicine*, **21**, 1331–1335. [20]

Bonett DG and Wright TA (2000). Sample size requirements for estimating Pearson, Kendall and Spearman correlations. *Psychometrika*, **65**, 23–28. [19]

Booth CM, Calvert AH, Giaccone G, Lobbezoo MW, Eisenhauer EA and Seymour LK (2008). Design and conduct of phase II studies of targeted anticancer therapy: Recommendations from the task force on methodology for the development of innovative cancer therapies (MDICT). *European Journal of Cancer*, **44**, 25–29. [17]

Borenstein M, Rothstein H and Cohen J (2005). *Power & Precision (Power Analysis): Version 4*. Biostat, Englewood, New Jersey, USA. [1]

Bristol DR (1989). Sample sizes for constructing confidence intervals and testing hypotheses. *Statistics in Medicine*, **8**, 803–811. [9]

Broderick JP, Palesch YY, Demchuk AM, Yeatts SD, Khatri P, Hill MD, Jauch EC, Jovin TG, Yan B, Silver FL, von Kummer R, Molina CA, Demaerschalk BM, Budzik R, Clark WM, Zaidat OO, Malisch TW, Goyal M, Schonwille WJ, Mazighi M, Engelter ST, Anderson G, Spilker J, Carrozzella J, Ryckborst KJ, Janis LS, Martin RH, Foster LD and Tomsick TA (2013). Endovascular therapy after intravenous t-PA versus t-PA alone for stroke. *New England Journal of Medicine*, **368**, 893–903. [4]

Brooker S, Bethony J, Rodrigues L, Alexander N, Geiger S and Hotez P (2005). Epidemiological, immunological and practical considerations in developing and evaluating a human hookworm vaccine. *Expert Review of Vaccines*, **4**, 35–50. [6]

Brown SR, Gregory WM, Twelves CJ, Buyse M, Collinson F, Parmar M, Seymour MT and Brown JM (2011). Designing phase II trials in cancer: a systematic review and guidance. *British Journal of Cancer*, **105**, 194–199. [17]

Browne RH (1995). On the use of a pilot study for sample size determination. *Statistics in Medicine*, **14**, 1933–1940. [16]

Bryant J and Day R (1995). Incorporating toxicity considerations into the design of two-stage Phase II clinical trials. *Biometrics*, **51**, 1372–1383. [18]

Burgess IF, Brown CM and Lee P (2005). Treatment of head louse infestation with 4% dimeticone lotion: randomised controlled equivalence trial. *British Medical Journal*; **330**, 1423–1425. [11]

Butenas S, Cawthern KM, van't Meer C, DiLorenzo ME, Lock JB and Mann KG (2001). Antiplatelet agents in tissue factor-induced blood coagulation. *Blood*, **97**, 2314–2322. [8]

Calverley P, Pauwels R, Vestbo J, Jones P, Pride N, Gulsvik A, Anderson J and Maden C (2003). Combined salmeterol and fluticasone in the treatment of chronic obstructive pulmonary disease: a randomised controlled trial. *Lancet*, **361**, 449–456. [14]

Campbell MJ (2013). Doing clinical trials large enough to achieve adequate reductions in uncertainties about treatment effects. *Journal of the Royal Society of Medicine*, **106**, 68–71. [2]

Campbell MJ (2014). Challenges of cluster randomised trials. *Journal of Comparative Effectiveness*, **3**, 271–278. [12]

Campbell MJ and Gardner MJ (2000). Medians and their differences. In: Altman DG, Machin D, Bryant TN and Gardner MJ (eds) *Statistics with Confidence*, 2nd edn. British Medical Journal Books, London, 171–190. [21]

Campbell MJ, Machin D and Walters SJ (2007). *Medical Statistics: A Textbook for the Health Sciences*, (4th edn.) Wiley, Chichester. [1, 3, 4, 18]

Campbell MJ and Walters SJ (2014). *How to Design, Analyse and Report Cluster Randomised Trials in Medicine and Health Related Research*. Chichester, Wiley. [12]

Campbell MK, Piaggio G, Elbourne DR and Altman DG (2012). Consort 2010 statement: extension to cluster randomized trials. *British Medical Journal*; **345**, e5661. doi:10.1136/bmj.e5661. [12]

Cantor AB (1996). Sample size calculations for Cohen's kappa. *Psychological Methods*, **2**, 150–153. [20]

Carter B (2010). Cluster size variability and imbalance in cluster randomized controlled trials. *Statistics in Medicine*; **29**, 2984–2993. [12]

Casagrande JT, Pike MC and Smith PG (1978). An improved approximate formula for comparing two binomial distributions. *Biometrics*, **34**, 483–486. [3]

Case LD and Morgan TM (2003). Design of Phase II cancer trials evaluating survival probabilities. *BMC Medical Research Methodology*, **3**, 6. [18]

Chao Y, Chan W-K, Birkhofer MJ, Hu OY-P, Wang S-S, Huang Y-S, Liu M, Whang-Peng J, Chi K-H, Lui W-Y and Lee S-D (1998). Phase II and pharmacokinetic study of paclitaxel therapy for unresectable hepatocellular carcinoma patients. *British Journal of Cancer*, **78**, 34–39. [16]

Chapman KL, Hardin-Jones MA, Goldstein JA, Halter KA, Havlik J and Schulte J (2008). Timing of palatal surgery and speech outcome. *Cleft Palate-Cranofacial Journal*, **45**, 297–308. [9]

Chen CLH, Venketasubramanian N, Lee C-F, Wong L and Bousser M-G (2013). Effects of ML601 on early vascular events in patients after stroke: The CHIMES study. *Stroke*, **44**, 3580–3583. [7]

Chen CLH, Young SHY, Gan HH, Singh R, Lao AY, Baroque AC, Chang HM, Hiyadan JHB, Chua CL, Advincula JM, Muengtaweeppongsa S, Chan BPL, de Silva HA, Towanabut S, Suwawela NC, Poungvarin N, Chankrachang S, Wong L, Eow GB, Navarro JC, Venketasubramanian N, Lee CF, Wong L and Bousser M-G (2013). Chinese medicine neuroaid efficacy on stroke recovery: A double-blind, placebo controlled, randomized study. *Stroke*, **44**, 2093–2100. [4]

Cheng J, Cho M, Cen J-M, Cai M-Y, Xu S, Ma Z-W, Liu X, Yang X-L, Chen C, Suh Y and Xiong X-D (2015). A tagSNP in *SIRT1* gene confers susceptibility to myocardial infarction in a Chinese Han population. PLoS ONE, **10**, e.0115339. [3]

Cheung YK and Thall PF (2002). Monitoring the rates of composite events with censored data in phase II clinical trials. *Biometrics*, **58**, 89–97. [18]

Chisholm JC, Machin D, McDowell H, McHugh K, Ellershaw C, Jenney M, Foot ABM (2007). Efficacy of carboplatin in a phase II window study to children and adolescents with newly diagnosed metastatic soft tissue sarcoma. *European Journal of Cancer*, **43**, 2537–2544. [1]

Chong S-A, Tay JAM, Subramaniam M, Pek E and Machin D (2009). Mortality rates among patients with schizophrenia and tardive dyskinesia. *Journal of Clinical Psychopharmacology*, **29**, 5–8. [6]

Chow PK-H, Tai B-C, Tan C-K, Machin D, Johnson PJ, Khin M-W and Soo K-C (2002). No role for high-dose tamoxifen in the treatment of inoperable hepatocellular carcinoma: An Asia-Pacific double-blind randomised controlled trial. *Hepatology*, **36**, 1221–1226. [1]

Chow SC, Shao J and Wang H (2002). A note on sample size calculations for mean comparisons based on non central t-statistics. *Journal of Pharmaceutical Statistics*, **12**, 441–456. [5]

Chow S-C and Wang H (2001). On sample size calculation in bioequivalence trials. *Journal of Pharmacokinetics and Pharmacodynamics*, **28**, 155–169. [11]

Cicchetti DV (2001). The precision of reliability and validity estimates re-visited: distinguishing between clinical and statistical significance of sample size requirements. *Journal of Clinical and Experimental Neuropsychology*, **23**, 695–700. [20]

Cohen J (1988). *Statistical Power Analysis for the Behavioral Sciences*, (2nd edn) Lawrence Earlbaum, New Jersey. [5, 8, 17, 19]

Cömert Kiliç S, Kiliç N and Sümbüllü MA (2015). Temporomandibular joint osteoarthritis: cone beam computed tomography findings, clinical features, and correlations. *International Journal of Oral & Maxillofacial Surgery*, **44**, 1268–1274. [19]

Connett JE, Smith JA and McHugh RB (1987). Sample size and power for pair-matched case-control studies. *Statistics in Medicine*, **6**, 53–59. [8]

Cook JA, Hislop J, Altman DG, Fayers P, Briggs AH, Ramsay CR, Norrie JD, Harvey IM, Buckley B, Fergusson D and Ford I (2015). Specifying the target difference in the primary outcome for a randomised controlled trial: guidance for researchers. *Trials*, **16**, 12. [1]

Cousineau D and Laurencelle L (2011). Non-central *t* distribution and the power of the *t* test: A rejoinder. *Tutorials in Quantitative Methods in Psychology*, **7**, 1–4. [11]

CPMP Working Party on Efficacy of Medicinal Products (1995). Biostatistical methodology in clinical trials in applications for marketing authorizations for medical products. *Statistics in Medicine*, **14**, 1659–1682. [1]

CPMP (2000) *Points to Consider on Switching between Superiority and Non-Inferiority*. EMEA, London. [11]

CPMP (2005). *Guideline on the Choice of the Non-inferiority Margin*. EMEA, London. [11]

CPMP (2010). *Guideline on the Investigation of Bioequivalence*. EMEA, London. [11]

Crisp A and Curtis P (2008). Sample size estimation for non-inferiority trials of time-to-event data. *Pharmaceutical Statistics*, **7**, 236–244. [11]

Cruciani RA, Dvorkin E, Homel P, Malamud S, Culliney B, Lapin J, Portenoy RK and Esteban-Cruciani N (2006). Safety, tolerability and symptom outcomes associated with L-carnitine supplementation in patients with cancer, fatigue, and carnitine deficiency: a phase I/II study. *Journal of Pain and Symptom Management*, **32**, 551–559. [8]

Cuschieri A, Weeden S, Fielding J, Bancewicz J, Craven J, Joypaul V, Sydes M and Fayers P (1999). Patient survival after D1 and D2 resections for gastric cancer: long-term results of the MRC randomized surgical trial. *British Journal of Cancer*, **79**, 1522–1530. [2]

Davies MJ, Heller S, Skinner TC, Campbell MJ, Carey ME, Cradock S, Dallosso HM, Daly H, Doherty Y, Eaton S, Fox C, Oliver L, Rantell K, Rayman G and Khunti K (2008) Effectiveness of the diabetes education and self management for ongoing and newly diagnosed (DESMOND) programme for people with newly diagnosed type 2 diabetes: cluster randomised controlled trial. *British Medical Journal*, **336**, 491–495. [10]

Day AC, Machin D, Aung T, Gazzard G, Husain R, Chew PTK, Khaw PT, Seah SKL and Foster PJ (2011). Central corneal thickness and glaucoma in East Asian people. *Investigative Ophthalmology & Visual Science*, **52**, 8407–8412. [2]

Day S (2007). *Dictionary for Clinical Trials*. (2nd edition). Wiley, Chichester. [13]

Demidenko E (2007). Sample size determination for logistic regression revisited. *Statistics in Medicine*, **26**, 3385–3397. [3]

D'Haens G, Löwenberg M, Samaan MA, Franchimont D, Ponsioen C, van den Brink GR, Fockens P, Bossuyt P, Amininejad L, Rafamannar G, Lensink EM and Van Gossum AM (2015). Safety and feasibility of using the second-generation pillcam colon capsule to assess active colonic Crohn's disease. *Clinical Gastoenterology and Hepatology*, **13**, 1480–1486. [20]

Diggle PJ, Heagerty P, Liang KY and Zeger AL (2002). *Analysis of Longitudinal Data* (2nd ed). Oxford University Press. [10]

Dite W, Langford ZN, Cumming TB, Churilov L, Blennerhassett JM and Bernhardt J (2015). A Phase 1 exercise dose escalation study for stroke survivors with impaired walking. *International Journal of Stroke*, **10**, 1051–1056. [15]

Donner A and Eliasziw M (1992). A goodness-of-fit approach to inference procedures for the kappa statistic: confidence interval construction, significance-testing and sample size estimation. *Statistics in Medicine*, **11**, 1511–1519. [20]

Draper B, Brodaty H, Low L-F, Richards V, Paton H and Lie D (2002). Self-destructive behaviors in nursing home residents. *Journal of the American Geriatrics Society*, **50**, 354–358. [19]

Dresser GK, Nelson SA, Mahon JL, Zou G, Vandervoort MK, Wong CJ, Feagan BG and Feldman RD (2013). Simplified therapeutic intervention to control hypertension and hypercholesterolemia: a cluster randomized controlled trial (STITCH2). *Journal of Hypertension*, **31**, 1702–1713. [12]

Drummond M and O'Brien B (1993). Clinical importance, statistical significance and the assessment of economic and quality-of-life outcomes. *Health Economics*, **2**, 205–212. [1]

Edwardes MD (2001). Sample size requirements for case-control study designs. *BMC Medical Research Methodology*, **1**, 11. [6]

Eldridge SM, Ashby D and Kerry S (2006). Sample size for cluster randomized trials: effect of coefficient of variation of cluster size and analysis method. *International Journal of Epidemiology*, **35**, 1202–1300. [12]

Eldridge SM, Chan CL, Campbell MJ, Bond CM, Hopewell S, Thabane L, Lancaster GA on behalf of the PAFS Consensus group (2016). CONSORT 2010 statement: extension to randomised pilot and feasibility trials. *British Medical Journal*, 355:i5239 | doi: 10.1136/bmj.i5239. [16]

Eldridge SM and Kerry S (2012). *A Practical Guide to Cluster Randomised Trials in Health Services Research*. Chichester, Wiley-Blackwell. [12]

Eldridge SM, Lancaster GA, Campbell MJ, Thabane L, Hopewell S, Coleman CL and Bond CM (2016). Defining feasibility and pilot studies in preparation for randomised controlled trials: development of a conceptual framework. *PLoS One*, **11**: doi:19.1371/journal.pone.0150205. [16]

Eranti S, Mogg A, Pluck G, Landau S, Purvis R, Brown RG, Howard R, Knapp M, Philpot M, Rabe-Hesketh S, Romeo R, Rothwell J, Edwards D and McLoughlin DM (2007). A randomized, controlled trial with 6-month follow-up of repetitive transcranial magnetic stimulation and electroconvulsive therapy for severe depression. *American Journal of Psychiatry*, **164**, 73–81. [11]

Eron J, Yeni P, Gathe J, Estrada V, DeJesus E, Staszewski S, Lackey P, Katlama C, Young B, Yau L, Sutherland-Phillips D, Wannamaker P, Vavro C, Patel L, Yeo J and Shaefer M, (2006). The KLEAN study of fosamprenavir-ritonavir versus lopinavir-ritonavir, each in combination with abacavir-lamivudine, for initial treatment of HIV infection over 48 weeks: a randomised non-inferiority trial. *Lancet*, **368**, 476–482. [11]

Etxeberria A, Pérez I, Alcorta I, Emparanza JI, Ruiz de Velasco E, Iglesias MT, Orozco-Beltrán D and Rotaeche R (2013). The CLUES study: a cluster randomized clinical trial for the evaluation of cardiovascular guideline implementation in primary care. *BMC Health Services Research*, **13**, 438. [2]

Farid M, Chowbay B, Chen X, Tan S-H, Ramasamy S, Koo W-H, Toh H-C, Choo S-P and Ong SY-K (2012). Phase I pharmacokinetic study of chronomodulated dose-intensified combination of capecitabine and oxaliplatin (XELOX) in metastatic colorectal cancer. *Cancer Chemotherapy and Pharmacology*, **70**, 141–150. [15]

Farrington CP and Manning G (1990). Test statistics and sample size formulae for comparative binomial trials with null hypothesis of non-zero risk difference or non-unity relative risk. *Statistics in Medicine*, **9**, 1447–1454. [11]

Fayers PM and Machin D (2016). *Quality of Life: The Assessment, Analysis and Reporting of Patient-reported Outcomes*, (3rd edn) Wiley-Blackwell, Chichester. [2, 4, 20]

FDA (1988). *Guidelines for the Format and Content of the Clinical and Statistics Section of New Drug Applications*. US Department of Health and Human Services, Public Health Service, Food and Drug Administration. [1]

FDA (1996). *Statistical Guidance for Clinical Trials of Non Diagnostic Medical Devices (Appendix VIII)*. US Department of Health and Human Services, Public Health Service, Food and Drug Administration. http://www.fda.gov/RegulatoryInformation/Guidances/ucm106757.htm. [1]

FDA (2003). *Guidance for Industry. Bioavailability and Bioequivalence Studies for Orally Administered Drug Products – General Considerations*. Food and Drug Administration, Rockville, MD. [11]

FDA (2010). *Guidance for Industry, Non-inferiority Clinical Trials*. Food and Drug Administration, Rockville, MD. [11]

Fiore J (1988). *Statistical Power Analysis for the Behavioral Sciences*, 2nd edn. Lawrence Earlbaum, New Jersey. [5, 8, 16, 19]

Fiore JF, Faragher IG, Bialocerkowski A, Browning L and Denehy L (2103). Time to readiness for discharge is a valid and reliable measure of short-term recovery after colorectal surgery. *World Journal of Surgery*, **37**, 2927–2934. [5, 7]

Fitzmaurice GM, Laird NM and Ware JH (2011). *Applied Longitudinal Analysis*. (2nd ed) Wiley, Hoboken. [10]

Fleis JL, Tytun A and Ury HK (1980). A simple approximation for calculating sample sizes for comparing independent proportions. *Biometrics*, **36**, 343–346. [3]

Fleiss JL (1986). *The Design and Analysis of Clinical Experiments*. Wiley, New York. [14]

Fleiss JL, Levin B and Paik MC (2003). *Statistical Methods for Rates and Proportions*. Wiley, Chichester. [3]

Fleming TR (1982). One-sample multiple testing procedure for Phase II clinical trials. *Biometrics*, **38**, 143–151. [2, 17]

Flinn IW, Goodman SN, Post L, Jamison J, Miller CB, Gore S, Diehl L, Willis C, Ambinder RF and Byrd JC (2000). A dose-finding study of liposomal daunorubicin with CVP (COP-X) in advanced NHL. *Annals of Oncology*, **11**, 691–695. [15]

Foo K-F, Tan E-H, Leong S-S, Wee JTS, Tan T, Fong K-W, Koh L, Tai B-C, Lian L-G and Machin D (2002). Gemcitabine in metastatic nasopharyngeal carcinoma of the undifferentiated type. *Annals of Oncology*, **13**, 150–156. [17]

Freedman LS (1982). Tables of the number of patients required in clinical trials using the logrank test. *Statistics in Medicine*, **1**, 121–129. [7]

Freedman LS, Parmar MKB and Baker SG (1993). The design of observer agreement studies with binary assessments. *Statistics in Medicine*, **12**, 165–179. [20]

Freidlin B, Jiang W and Simon R (2010). The cross-validated adaptive signature design for predictive analysis of clinical trials. *Clinical Cancer Research*, **16**, 691–698. [15]

Freidlin B, McShane LM, Polley MY and Korn EL (2012). Randomised Phase II trial designs with biomarkers. *Journal of Clinical Oncology*, **30**, 3304–3309. [18]

Freidlin B and Simon R (2005). Adaptive signature design: An adaptive clinical trial design for generating and prospectively testing a gene expression signature for sensitive patients. *Clinical Cancer Research*, **11**, 7872–7878. [15]

Frison L and Pocock SJ (1992). Repeated measures in clinical trials: analysis using mean summary statistics and its implications for design. *Statistics in Medicine*, **11**, 1685–1704. [10]

Frison L and Pocock SJ (1997). Linearly divergent treatment effects in clinical trials with repeated measures: efficient analysis using summary statistics, *Statistics in Medicine* **16**, 2855–2872. [10]

Gajewski BJ and Mayo MS (2006). Bayesian sample size calculations in phase II clinical trials using a mixture of informative priors. *Statistics in Medicine*. **25**, 2554–2566. [17]

Gandhi M, Tan S-B, Chung AY-F, and Machin D (2015). On developing a pragmatic strategy for clinical trials: A case study of hepatocellular carcinoma. *Contemporary Clinical Trials*, **43**, 252–259. [1]

Ganju J, Izu A and Anemona A (2008). Sample size for equivalence trials: A case study from a vaccine lot consistency trial. *Statistics in Medicine*, **27**, 3743–3754. [11]

Gao F, Earnest A, Matchar DB, Campbell MJ and Machin D (2015). Sample size calculations for the design of cluster randomized trials: a review. *Contemporary Clinical Trials*, **42**, 41–50. [12]

George SL and Desu MM (1974). Planning the size and duration of a clinical trial studying the time to some critical event. *Journal of Chronic Diseases*, **27**, 15–24. [7]

Ghisi GL, dos Santos RZ, Bonin CBD, Roussenq S, Grace SL, Oh P and Benetti M (2014). Validation of a Portuguese version of the Information Needs in Cardiac Rehabilitation (INCR) scale in Brazil. *Heart & Lung*, **43**, 192–197. [20]

Giraudeau B, Ravaud P and Donner A (2008, 2009). Sample size calculation for cluster randomized cross-over trials. *Statistics in Medicine*; **27**, 5578–5585 (Correction, **28**, 720). [12]

González-Martín A, Crespo C, García-López JL, Pedraza M, Garrido P, Lastra E and Moyano A (2002). Ifosfamide and vinorelbine in advanced platinum-resistant ovarian cancer: excessive toxicity with a potentially active regimen. *Gynecologic Oncology*, **84**, 368–373. [18]

Goodman SN, Zahurak ML and Piantadosi S (1995). Some practical improvements in the continual reassessment method for phase I studies. *Statistics in Medicine*, **14**, 1149–1161. [15]

GRIT Study Group, The (2004). Infant wellbeing at 2 years of age in the Growth Restriction Intervention Trial (GRIT): multicentred randomised controlled trial. *Lancet*, **364**, 513–520. [5]

Grundy RG, Wilne SA, Weston CL, Robinson K, Lashford LS, Ironside J, Cox T, Chong WK, Campbell RHA, Bailey CC, Gattamaneni R, Picton S, Thorpe N, Mallucci C, English MW, Punt JAG, Walker DA, Ellison DW and Machin D (2007). Primary postoperative chemotherapy without radiotherapy for intracranial ependymoma in children: the UKCCSG / SIOP prospective study. *Lancet Oncology*, **8**, 696–705. [7]

Guenther WC (1981). Sample size formulas for normal theory *t*-tests. *The American Statistician*, **35**, 243–244. [5, 8]

Gupta SK (2011). Non-inferiority clinical trials: Practical issues and current regulatory perspective. *Indian Journal of Pharmacology*, **43**, 371–374. [11]

Gwadry-Sridhar F, Guyatt G, O'Brien B, Arnold JM, Walter S, Vingilis E and MacKeigan L (2008). TEACH: Trial of Education And Compliance in Heart dysfunction chronic disease and heart failure (HF) as an increasing problem. *Contemporary Clinical Trials*, **29**, 905–918. [12]

Haanen, H Hellriegel K and Machin D (1979). EORTC protocol for the treatment of good-risk patients with chronic myelogenous leukaemia. A randomized trial. *European Journal of Cancer*, **15**, 803–809. [2]

Hade EM, Murray DM, Pennell ML, Rhoda D, Paskett ED, Champion VL, Crabtree BF, Dietrich A, Dignan MB, Farmer M, Fenton JJ, Flocke S, Hiatt RA, Hudson SV, Mitchell M, Monahan P, Shariff-Marco S, Slone SL, Stange K, Stewart SL and Strickland PAO (2010). Intraclass correlation estimates for cancer screening outcomes: estimates and applications in the design of group-randomized cancer screening studies. *Journal of the National Cancer Institute Monographs*, **40**, 90–107. [12]

Halpern SD, Karlawish JHT and Berlin JA (2002). The continuing unethical conduct of underpowered clinical trials. *Journal of the American Medical Association*, **288**, 358–362. [2]

Hancock MJ, Maher CG, Latimer J, McLachlan AJ, Cooper CW, Day RO, Spindler MF and McAuley JH (2007). Assessment of diclofenac or spinal manipulative therapy, or both, in addition to recommended first-line treatment for acute low back pain: a randomised controlled trial. *Lancet*, **370**, 1638–1643. [14]

Harris EK and Boyd JC (1995). *Statistical Bases of Reference Values in Laboratory Medicine*. Marcel Dekker, New York. [21]

Hayes RJ and Moulton L (2009). *Cluster Randomised Trials*. Boca Raton, Chapman and Hall/CRC. [12]

Hegarty K, O'Doherty L, Taft A, Chondros P, Brown S, Valpied J, Astbury J, Taket A, Gold L, Feder G and Gunn J (2013). Screening and counselling in the primary care setting for women who have experienced intimate partner violence (WEAVE): a cluster randomised controlled trial. *Lancet*, **382**, 249–258. [4, 12]

Hemming K and Marsh J (2013). A menu-driven facility for sample-size calculations in cluster randomized controlled trials. *The Stata Journal*, **13**, 114–135. [12]

Hemming K, Eldridge S, Forbes G, Weijer C, Taljaard M (2017). How to design efficient cluster randomised trials. *British Medical Journal*, **358**:j3064

Hemming K and Taljaard M (2017). Sample size calculations for stepped wedge and cluster randomised trials: a unified approach. *Journal of Clinical Epidemiology*, **69**, 137–146. [11, 12]

Home PD, Pocock SJ, Beck-Nielson H, Curtis PS, Gomis R, Hanefeld M, Jones NP, Komajda M, McMurray JJV for the RECORD Study Team (2009). Rosiglitazone evaluated for cardiovascular outcomes in oral agent combination therapy for type 2 diabetes (RECORD): a multicentre, randomised, open-label trial. *Lancet*, **373**, 2125–2135. [11]

Hoo WL, Stavroulis A, Pateman K, Saridogan E, Cutner A, Pandis G, Tong ENC and Jurkovic D (2014). Does ovarian suspension following laparoscopic surgery for endometriosis reduce postoperative adhesions? An RCT. *Human Reproduction*, **29**, 670–676. [16]

Hooper R, Teerenstra S, de Hoop E and Eldridge S (2016). Sample size calculation for stepped wedge and other longitudinal cluster randomized trials. *Statistics in Medicine*, **35**, 4718–4728. [13]

Hosmer DW and Lemeshow S (2000). *Applied Logistic Regression*, (2nd edn.) Wiley, Chichester. [3]

Hosselet J-J, Ayappa I, Norman RG, Krieger AC and Rapoport DM (2001). Classification of sleep-disordered breathing. *American Journal of Respiratory Critical Care Medicine*, **163**, 398–405. [21]

Iaffaioli RV, Formato R, Tortoriello A, Del Prete S, Caraglia M, Pappagallo G, Pisano A, Fanelli F, Ianniello G, Cigolari S, Pizza C, Marano O, Pezzella G, Pedicini T, Febbraro A, Incoronato P, Manzione L, Ferrari E, Marzano N, Quattrin S, Pisconti S, Nasti G, Giotta G, Colucci G and other Goim authors (2005) Phase II study of sequential hormonal therapy with anastrozole/exemestane in advanced and metastatic breast cancer. *British Journal of Cancer*, **92**, 1621–1625. [2, 17]

IBM Corp (2013). IBM SPSS Statistics for Windows, Version 22, Armonk, New York: IBM Corp. [12]

Ilisson J, Zagura M, Zilmer K, Salum E, Heilman K, Piir A, Tillmann V, Kals J, Zilmer M and Pruunsild C (2015). Increased carotid artery intima-media thickness and myeloperoxidase level in children with newly diagnosed juvenile idiopathic arthritis. *Arthritis Research & Therapy*, **17**, 180. [5]

International Conference on Harmonisation of Technical Requirements for Registration of Pharmaceuticals for Human Use (1998). *ICH Harmonised Tripartite Guideline - Statistical Principles for Clinical Trials E9*. http://www.ich.org/products/guidelines/efficacy/efficacy-single/article/statistical-principles-for-clinical-trials.html. [1]

Itoh K, Ohtsu T, Fukuda H, Sasaki Y, Ogura M, Morishima Y, Chou T, Aikawa K, Uike N, Mizorogi F, Ohno T, Ikeda S, Sai T, Taniwaki M, Kawano F, Niimi M, Hotta T, Shimoyama M and Tobinai K (2002). Randomized phase II study of biweekly CHOP and dose-escalated CHOP with prophylactic use of lenograstim (glycosylated G-CSF) in aggressive non-Hodgkin's lymphoma: Japan Clinical Oncology Group Study 9505. *Annals of Oncology*, **13**, 1347–1355. [18]

Ivers NM, Taljaard M, Dixon S, Bennett C, McRae A, Taleban J, Skea Z, Brehaut JC, Boruch RF, Eccles MP, Grimshaw JM, Weijer C, Zwarenstein M and Donner A (2011). Impact of CONSORT extension for cluster randomized trials on quality of reporting and study methodology: review of random sample of 300 trials, 2000-8. *British Medical Journal*, **343**, d5886. [12]

Jackson L, Cohen J, Sully B and Julious S (2015). NOURISH, Nutritional OUtcomes from a Randomised Investigation of Intradialytic oral nutritional Supplements in patients receiving Haemodialysis: a pilot randomised controlled trial. *Pilot and Feasibility Studies*, **1**, 11. [16]

Jiang W, Freidlin B and Simon R (2007). Biomarker adaptive threshold design: A procedure for evaluating treatment with possible biomarker-defined subset effect. *Journal of the National Cancer Institute*, **99**, 1036–1043. [15]

Johnson VE and Cook JD (2009). Bayesian design of single-arm phase II clinical trials with continuous monitoring. *Clinical Trials*, **6**, 217–226. [17, 18]

Johnson VE and Rossell D (2010). On the use of non-local prior densities in Bayesian hypothesis tests. *Journal of the Royal Staistical Society B*, **72**, 143–170. [17]

Jones B, Jarvis P, Lewis JA and Ebbutt AF (1996). Trials to assess equivalence: the importance of rigorous methods. *British Medical Journal*, **313**, 36–39. [11]

Jones CL and Holmgren E (2007). An adaptive Simon two-stage design for Phase 2 studies of targeted therapies. *Contemporary Clinical Trials*, **28**, 654–661. [18]

Julious (2004). Sample sizes for clinical trials with Normal data. *Statistics in Medicine*, **23**, 1921–1986. [11]

Julious SA (2005a). Two-sided confidence intervals for the single proportion: comparison of seven methods. *Statistics in Medicine*, **24**, 3383–3384. [1]

Julious SA (2005b). Sample Size of 12 per Group Rule of Thumb for a Pilot Study. *Pharmaceutical Statistics*, **4**, 287–291. [16]

Julious SA and Campbell MJ (1996). Sample size calculations for ordered categorical data (letter). *Statistics in Medicine*, **15**, 1065–1066. [3]

Julious SA and Campbell MJ (1998). Sample sizes for paired or matched ordinal data. *Statistics in Medicine*, **17**, 1635–1642. [8]

Julious SA and Campbell MJ (2012). Tutorial in biostatistics: sample sizes for parallel group clinical trials with binary data. *Statistics in Medicine*, **31**, 2904–2936. [3, 11]

Julious SA. and Owen NRJ (2006). Sample size calculations for clinical studies allowing for uncertainty about the variance. *Pharmaceutical Statistics*, **5**, 29–37. [16]

Julious SA, Tan S-B and Machin D (2010). *An Introduction to Statistics in Early Phase Trials*. Wiley-Blackwell, Chichester. [11]

Kahn RS, Fleischhacker WW, Boter H, Davidson M, Vergouwe Y, Keet IPM, Gheorghe MD, Rybakowski JZ, Galderisi S, Libiger J, Hummer M, Dollfus S, López-Ibor JJ, Hranov KG, Gaebel W, Peuskins J, Lindfors N, Riecher-Rössler A and Grobbee DE (2008). Effectiveness of antipsychotic drugs in first-episode schizophrenia and schizophreniform disorder: an open randomised clinical trial. *Lancet*, **371**, 1085–1097. [14]

Kasliwal R, Wilton LV and Shakir SAW (2008). Monitoring the safety of pioglitazone. *Drug Safety*, **31**, 839–850. [6]

Keene ON, Jones MRK, Lane PW and Anderson J (2007). Analysis of exacerbation rates in asthma and chronic obstructive pulmonary disease: example from the TRISTAN study. *Pharmaceutical Statistics*, **6**, 89–97. [6]

Kieser M and Wassmer G (1996). On the use of the upper confidence limit for the variance from a pilot sample for sample size determination. *Biometrical Journal*, **8**, 941–949. [16]

Kim ES, Herbst JJ, Wistuba II, Lee JJ, Blumenschein GR, Tsao A, Stewart DJ, Hicks ME, Erasmus J, Gupta S, Alden CM, Liu S, Tang X, Khuri FR, Tran HT, Johnson BE, Heymach JV, Mao L, Fossella F, Kies MS, Papadimitrakopoulou V, Davis SE, Lippman SM and Hong WK. (2011). The BATTLE trial: personalizing therapy for lung cancer. *Cancer Discovery*, **1**, 44–53. [18]

King (2009). Once-daily insulin detemir is comparable to once-daily insulin glargine in providing glycaemic control over 24 h in patients with type 2 diabetes: a double-blind, randomized, crossover study. *Diabetes, Obesity and Metabolism*, **11**, 69–71. [11]

Kinmonth A-L, Fulton Y and Campbell MJ (1992). Management of feverish children at home. *British Medical Journal*, **305**, 1134–1136. [4]

Kopec JA, Abrahamowicz M and Esdaile JM (1993). Randomised discontinuation trials: utility and efficiency. *Journal of Clinical Epidemiology*, **46**, 959–971. [18]

Korn EL, Midthune D, Chen TT, Rubinstein LV, Christian MC and Simon RM (1994). A comparison of two Phase I trial designs. *Statistics in Medicine*, **13**, 1799–1806. [15]

Kraemer HC, Mintz J, Nosa A, Tinklenberg J and Yesavage JA (2006). Caution regarding the use of pilot studies to guide power calculations for study purposes. *Archives of General Psychiatry*, **63**, 484–489. [16]

Kwak M and Jung S (2014). Phase II clinical trials with time-to-event endpoints: optimal two-stage designs with opne sample log-rank test. *Statistics in Medicine*, **33**, 2004–2016. [18]

Lachenbruch PA (1992). On the sample size for studies based upon McNemar's test. *Statistics in Medicine*, **11**, 1521–1525. [11]

Lachin JM (1992). Power and sample size evaluation for the McNemar test with application to matched case-control studies. *Statistics in Medicine*, **11**, 1239–1251. [8]

Lancaster GA, Dodd S and Williamson PR (2004). Design and analysis of pilot studies: recommendations for good practice. *Journal of Evaluation in Clinical Practice*, **10**, 307–312. [16]

Latouche A, Porcher R and Chevret S (2004). Sample size formula for proportional hazards modelling of competing risks. *Statistics in Medicine*, **23**, 3263–3274. [7]

Latouche A and Porcher R (2007). Sample size calculations in the presence of competing risks. *Statistics in Medicine*, **26**, 5370–5380. [7]

Lehman EL (1975). *Nonparametric Statistical Methods Based on Ranks.* Holden-Day, San Francisco. [5]

Lehnert M, Mross K, Schueller J, Thuerlimann B, Kroeger N and Kupper H (1998). Phase II trial of dexverapamil and epirubicin in patients with non-responsive metastatic breast cancer. *British Journal of Cancer,* **77**, 1155–1163. [16]

Lemeshow S, Hosmer DW and Klar J (1988). Sample size requirements for studies estimating odds ratios or relative risks. *Statistics in Medicine,* **7**, 759–764. [9]

Lenth RV (2006-9). *Java Applets for Power and Sample Size.* http://www.stat.uiowa.edu/~rlenth/Power. [1]

Leong SS, Wee J, Tay MH, Toh CK, Tan SB, Thng CH, Foo KF, Lim WT, TanT and Tan EH (2005). Paclitaxel, carboplatin and gemcitabine in metastatic nasopharyngeal carcinoma: A phase II trial using a triplet combination. *Cancer,* **103**, 569–575. [17]

Leong SS, Toh CK, Lim WT, Lin X, Tan SB, Poon D, Tay MH, Foo KF, Ho J and Tan EH (2007) A randomized phase II trial of single agent Gemcitabine, Vinorelbine or Docetaxel in patients with advanced non-small cell lung cancer who have poor performance status and/or are elderly. *Journal of Thoracic Oncology,* **2**, 230–236. [18]

Levy HL, Milanowski A, Chakrapani A, Cleary M, Lee P, Trefz FK, Whitley CB, Feillet F, Feigenbaum AS, Bebchuk JD, Christ-Schmidt H and Dorenbaum A (2007). Efficacy of sepropterin dihydrochloride (tetrahydrobiopterin, 6R-BH4) for reduction of phenylalanine concentration in patients with phenylketonuria: a phase III randomised placebo-controlled study. *Lancet,* **370**, 504–510. [10]

Lewis JA (1981). Post-marketing surveillance: how many patients? *Trends in Pharmacological Sciences,* **2**, 93–94. [6]

Lewis JA (1983). Clinical trials: statistical developments of practical benefit to the Pharmaceutical Industry. *Journal of the Royal Statistical Society* (A), **146**, 362–393. [6]

Li J and Fine J (2004). On sample size for sensitivity and specificity in prospective diagnostic accuracy studies. *Statistics in Medicine,* **23**, 2537–2550. [21]

Lie S-FDJ, Ozcan M, Verkerke GJ, Sandham A and Dijkstra PU (2008). Survival of flexible, braided, bonded stainless steel lingual retainers: a historic cohort study. *European Journal of Orthodontics,* **30**, 199–204. [3, 6]

Linnet K (1987). Two-stage transformation systems for normalization of reference distributions evaluated. *Clinical Chemistry,* **33**, 381–386. [21]

Liu PY (2001). Phase II selection designs. In: Crowley J (ed) *Handbook of Statistics in Clinical Oncology,* Marcel Dekker Inc, New York, pp 119–127. [18]

Lo ECM, Luo Y, Fan MW and Wei SHY (2001). Clinical investigation of two glass-ionomer restoratives used with the atraumatic restorative treatment approach in China: Two-years results. *Caries Research,* **35**, 458–463. [8]

Low JG, Sung C, Wijaya L, Wei Y, Rathore APS, Watanabe S, Tan BH, Toh L, Chua LT, Hou Y, Chow A, Howe S, Chan WK, Tan KH, Chung JS, Cherng BP, Lye DC, Tambayah PA, Ng LC, Connolly J, Hibberd ML, Leo YS, Cheung YB, Ooi EE and Vasudevan SG (2014). Efficacy and safety of celgosivir in patients with dengue fever (CELADEN): a phase 1b, randomised, double-blind, placebo-controlled, proof-of-concept trial. *Lancet Infectious Diseases,* **14**, 706–715. [18]

Lowrie R, Mair FS, Greenlaw N, Forsyth P, Jhund PS, McConnachie A, Rae B, and McMurray JJV (2012). Pharmacist intervention in primary care to improve outcomes in patients with left ventricular systolic dysfunction. *European Heart Journal,* **33**:314–324. [12]

Lu Y and Bean JA (1995). On the sample size for one-sided equivalence of sensitivities based upon McNemar's test. *Statistics in Medicine,* **14**, 1831–1839. [11]

Machin D and Campbell MJ (2005). *Design of Studies for Medical Research*, Wiley, Chichester. [1, 2, 16]

Machin D, Campbell MJ, Fayers PM and Pinol A (1997). *Statistical Tables for the Design of Clinical Studies*, 2nd edn. Blackwell Scientific Publications, Oxford. [2]

Machin D and Fayers PM (2010). *Randomized Clinical Trials*. Wiley-Blackwell, Chichester. [18]

Matthews JNS, Altman DG, Campbell MJ and Royston JP (1990). Analysis of serial measurements in medical research. *British Medical Journal*, **300**, 230–235. [10]

Mayo MS and Gajewski BJ (2004). Bayesian sample size calculations in phase II clinical trials using informative conjugate priors. *Controlled Clinical Trials*, **25**, 157–167. [17]

Mhurchu CN, Gorton D, Turley M, Jiang Y, Michie J, Maddison R and Hattie J (2013). Effects of a free school breakfast programme on children's attendance, academic achievement and short-term hunger: results from a stepped-wedge, cluster randomised controlled trial. *J Epidemiology & Community Health*, **67**, 257–264. [13]

Mick R, Crowley JJ and Carroll RJ (2000). Phase II clinical trial design for noncytotoxic anticancer agents for which time to disease progression is the primary endpoint. *Controlled Clinical Trials*, **21**, 343–359. [16, 17]

Mick R, Crowley JJ and Carroll RJ (2000). Phase II clinical trial design for noncytotoxic anticancer agents for which time to disease progression is the primary endpoint. *Controlled Clinical Trials*, **21**, 343–359. [18]

Moberg J and Kramer M (2015). A brief history of the cluster randomised design. *Journal of the Royal Society of Medicine*, **108**, 192–198. [12]

Moinester M and Gottfried R (2014). Sample size estimation for correlations with pre-specified confidence interval. *The Quantitative Methods for Psychology*, **19**, 124–130. [19]

Morrison JM, Gilmour H and Sullivan F (1991). Children seen frequently out of hours in one general practice. *British Medical Journal*, **303**, 1111–1114. [8]

Motzer RJ, Escudier B, Oudard S, Hutson TE, Porta C, Bracardo S, Grünwald V, Thompson JA, Figlin RA, Hollaender N, Urbanowitz G, Berg WJ, Kay A, Lebwohl D and Ravaud A (2008). Efficacy of everolimus in advanced renal cell carcinoma: a double-blind, randomised, placebo-controlled phase III trial. *Lancet*, **372**, 449–456. [7]

Mountain GA, Hind D, Gossage-Worrall R, Walters SJ, Duncan R, Newbould L, Rex S, Jones C, Bowling A, Cattan M, Cairns A, Cooper C, Tudor Edwards R and Goyder EC (2014). 'Putting Life in Years' (PLINY) telephone friendship groups research study: pilot randomised controlled trial. *Trials*, **15**, 141–152. [16]

Mühlhauser I, Bender R, Bott U, Jörgens V, Grüsser M, Wagener W, Overmann H and Berger M (1996). Cigarette smoking and progression of retinopathy and nephropathy in type 1 diabetes. *Diabetic Medicine*, **13**, 536–543. [4]

Munro JF, Nicholl JP, Brazier JE, Davey R and Cochrane T (2004). Cost effectiveness of a community based exercise programme in over 65 year olds: cluster randomised trial. *Journal of Epidemiology and Community Health*, **58**, 1004–1010. [12]

Naylor CD and Llewellyn-Thomas HA (1994). Can there be a more patients-centred approach to determining clinically important effect size for randomized treatments? *Journal of Clinical Epidemiology*, **47**, 787–795. [1]

NCSS, LC (2017). *Pass 15 Power Analysis and Sample Size Software (PASS 15): Kaysville*, Utah, USA. [1]

Nejadnik H, Hui JH, Choong EPF, Tai B-C and Lee EH (2011). Autologous bone marrow-derived mesenchymal stem cells versus autologous chondrocyte implantation: An observational cohort study. *The American Journal of Sports Medicine*, **38**, 1110–1116. [5]

Newcombe RG and Altman DG (2000). Proportions and their differences. In Altman DG, Machin D, Bryant TN and Gardner MJ (eds). *Statistics with Confidence*, 2nd edn. British Medical Journal Books, London, pp 45–56. [1, 9, 20]

Ngo CS, Pan C-W, Finkelstein EA, Lee C-F, Wong IB, Ong J, Ang M, Wong T-Y and Saw S-M (2014). A cluster randomized controlled trial evaluating an incentive-based outdoor physical activity programme to increase outdoor time and prevent myopia in children. *Opthalmic & Physiological Optics*, **34**, 362–368. [12]

Noether GE (1987). Sample size determination for some common nonparametric tests. *Journal of the American Statistical Association*, **82**, 645–647. [5]

Nomura Y, Tamaki Y, Tanaka T, Arakawa H, Tsurumoto A, Kirimura K, Sato T, Hanada N and Kamoi K (2006). Screening of periodontitis with salivary enzyme tests. *Journal of Oral Science*, **48**, 177–183. [21]

Novikov I, Fund N and Freedman LS (2010). A modified approach to estimating sample size for simple logistic regression with one continuous covariate. *Statistics in Medicine*, **29**, 97–107. [3]

Nthumba PM, Stepita-Poenaru E, Poenaru D, Bird P, Allegranzi B, Pittet D and Harbarth S (2010). Cluster-randomized, crossover trial of the efficacy of plain soap and water *versus* alcohol-based rub for surgical hand preparation in a rural hospital in Kenya. *British Journal of Surgery*, **97**, 1621–1628. [12]

Nwaru BI and Sheikh A (2015). Hormonal contraceptives and asthma in women of reproductive age: analysis of data from serial national Scottish Health Surveys. *Journal of the Royal Society of Medicine*, **108**, 358–371. [3]

Obuchowski NA and McClish DN (1997). Sample size determination for diagnostic accuracy studies involving binormal ROC curve indices. *Statistics in Medicine*, **16**, 1529–1542. [21]

O'Quigley J (2001). Dose-finding designs using continual reassessment method. In: Crowley J (ed) *Handbook of Statistics in Clinical Oncology*, Marcel Dekker Inc, New York, pp 35–72. [15]

O'Quigley J, Pepe M and Fisher L (1990). Continual reassessment method: a practical design for phase I clinical trials in cancer. *Biometrics*, **46**, 33–48. [15]

Ornetti P, Gossec L, Laroche D, Combescure C, Dougados M and Maillfert J-F (2015) Impact of repeated measures of joint space width on the sample size calculation: An application of hip osteoarthritis. *Joint Bone Spine*, **82**, 172–176. [10]

Palacios CRF, Haugen EN, Thompson AM, Rasmussen RW, Goracke N and Goyal P (2016). Clinical outcomes with a systolic blood pressure lower than 120 mmHg in older patients with high disease burden. *Renal Failure*, **38**, 1364–1369. [5]

Pandis N (2012). Sample calculations for comparing proportions. *American Journal of Orthodontics and Dentofacial Orthopedics*, **141**, 666–667. [3]

Pandis N and Machin D (2012). Sample calculations for comparing rates. *American Journal of Orthodontics and Dentofacial Orthopedics*, **142**, 565–567. [6]

Pandis N, Polychronopoulou A and Eliades T (2007). Self-ligating vs conventional brackets in the treatment of mandibular crowding: a prospective clinical trial of treatment duration and dental effects. *American Journal of Orthodontics and Dentofacial Orthopedics*, **132**, 208–215. [5]

Papp K, Bissonnette R, Rosoph L, Wasel N, Lynde CW, Searles G, Shear NH, Huizinga RB and Maksymowych WP (2008). Efficacy of ISA247 in plaque psoriasis: a randomised multicentre, double-blind, placebo-controlled phase III study. *Lancet*, **371**, 1337–1342. [14]

Parikh NA, Kennedy KA, Lasky RE, McDavid GE and Tyson JE (2013). Pilot randomized trial of hydrocortisone in ventilator-dependent extremely preterm infants: effects on regional brain volumes. *The Journal of Pediatrics*, **162**, 685–690. [1, 16]

Piaggio G, Carolli G, Villar J, Pinol A, Bakketeig L, Lumbiganon P, Bergsjø P, Al-Mazrou Y, Ba'aqeel H, Belizán JM, Farnot U and Berendes H (2001). Methodological considerations on the design and analysis of an equivalence stratified cluster randomization trial. *Statistics in Medicine*, **20**, 401–416. [11]

Piaggio G, Elbourne DR, Pocock SJ, Evans SJW and Altman DG for the CONSORT Group (2012). Reporting of noninferiority and equivalence randomized trials: Extension of the CONSORT 2010 statement. *Journal of the American Medical Association*, **308**, 2594–2604. doi:10.001/jama.2012.87802. [11]

Piaggio G and Pinol APY (2001). Use of the equivalence approach in reproductive health trials. *Statistics in Medicine*, **20**, 3571–3587. [11]

Pintilie M (2002). Dealing with competing risks: testing covariates and calculating sample size. *Statistics in Medicine*, **21**, 3317–3324. [7]

Poldervaart JM, Reitsma JB, Koffijberg H, Backus BE, Six AJ, Doevendans PA and Hoes AW (2013). The impact of the HEART risk score in the early assessment of patients with acute chest pain: design of a stepped wedge, cluster randomised trial. *BMC Cardiovascular Disorders*, **13**, 77. [13]

Poon CY, Goh BT, Kim M-J, Rajaseharan A, Ahmed S, Thongprasom K, Chaimusik M, Suresh S, Machin D, Wong-HB and Seldrup J (2006). A randomised controlled trial to compare steroid with cyclosporine for the topical treatment of oral lichen planus. *Oral Surg Oral Med Oral Path Oral Radiol Endod*, **102**, 47–55. [2]

Pusztai L and Hess KR (2004). Clinical trial design for microarray predictive marker discovery and assessment. *Annals of Oncology*, **15**, 1731–1737. [18]

Rahardja D, Zhao YD and Qu Y (2012). Sample size determination for the Wilcoxon-Mann-Whitney test. A comprehensive review. *Statistics in Pharmaceutical Research*, **1**, 317–322. [5]

Ravaud A, Hawkins R, Gardner JP, von der Maase H, Zantl N, Harper P, Rolland F, Audhuy B, Machiels JP, Pétavy F, Gore M, Schöffski P and El-Hariry I (2008). Lapatinib versus hormone therapy in patients with advanced renal cell carcinoma: a randomized phase III clinical trial. *Journal of Clinical Oncology*, **26**, 2285–2291. [15]

Realini TD (2009. A prospective, randomized, investigator-masked evaluation of the monocular trial in ocular hypertension or open-angle glaucoma. *Opthalmology*, **116**, 1237–1242. [8]

Richards B, Parmar MKB, Anderson, CK, Ansell ID, Grigor K, Hall RR, Morley AR, Mostofi FK, Risdon RA and Uscinska BM (1991). Interpretation of biopsies of "normal" urothelium in patients with superficial bladder cancer. *British Journal of Urology*, **67**, 369–375. [20]

Roebruck P and Kühn A (1995). Comparison of tests and sample size formulae for proving therapeutic equivalence based on the difference of binomial probabilities. *Statistics in Medicine*, **14**, 1583–1594. [11]

Rotondi M and Donner A (2012). Sample size estimation in cluster randomized trials: An evidence-based perspective. *Computation Statistics and Data Analysis*, **56**, 1174–1187. [12]

SAS Institute (2004). *Getting Started with the SAS Power and Sample Size Application: Version 9.1*, SAS Institute, Cary, NC. [1]

Saville DJ (1990). Multiple comparison procedures: The practical solution. *The American Statistician*, **44**, 174–180. [14]

Schoenfeld DA (1983). Sample-size formula for the proportional hazards regression model. *Biometrics*, **39**, 499–503. [7]

Schouten HJA (1999). Sample size formula with a continuous outcome for unequal group sizes and unequal variances. *Statistics in Medicine*, **18**, 87–91. [5]

Schulz KF and Grimes DA (2005). Sample size calculations in randomised trials: mandatory and mystical. *Lancet*, **365**, 1348–1353. [2]

Sedgwick P (2013). Equivalence trials. *British Medical Journal*; **346**::f184 doi:10.1136/bmj.f184. [11]

Shimodera S, Kato T, Sato H, Miki K, Shinagawa Y, Kondo M, Fujita H, Morokuma I, Ikeda Y, Akechi T, Watanabe N, Yamada M, Inagaki M, Yonemoto N and Furukawa TA (2012). The first 100 patients in the SUN(^_^)D trial (strategic use of new generation antidepressants for depression): examination of feasibility and adherence during the pilot phase. *Trials*, **13**, 80. http:/www.trialsjournal.com/content/30/1/80. [16]

Silverstein FE, Faich G, Goldstein JL, Simon LS, Piincus T, Whelton A, Makuch R, Eisen G, Agrawal NM, Stenson WF, Burr AM, Zhao WW, Kent JD, Lefkowith JB, Verburg KM and Geis GS (2000). Gastrointestinal toxicity with celecoxib vs nonsteroidal anti-inflammatory drugs for osteoarthritis and rheumatoid arthritis. *Journal of the American Medical Association*, **284**, 1247–1255. [6]

Sim J and Lewis M (2011). The size of a pilot study for a clinical trial should be calculated in relation to considerations of precision and efficiency. *Journal of Clinical Epidemiology*, **65**, 301–308. [16]

Simon R (1989). Optimal two-stage designs for phase II clinical trials. *Controlled Clinical Trials*, **10**, 1–14. [17]

Simon R (2005). A roadmap for developing and validating therapeutically relevant genomic classifiers. *Journal of Clinical Oncology*, **23**, 7332–7341. [15]

Simon R (2008a). Using genomics in clinical trial design. *Clinical Cancer Research*, **14**, 5984–5993. [15]

Simon R (2008b). Designs and adaptive analysis plans for pivotal clinical trials of therapeutics and companion diagnostics. *Expert Opinion of Molecular Diagnostics*, **2**, 721–729. [15]

Simon R (2010). Clinical trial designs for evaluating the medical utility of prognostic and predictive biomarkers in oncology. *Personalized Medicine*, **7**, 33–47. [15]

Simon R (2012). Clinical trials for predictive medicine. *Statistics in Medicine*, **31**, 3031–3040. [15]

Simon R and Wang SJ (2006). Use of genomic signatures in therapeutics development. *The Pharmacogenomcs Journal*, **6**, 167–173. [15]

Simon R, Wittes RE and Ellenberg SS (1985). Randomized phase II clinical trials. *Cancer Treatment Reports*, **69**, 1375–1381. [18]

Smith PG and Morrow R (1996). *Field Trials of Health Interventions in Developing Countries: A Toolbox*. Macmillan, London. [6]

Smolen JS, Beaulieu A, Rubbert-Roth A, Ramos-Remus C, Rovensky J, Alecock E, Woodworth T and Alten R (2008). Effect of interleukin-6 receptor inhibition with tocilizumab in patients with rheumatoid arthritis (Option study): a double-blind, placebo-controlled, randomised trial. *Lancet*, **371**, 987–997. [14]

Sng BL, Wang H, Assam PN and Sia AT (2015). Assessment of an updated double-vasopressor automated system using Nexfin™ for the maintenance of haemodynamic stability to improve peri-operative outcome during spinal anaesthesia for caesarean section. *Anaesthesia*, **70**, 691–698. [3]

Sng BL, Woo D, Leong WL, Wang H, Assam PN and Sia AT (2014). Comparison of computer-integrated patient-controlled epidural analgesia with no initial basal infusion versus moderate basal infusion for labor and delivery: A randomized controlled trial. *Journal of Anaesthesiology Clinical Pharmacology*, **30**, 496–501. [9]

Soria J-C, Felip E, Cobo M, Lu S, Syrigos K, Lee KH, Goker E, Georgoulias V, Li W, Isla D, Guclu SZ, Morabito A, Min YJ, Ardizonni A, Gadgeel SM, Wang B, Chand VK, and Goss GD (2015). Afatinib versus erlotinib as second-line treatment of patients with advanced squamous cell carcinoma of the lung (LUX-Lung 8): an open-label randomised controlled phase 3 trial. *Lancet Oncology*, **16**, 897–907. [7]

Sridhar SC, Shao J and Wang H (2002). A note on sample size calculations for mean comparisons based on non central t-statistics. *Journal of Pharmaceutical Statistics*, **12**, 441–456. [5]

Sridhar T, Gore A, Boiangiu I, Machin D and Symonds RP (2009). Concomitant (without adjuvant) temozolomide and radiation to treat glioblastoma: A retrospective study. *Journal of Oncology*, **21**, 19–22. [1]

Stadler WM, Rosner G, Small E, Hollis D, Rini B, Zaentz SD, Mahony J and Ratain MJ (2005). Successful implementation of the randomized discontinuation trial design: an application to the study of the putative antiangiogenic agent carboxyaminoimidazole in renal cell carcinoma-CALGB 69901. *Journal of Clinical Oncology*, **23**, 3726–3732. [18]

Stadler WM (2007). The randomized discontinuation trial: a phase II design to assess growth-inhibitory agents. *Molecular Cancer Therapeutics*, **6**, 1180–1185. [18]

StataCorp (2014). *Stata Statistical Software: Release 14*. College Station, Texas, USA. [1]

Statistical Solutions (2015). *nQuery Adviser + nTerim: Users Guide*. Cork, Ireland. [1]

Storer BE (2001). Choosing a Phase I design. In: Crowley J (ed) *Handbook of Statistics in Clinical Oncology*, Marcel Dekker Inc, New York, pp 73–91. [15]

Strom BL (2013). Sample size considerations for pharmacoepidemiology studies. In Strom BL, Kimmel SE and Hennessy S (eds) *Pharmacoepidemiology*, (5th edn) Wiley, Chichester. [6]

Tai BC, Chen ZJ and Machin D (2018). Estimating sample size in the presence of competing risks – Cause-specific hazard or cumulative incidence approach? *Statistical Methods in Medical Research*, **27**, 114–125. [7]

Tai BC, Grundy R and Machin D (2011). On the importance of accounting for competing risks in paediatric brain cancer: II. Regression modeling and sample size. *International Journal of Radiation Oncology, Biology and Physics*, **79**, 1139–1146. [7]

Tai BC and Machin D (2014) *Regression Methods for Medical Research*. Wiley-Blackwell, Chichester. [2, 7]

Tai B-C, Wee J and Machin D (2011). Analysis and design of randomised clinical trials involving competing risks endpoints. *Trials*, **12**, 127. [7]

Tan SB and Machin D (2002). Bayesian two-stage designs for phase II clinical trials. *Statistics in Medicine*, **21**, 1991–2012. [17]

Tan SB, Wong EH and Machin D (2004). Bayesian two-stage design for phase II clinical trials. In *Encyclopedia of Biopharmaceutical Statistics*, 2nd edn (online) (Ed: Chow SC). http://www.dekker.com/servlet/product/DOI/101081EEBS120023507. Marcel Dekker, New York. [17]

Tan S-H, Machin D and Tan S-B (2012). Sample sizes for estimating differences in proportions – Can we keep things simple? *Journal of Biopharmaceutical Statistics*, **22**, 133–140. [9]

Teare MD, Dimairo M, Shephard N, Hayman A, Whitehead A and Walters SJ (2014). Sample size requirements to estimate key design parameters from external pilot randomised controlled trials: A simulation study. *Trials*, **15**, 264. [16]

Teerenstra S, Eldridge S, Graff M, de Hoop E and Born GF (2012). A simple sample size formula for analysis of covariance in cluster randomized. *Statistics in Medicine*, **31**, 2169–2178. [12]

Thabane L, Ma J, Chu R, Cheng J, Ismaila A, Rios LP, Robson R, Thabane M, Giangregorio L and, Goldsmith CH (2010). A tutorial on pilot studies: The what, why and how. *BMC Medical Research Methodology*, **10**, 1. [16]

Thall P and Simon R (1994). A Bayesian approach to establishing sample size and monitoring criteria for phase II clinical trials. *Controlled Clinical Trials* **15**, 463–481. [17]

Travers DA, Waller AE, Bowling JM, Flowers D and Tintinalli J (2002). Five-level triage system more effective than Three-level in tertiary emergency department. *Journal of Emergency Nursing*, **28**, 395–400. [20]

Tubert-Bitter P, Begaud B, Moride Y and Abenhaim L (1994). Sample size calculations for single group post-marketing cohort studies. *Journal of Clinical Epidemiology*, **47**, 435–439. [6]

Vaidya JS, Joseph DJ, Tobias JS, Bulsara M, Wenz F, Saunders C, Alvarado M, Flyger HL, Massarut S, Eiermann W, Keshtgar M, Dewar J, Kraus-Tiefenbacher U, Süttterlin M, Esserman L, Holtveg HMR, Roancadin M, Pigorsch S, Metaxas M, Falzon M, Matthews A, Corica T, Williams NR and Baum M (2010). Targeted intraoperative radiotherapy versus whole breast radiotherapy for breast cancer (TARGIT-A trial): an international, prospective, randomised, non-inferiority phase 3 trial. *Lancet*, **376**, 91–102. [11]

Van Breukelen GJP and Candel MJJM (2012). Comments on 'Efficiency loss because of varying cluster size in cluster randomized trials is smaller than literature suggests'. *Statistics in Medicine*, **31**, 397–400. [12]

Walker E and Nowcki AS (2010). Understanding equivalence and noninferiority testing. *Journal of General Internal Medicine*, **26**, 192–196. [11]

Wallentin L, Wilcox RG, Weaver WD, Emanuelsson H, Goodvin A, Nyström P and Bylock A (2003). Oral ximelagatran for secondary prophylaxis after myocardial infarction: the ESTEEM randomised controlled trial. *Lancet*, **362**, 789–797. [14]

Walter SD, Eliasziw M and Donner A (1998) Sample size and optimal designs for reliability studies. *Statistics in Medicine*, **17**, 101–110. [20]

Walters SJ (2009). *Quality of Life Outcomes in Clinical Trials and Health Care Evaluation*. Wiley, Chichester. [5]

Wang SJ, O'Neill RT and Hung HMJ (2007). Approaches to evaluation of treatment effect in randomised clinical trials with genomic subset. *Pharmaceutical Statistics*, **6**, 227–244. [15]

Wang YG, Leung DHY, Li M and Tan SB (2005). Bayesian designs for frequentist and Bayesian error rate considerations. *Statistical Methods in Medical Research* **14**, 445–456. [17]

Watson REB, Ogden S, Cotterell LF, Bowden JJ, Bastrilles JY, Long SP and Griffiths CEM (2009). A cosmetic 'anti-aging' product improves photoaged skin: a double-blind, randomized controlled trial. *British Journal of Dermatology*, **161**, 419–426. [5]

Weng J, Li Y, Xu W, Shi L, Zhang Q, Zhu D, Hu Y, Zhou Z, Yan X, Tian H, Ran X, Luo Z, Xian J, Yan L, Li F, Zeng L, Chen Y, Yang L, Yan S, Liu J, Li M, Fu Z and Cheng H (2008). Effect of intensive insulin therapy on β-cell function and glycaemic control in patients with newly diagnosed type 2 diabetes: a multicentre randomised parallel-group trial. *Lancet*, **371**, 1753–1760. [14]

Whatley J, Street R, Kay S and Harris PE (2016). Use of reflexology in managing secondary lymphoedema for patients affected by treatments for breast cancer: A feasibility study. *Complementary Therapies in Clinical Practice*, **23**, 1–8. [16]

White A and Ernst E (2001). The case for uncontrolled clinical trials: A starting point for the evidence base for CAM. *Complementary Therapies in Medicine*, **9**, 111–115. [16]

Whitehead AL, Julious SA, Cooper CL and Campbell MJ (2015). Estimating the sample size for a pilot randomised trial to minimise the overall trial sample size for the external pilot and main trial for a continuous outcome variable. *Statistical Methods in Medical Research*. **25**, 1057–1073. [16]

Whitehead AL, Sully BGO and Campbell MJ (2014). Pilot and feasibility studies: Is there a difference from each other and from a randomised controlled trial? *Contemporary Clinical Trials*, **38**, 130–133. [16]

Whitehead J (1993). Sample size calculations for ordered categorical data. *Statistics in Medicine*, **12**, 2257–2272. [4]

Whitehead J (2014). One stage and two stage designs for phase II clinical trials with survival endpoints. *Statistics in Medicine*, **33**, 3830–3843. [18]

Whiteley W, Al-Shahi R, Warlow CP, Zeideler M and Lueck CJ (2006). CSF opening pressure: Reference interval and the effect of body mass index. *Neurology*, **67**, 1690–1691. [21]

Wight J, Jakubovic M, Walters S, Maheswaran R, White P and Lennon V (2004). Variation in cadaveric organ donor rates in the UK. *Nephrology Dialysis Transplantation*; **19**, 963–968. [1]

Williamson P, Hutton JL, Bliss J, Blunt J, Campbell MJ and Nicholson R (2000). Statistical review by research ethics committees. *Journal of the Royal Statistical Society A*, **163**, 5–13. [2]

Woertman W, de Hoop E, Moerbeek M, Zuidema SU, Gerritsen DL and Teerenstra S (2013). Stepped wedge designs could reduce the required sample size in cluster randomized trials. *Journal of Clinical Epidemiology*, **66**, 752–758. [13]

Wolbers M, Koller MT, Stel VS, Schaer B, Jager KJ, Leffondré K and Heinze G (2014). Competing risks analyses: objectives and approaches. *European Heart Journal*, **35**, 2936–2941. [7]

Xie T and Waksman J (2003). Design and sample size estimation in clinical trials with clustered survival times as the primary endpoint. *Statistics in Medicine*, **22**, 2835–2846. [12]

Zhao YD, Rahardja D and Qu Y (2008). Sample size calculation for the Wilcoxon-Mann-Whitney test adjusting for ties. *Statistics in Medicine*, **27**, 462–468. [4]

Zhu H and Lakkis H (2014). Sample size calculation for comparing two negative binomial rates. *Statistics in Medicine*, **33**, 376–387. [6]

Zinman B, Harris SB, Neuman J, Gerstein HC, Retnakaran RR, Raboubd J, Qi Y and Hanley AJG (2010). Low-dose combination therapy with rosiglitazone and metformin to prevent type 2 diabetes mellitus (CANOE trial): a double-blind randomised controlled study. *Lancet*, **376**, 103–111. [4, 7]

Zodpey SZ, Tiwari RR and Kulkarni HR (2000). Risk factors for haemorrhagic stroke: a case-control study. *Public Health*, **114**, 177–182. [8]

Zongo I, Dorsey G, Rouamba N, Tinto H, Dokomajilar C, Guiguemde RT, Rosenthal P and Ouedraogo JB (2007). Artemether-lumefantrine versus amodiaquine plus sulfadoxine-pyrimethamine for uncomplicated falciparum malaria in Burkina Faso: a randomised no-inferiority trial. *Lancet*, **369**, 491–498. [11]

Index

Page numbers in *italics* refer to illustrations; those in **bold** refer to tables

Sample Sizes for Clinical, Laboratory and Epidemiology Studies, Fourth Edition. David Machin, Michael J. Campbell,
Say Beng Tan and Sze Huey Tan.
© 2018 John Wiley & Sons Ltd. Published 2018 by John Wiley & Sons Ltd.